CLINICAL APPLICATION OF RADIOLABELLED PLATELETS

Developments in Nuclear Medicine

VOLUME 17

Series Editor: Peter H. Cox

Consulting Editor: Henry N. Wagner

The titles published in this series are listed at the end of this volume.

Clinical Application of Radiolabelled Platelets

edited by

Ch. KESSLER
Department of Neurology, Medical University Lübeck, Lübeck, F.R.G.

M. R. HARDEMAN
Department of Internal Medicine, Academic Medical Center,
University of Amsterdam, Amsterdam, The Netherlands

H. HENNINGSEN
Department of Neurology, University of Heidelberg, Heidelberg, F.R.G.

and

J.-N. PETROVICI
Department of Neurology, Cologne-Merheim Hospital, Cologne, F.R.G.

KLUWER ACADEMIC PUBLISHERS
DORDRECHT / BOSTON / LONDON

Library of Congress Cataloging in Publication Data

Clinical application of radiolabelled platelets / edited by Ch.
  Kessler ... [et al.].
       p.   cm. -- (Developments in nuclear medicine)
    Based on the Cologne-Symposium on Radiolabelled Platelets, held in
  1987, and organized by the Departments of Neurology and Nuclear
  Medicine at Cologne-Merheim Hospital.

    1. Radiolabeled blood platelets--Diagnostic use--Congresses.
  I. Kessler, Ch. (Christoff) II. Cologne-Symposium on Radiolabelled
  Platelets (1987) III. Cologne-Merheim Hospital. Dept. of
  Neurology. IV. Cologne-Merheim Hospital. Dept. of Nuclear
  Medicine. V. Series.
    [DNLM: 1. Blood Platelets--radionuclide imaging--congresses.
  2. Indium Radioisotopes--diagnostic use--congresses. 3. Monitoring,
  Physiologic--congresses.   W1 DE998KF / WH 300 C641 1987]
  RC670.5.R34C55   1990
  616.1--dc20
  DNLM/DLC
  for Library of Congress   90-4308

ISBN-13: 978-94-010-6749-2   e-ISBN-13: 978-94-009-0581-8
DOI: 10.1007/978-94-009-0581-8

Published by Kluwer Academic Publishers,
P.O. Box 17, 3300 AA Dordrecht, The Netherlands.

Kluwer Academic Publishers incorporates
the publishing programmes of
D. Reidel, Martinus Nijhoff, Dr W. Junk and MTP Press.

Sold and distributed in the U.S.A. and Canada
by Kluwer Academic Publishers,
101 Philip Drive, Norwell, MA 02061, U.S.A.

In all other countries, sold and distributed
by Kluwer Academic Publishers Group,
P.O. Box 322, 3300 AH Dordrecht, The Netherlands.

.

Printed on acid-free paper

Acknowledgements

The Editors would like to record their gratitude to the following sponsors:

Amersham Buchler Braunschwieg

Bayer AG Leverkusen

Fresenius AG Oberurssel

Hanssen GmbH Dusseldorf

Mallinckrodt Diagnostica GmbH Dietzenbach 2

And especially LIPHA Arnzeimittel GmbH Essen for their generous financial support.

CONTENTS

MONITORING OF ANTIPLATELET THERAPY

PLATELET SCINTIGRAPHY IN STROKE PATIENTS

PLATELET SCINTIGRAPHY IN ANGIOLOGY

HEMATOLOGY AND OTHER CLINICAL APPLICATIONS

INTRODUCTION

AIMS OF THE COLOGNE-SYMPOSIUM ON RADIOLABELLED PLATELETS

In 1976, M. Thakur et al (1) were the first to publish a paper concerning the in vivo thrombus detection with 111-In-labelled platelets. Previous attempts at scintigraphic thrombus localisation had been disappointing because of the unspecific binding of a number of the isotopes used, as well as the poor labelling efficiency or an insufficient low gamma-emitting property. Because of its physical characteristics (2.8 days half-life, 94% gamma emission) 111 Indium turned out to be the best isotope for platelet kinetic studies as well as for the measurement of platelet incorporation by Thrombi to be used up until now.
The lipophile complexes of 111-In (8-hydroxyquinoline, acetylacetone, tropolone) diffuse passively into the platelets without altering the function or the life span of the platelets. This advantage has let to an increase in the clinical applications of 1211-In labelled platelets.
Today, radiolabelled platelets are used for thrombus detection in several different medical areas such as cardiology, nephrology. angiology or neurology. Even though many scientists and hospital doctors now routinely use radiolabelled platelet as a diagnostic tool, there is as yet not a standardized labelling method. In addition to this, there are neither standardized image procedures for the different clinical applications nor an agreement about specificity and sensitivity of the method.
In 1983, a symposium on Radiolabelled Cellular Blood Elements was organized by M.Thakur, M.R.Hardeman and M.D. Ezekowitz with the assistance of the NATO Advanced Study Institute. The symposium took place in Maratea near Naples in Italy. During this meeting, many scientists has the opportunity to present the results of recent investigations. Since then, there have been a number of developments in this field as e.g. the introduction of several dual radiotracer methods or platelet labelling with monoclonal antibodies.
Four years after the Maratea meeting the Departments of Neurology and Nuclear Medicine at the Cologne-Merheim Hospital, Cologne, West Germany organized a symposium on the clinical applications of radiolabelled platelet, the aim of which was to discuss the current state of scientific and clinical work in this particular area; and indeed the symposium was characterised by extraordinarily lively discussions and intensive debates of controversial points. It is to be hoped that some agreements were achieved between the participants in the theoretical problems as well as in

technical procedures. The "Round Table Discussion" included in this volume gives a vivid impression of the productive atmosphere of the two days at the Cologne meeting.

I would like to thank all the speakers and also to thank those who took part in the discussion for their commitment to the subject. Many thanks are due to all who helped to make the meeting possible. Especially, I am indebted to Carlo Praetorius and Dieter Stoeffges from the Lipha Corporation for their organising skills and all sponsors (see page) who helped to finance the meeting.

LITERATURE

1. Thakur MI, Welch MJ, Joist JH, Coleman RE (1976(Indium-111 labelling platelets: studies in preparation and evaluation of In vitro and in vivo function. Throm Res. 9: 345-357.

Christoff Kessler
Lübeck.

THROMBOEMBOLISM AND RADIOLABELLED PLATELETS

Thakur M.C.

INTRODUCTION

Disorders caused by arterial and venous thromboemboli
can be life threatening. Coronary artery thrombosis (CAT)
leads to ischemia or infarction of myocardium and thrombotic
or embolic occlusions of cerebral arteries result in
ischemia or infarction of the central nervous system. Venous
thrombotic disorders are frequently associated with the
formation of emboli that may obscure otherwise smooth
pulmonary circulation and complicate the recovery from
primary illnesses.

In recent years years much of the basic research in
this field is focussed on the understanding of the
pathophysiology of these disorders and has obtained
considerable insight. Following initial vessel damage
subendothelial structures are exposed to the blood stream
and platelets begin to adhere and form aggregates on the
injury site. Coagulation proteins are then activated
sequentially and begin to generate the enzyme thrombin which
cleaves plasma fibrinogen in fibrin monomers. These
polymerize around the clumped platelets and hold them in
place thereby producing a partial or total occlusion of the
vessel. Detecting such occlusion calls for vigorous
anticoagulant therapy which may reduce patient morbidity and
mortality.

ROLE OF RADIOLABELLED PLATELETS:

Platelets labelled with a gamma emitting radionuclide
such as In-III have provided us with a tool to localize
these clots in vivo by external scintigraphy. While the
techniques of labelling platelets and results of preliminary
evaluation have appeared elsewhere (1, 2, 3, 4, 5(, this
monograph describes many such excellent clinical and
experimental applications in which radiolabelled platelets
have been instrumental. Although this is rewarding and
gratifying, we have been only partially successful in
imaging clots situated in certain vital organs such as the
heart (CAT) or the lungs. This could be attributed to
several important reasons.

During labelling, we try to make sure to use mild
procedures, so that the platelets labelled with In-III would
maintain adequate aggregability in vitro, and have the
proper survival of 8-10 days in vivo. Although it is
important that the labelling procedures are innocuous to

1

Ch. Kessler et al. (eds.), Clinical Application of Radiolabelled Platelets, 1–6.
© 1990 *Kluwer Academic Publishers.*

platelets and do not alter either their viability or the pathophysiologic functional ability, the unaltered radiolabelled platelets cause extensive high blood background and thereby obscure the visualization of thrombi particularly in the high blood pool areas. Examples of these are thrombi in coronary artery or lesions of bacterial endocarditis (6). Feasibility of these procedures were studied using experimental lesions induced in animals. Such lesions normally are large in size. These result in high lesion to blood radioactivity ratios and are visualized unequivocally by external scintigraphy even at the early hours after the administration of labelled platelets (7, 8). Clinical lesions, although highly symptomatic, tend to the small in living patients and have been only rarely visualized (9). Subtracting the blood background activity using Tc-99m erythrocytes has not been reliably successful (10).

In addition to the high blood back ground radioactivity, the size of such lesions in patients are frequently so small that they cannot be resolved by the intrinsic low resolution of an Anger gamma camera. Single photon emission tomographic (SPECT) imaging may be helpful, but as yet such systematic studies are almost non-existent.

The effect of anticoagulation therapy has reportedly prevented visualization of pulmonary emboli in patients, but they have been visualised when heparin therapy had been curtailed for 2 hr. prior to and 2 hr. post In-III platelet administration. Physicians in certain institutions regard such practice as unsafe, unethical and may complicate the clinical management of the patient population.

In patients suffering from idiopathic thrombocytic purpura (ITP), clinicians frequently need to know as to what extent the spleen is involved in destroying platelets. One way to determine this would be to label patient's platelets with In-III and to quantify the radioactivity accumulated in the spleen. Due to the heterogenity of platelet labelling procedures and the labelling reagent media, the accumulation of radiolabelled platelets in the normal spleen has been reported to be between 25%-45% (12). At such a wide range of variation it has been frequently difficult to assess as to when, in an ITP patient, the spleen is actively involved and the spleen ectomy is warranted.

How could these problems be solved? Or as much as we would like, could they ever be solved? In order to minimize the platelet radioactivity background, it has been suggested that the viability of labelled platelets be purposefully reduced before administration to the patient. To me, personally, such an approach is unatractive, for it certainly would reduce the quantity of platelets deposited on the lesion, and would thereby reduce the lesion to background ratio and ultimately would knot offer any advantage. The risk of highly rapid platelet clearance could not be eliminated either. The resolution of gamma cameras has probably reached its maximum and the SPECT scanning may offer advantage for the better perception of small thrombi over a large blood pool activity. The use of perhaps the better methods, such as the one that allows us to label platelets selectively in vivo using radiolabelled monoclonal antibodies, may eliminate the heterogeneity that exists in our platelet labelling techniques and perhaps result in the narrow range of platelet quantity taken up by the normal spleen. Such results may provide us with a better guideline in the quantitative assessment of the role that the spleen may play in diseases such as ITP.

RADIOLABELLED MONOCLONAL ANTIBODIES:

All In-III agents known to label platelets in either the non-plasma of the plasma medium are non specific, and require to draw patients' blood and separate platelets free of other blood cells. The recent advances in hybridoma technology has offered investigators antibodies specific for platelet surface antigens, mainly glycoproteins, that would interact only with platelets, potentially even in vivo. Several such antibodies with different specificity have been prepared and tested; in animals in the U.S.A. (13, 14, 15) and in patients in England (16). Although at this time, several parameters are unknown and many questions remain unanswered, the preliminary results have been promising both in animals as well as in humans. Unless the antibodies in question interact with both human and animal platelets, answers to several questions can not be easily and reliably obtained.

None of the antibodies we have tested interact with human as well as animal platelets and require them to be tested in humans. In the United States, for evaluating antibodies in humans, food and drug research administrations' (FDA) approval must be obtained. Prior to applying for such a permission, antibodies to be used must be tested vigorously. The antibody production procedure must also be supplied, and strictly adhered to, so that the consistency and stability of the product could be evaluated and its sub classes tested. Some of the tests suggested are given below.

A.   Tests for viral and nucleic acid

CONTAMINATION:

1.   Lymphocytic choriomanengitis (LCM) virus by intracerebral inoculation into several healthy mice.
2.   Mouse antibody production (MAP) tests for murine viruses such as LCM, Reovirus type 3, pollyoma, mouse pneumonia virus, mouse adenovirus, mouse hepatitis etc.
3.   Tests for Murine leukemia viruses, preferably MCF type, viruses, the S + L - tests and the XC test.
4.   Tests for polynucleotides.

4

B.   Safety Study

    Safety study in a limited number of animals of the type other than mice. The use of additional species is encouraged.

    Animals should be watched for acute and chronic toxicity, behaviour and body weight. Vital and target organ histology should be performed. Blood counts, blood chemistry, during analysis, and tests for hepatic and renal toxicity should be carried out.

C.   Tests for human tissue cross-reactivity

1.   Immunohistological survey of adult humans vital organs, frozen quickly and fixed chemically.
2.   Similar histological tests and quick frozen or chemically fixed fetal vital organs.
3.   Immunohistology of blood and blood forming organs.

D.   Quality control of final product:

    Final product must be tested for :
        1. Sterility and a pyrogenicity.
        2. Specificity.
        3. Electropherectic migration.
        4. Lowry determination for antibody quantity.

    There are a few of the several tests required without which FDA approval cannot be obtained.

BIOMATERIALS AND ARTIFICIAL ORGANS

    The technological advances to replace damaged organs or blood vessels, totally or partly, has increased the life time of many. The basis for this success is improved quality of individual biomaterials. The thrombogenicity of these materials has been substantially reduced, but has not been totally eliminated. Although endothelial cells can be grown in culture, serious doubts remain if they can thrive on the surface of biomaterials. Radiolabelled platelet scintigraphy provides a sensitive and reliable technique to determine the thrombogenicity of a biomaterial in vitro and of the implanted artificial organs in vivo. It is for such reasons, radiolabelled platelets will continue to play even a greater role in the health care and in biomedical research.

    The author wishes to thank Profs. Petrovici, Kessler and Mödder for giving him the opportunity to participate in this symposium and is confident that this compendious monograph will serve as a useful guide to investigators involved in the diagnosis of thrombotic disorders and therapy.

REFERENCES

1. Thakur M.L., Welch M.J., Hoist J.H. et al. (1976) Indium-III labelled platelets: Studies on preparation and evaluation of in vitro and in vivo functions. Thrombosis Research, Vol. 9, 345-355.
2. Thakur M.L., McKenney S.L., Park C.H., (1985) Simplified and efficient labelling of human platelets in plasma using Indium-III-2-Mercaptopyridine-N-oxide: Preparation and Evaluation. J. Nucl. Med. 26, 510-517.
3. Indium-III labelled neutrophils, platelets, and lymphocytes, Ed. M.L. Thakur and A. Gottschalk, TRIVIRUM Publishing Co. (1980) (References therein).
4. Radiolabelled Cellular blood elements, Ed. M.L. Thakur, Plenum Publishing Co. (1983) (References therein).
5. Platelet kinetics and imaging, Vol. 1, Techniques and normal platelet kinetics. Eds. dA. duP. Heyns, P.N. Bandenhorst, M.G. Lotter, CRC Press (1985) (References therein).
6. Thakur M.L., Riba A.L., Zaret B.L., Imaging bacterial endocarditis in humans (unpublished work).
7. Riba A.L., Thakur M.L., Gottschalk A., Zaret B.L. (1979) Imaging experimental coronary artery thrombosis with In-III platelets. Circulation, Vol. 60, 767-775.
8. Riba A.L., Thakur M.L., Gottschalk A., Andriole V.T., Zaret B.L., (1979) Imaging experimental infective endocarditis with In-III labelled blood cellular components. Circulation Vol. 59, 336-343.
9. Raichlen J., Thakur M.L., Park C.H. Imaging coronary artery thrombosis with In-III labelled platelets in humans. (unpublished data).
10. Powers W.J., Siegel B.A. (1983) Thrombus imaging with In-III platelets, Seminars in thrombosis and hematosis, Vol. 9, 115-131.
11. Sostman H.D., Neumann R.D., Lok J. et al. (1982) The detection of pulmonary embolism in man with In-III labelled autologus platelets. M.J. Roentgenol., 138, 945-951.
12. Thakur M.L. and McKenney S. (1983) Techniques of cell labelling: In Radiolabelled cellular blood elements. M.L. Thakur, Plenum Publishing Company, page 67-87.
13. Som P., Oster Z.H., Samora P.O. et al.(1988) Radioimmunoimaging of experimental thrombi in dogs using Technetium-99m labelled monoclonal antibody fragments reactive with human platelets. J. Nucl. Med., 27, 1315-1320.
14. Oster Z.H., Srivastava, Som P. et al. (1985) Thrombus radioimmunoscintigraphy: An approach using monoclonal anti-platelet antibody. Proc. Natl. Acd. Sci. USA., 82, 3465-3468.
15. Thakur M.L., Thiagarajan P., White III F. et al. (1987) Monoclonal antibodies for specific cell labelling: Consideration, preparation and preliminary evaluation, Nucl. Med. and Biology, Vol. 14, 51-58.

16. Lavender and Peters M. Private communication and this monograph.

PLATELET ISOLATION TECHNIQUE AND VIABILITY TESTING

M.R.Hardeman

Dept of Internal Medicine, Academic Medical Centre, Meibergdreef 9, 1105 AZ Amsterdam. Netherlands

INTRODUCTION

Although platelet like corpuscles were first described in 1842 by Simon in Germany, Addison in England and Donne' in France, their existence was still denied a hundred years later. Even after Bizzozero in 1882 had observed the third type of formed element directly in the circulating blood of a living animal, these "paistrine" or "Blutplattchen", as they were called by him in Italian and German papers respectively, were considered to be artefacts[1] or simply designated as "blood dust", as Page [2] had been taught. The name "thrombocyte", first proposed by the Dutch Scientist Dekhuyzen [3], was initially used for the nucleus-containing platelet found in sub-mammalian species but was later accepted also for the nucleus-lacking mammalian platelets.

In 1953, when the existence of the platelets had become generally recognized, they were, nevertheless still considered as bits of cytoplasm rather than viable cells with metabolic activities [4].

As we all know now blood platelets are highly organised cells with a complicated ultra-structure [Fig.1] and they are indispensible to hemostasis and coagulation; their shortage or malfunction is the cause of the majority of bleeding disorders. Furthermore, they are involved in many other physiological or pathological processes. The reason why the platelets have been neglected for such a long time is probably best described by Tocantins [5]:

> " The platelet is elusive, inconspicuous, retiring, and attends to its chores without fanfare.
> Platelets have neither the strong individualism of a leukocyte, nosing and pushing its way everywhere, nor do they splash themselves with the gaudy colours of an erythrocyte."

In vitro manipulation and study has been seriously hampered by the fact that the very nature of the platelets is their high sensitivity to environmental changes; many experiments had to be stopped prematurely due to irreversible platelet aggregation. Although a few tricks are known now in order to avoid this unwanted aggregation [6,7], cautious handling is needed, especially when subsequent reinjection of viable cells is planned.

7

Ch. Kessler et al. (eds.), Clinical Application of Radiolabelled Platelets, 7–25.
© 1990 *Kluwer Academic Publishers.*

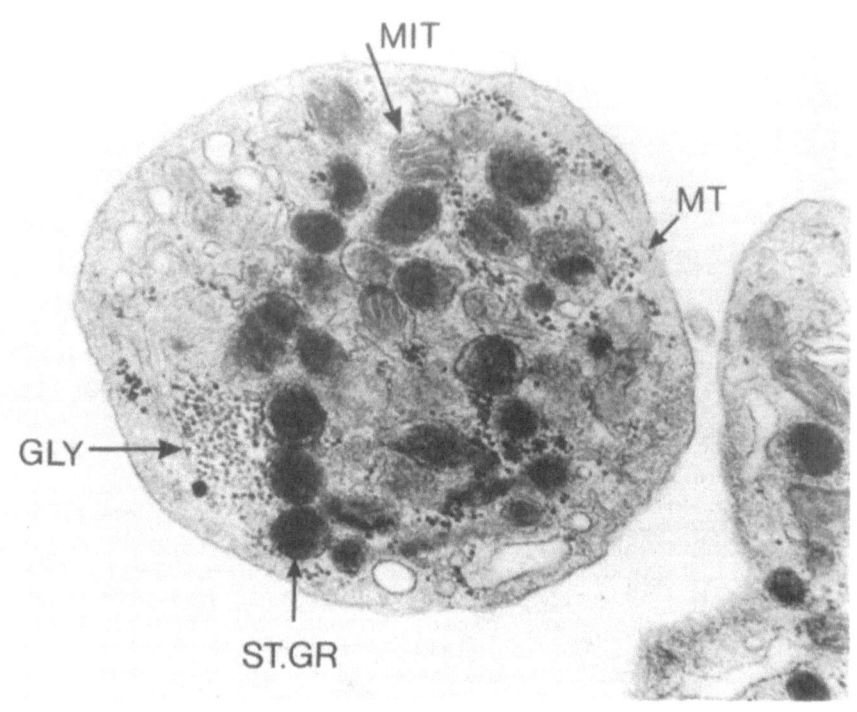

Fig. 1

Electron-micrograph showing some ultra-structural features of the human
thrombocyte (MIT= mitochondrion,MT= mictotubules, ST.GR= storage granule,
GLY= glycogen). Magnification: x 50.000

PLATELET ISOLATION TECHNIQUES

Since up till now no platelet-specific labelling procedure has been found satisfactory, we have to face the necessity to separate them from other, contaminating, cell types.

Existing blood-cell isolation techniques can be distinguished into three categories i.e. methods based on physical, functional and biological cell surface properties. The latter two techniques, however, interfere irreversibly with cell properties and are thus of no use for our purpose, i.e. reinjection of sterile, viable and functioning labelled cells. Fortunately, the first category offers offers satisfying possibilities for platelets. Methods based on differences in cell density are most popular, not in the least because of their simplicity. From Table 1 it can be deduced that platelets are easily separated from other blood cells, on basis of their density, by fractional centrifugation. Density is one of the factors influencing the sedimentation velocity, according to the Law of Stoke:

$$V = 2gr^2 \, \phi_d / \, 9nk$$

[V= terminal sedimentation velocity, g= acceleration owing to gravity or centrifugal force, r= particle radius, ϕ_d = difference of particle density from that of the medium, n = viscosity of the medium, k = factor depending on the shape of the particle.]

Simple centrifugation of blood for 15 min at 180g yields pure platelets [supernatant], rather crude preparations of white cells [buffy coat] and erythrocytes [sediment]. Although the platelets in the supernatant platelet rich plasma are pure with respect to other cell types, their population is probably not quite representative for the platelet population in whole blood, repeated washing of the sedimented buffy coat and red cell layer can increase the harvesting efficiency to 98% [8].

Table 1
Morphological dimensions, count and density of cellular blood elements

Cell Type	Volume (fl)	Diameter (um)	Count (ul^{-1})	Mean Density (g cm^{-3})
Erythrocyte	90	8	5.000.000	1.092
Thrombocyte	6	3	250.000	1.030
Granulocyte	450	10-15	4.300	1.089
Lymphocyte	210	7-18	2.200	1.070
Monocyte	470	12-20	500	1.069
Plasma				1.027

In the practice of clinical application of radiolabelled platelets, there are several manipulations, inherent to the isolation and labelling procedure [9] which have the potential for irreversible damage to the cells [Table 2].

Table 2

Manipulations (all at room temperature)	Result
1. venepuncture	WB
2. anticoagulation	ACD-WB
3. centrifugation	supernatant: PRP
4. acidification	ACD-PRP (pH 6.5)
5. centrifugation	platelet pellet
6. resuspension	PRS
7. labelling procedure	P'RS
8. wash (i.e. step 5 and 6 again)	P'RS
9. re-injection	?

The chance for "collection injury" can be minimised by several precautions. The whole isolation and labelling procedure should be performed at room temperature [10], shear stress activation can be avoided by using large bore needles and transporting the platelet suspension not too vigorously. ACD is the anti-coagulant of choice [11].

Most used labelling techniques employ a non-plasmatic medium, since plasma proteins, like transferrin, compete with the ligand for the label and thus will impair the labelling efficacy to levels below 80%, making extra wash steps necessary. New techniques have been developed which claim sufficient labelling efficiency in diluted or undiluted plasma. In all cases, however, the cells have to be concentrated which implies pelleting and resuspension.

Acidification of PRP with ACD to pH 6.5 enables an easier manipulation with a minimal chance for aggregation. The lowered pH does not affect their hemostatic activity after reinjection [6]. The lack of plasma during the short labelling procedure was felt as a serious problem by some investigators. From a physiological point of view, this problem is strongly exaggerated. Measuring liver sequestration, considered to be a highly sensitive method for the detection of manipulation injury [12], Peters et al indeed demonstrated hepatic sequestration early after reinjection of platelets labelled in saline. The phenomenon, however, was reversible within 30 min and not always consistent [13]. It may be true that a plasmatic environment protects the platelets better for possible manipulation injury; however, if this happens it is apparently repaired soon after re-injection, and this does not exclude normal in vivo kinetics or function [12][14] [fig 2.]. Even after prolonged storage in a non-plasma medium, these parameters

were at least as good as for platelets stored in plasma
[15]. On the other hand it can be argued that the prescence
of plasmatic coagulation proteins could trigger platelet
activation more or less during the labelling procedure.

From a practical point of view, however, the plasma
method would undoubtedly be preferable if the platelets
could be labelled directly in the PRP, but as has been
mentioned before, concentration of the platelets is
necessary in order to obtain satisfactory labelling
efficiency. The danger of irreversible cell damage lies
primarily in centrifugation to a pellet [16][19] and its
subsequent resuspension which should therefore be minimised
as much as possible. Therefore, a high labelling efficiency
[i.e. 80% or higher] contributes to the feasibility and
success of a labelling protocol since it enables to omit an
extra wash step.

In this respect another method for cell separation
should be mentioned. This method, counterflow centrifugation
or elutriation, exploits mainly differences in cell size,
contributing to the second power to the sedimentation
velocity [see Stoke's formula]. During centrifugation the
tendency of the cells to sedimentate under the influence of
the centrifugal force is offset by a liquid flowing in the
opposite, centripetal, direction [Fig 3]. When the
centrifugal and counterflow forces are balanced, a wide
range of particle sizes can be concentrated and kept in
separate bands in suspension. The shape of the sedimentation
chamber is important for efficient separation. Either by a
stepwise increase of the counterflow rate or a stepwise
decsease in the rotor speed, the various bands of cells can
be harvested. The elutriator rotor became commercially
available in 1973 [Beckman Instruments], since then the use
of this technique has increased rapidly. The advantages are
clear: any medium can be used, no foreign substances that
can activate or damage the cells are introduced, low g
forces are employed, no pelleting or resuspension is needed.
For cell labelling purposes the final suspension obtained
is, however, too diluted, impairing labelling efficiency to
an unacceptable level [20]. Various ways to solve this
specific problem have been reviewed earlier [20].

Recently, a multichamber counterflow centrifugal system
has been introduced [Dijkstra Vereenigde B.V. Amsterdam].
Apart from the fact that 4 different separations can be
performed at the same time, it is also possible to perform
with this system a procedure based on connecting two
chambers in series, using the first one for separation and
the second one for concentration. A further advantage is
that there are no rotation seals and that the closed tubing
and chamber system is delivered sterile and can be used
directly without disrupting sterility. A special gear
construction makes it possible not to rip the tubing.
Practical testing of this system is now underway.

It can be concluded that, dealing with platelet
isolation, no significant problems are encountered.
Acidification [pH 6.5] of PRP with some ACD enables easier
resuspension after centrifugation. This and a nonplasma
environment during the labelling procedure does not normally
result in irreversible loss of platelet function and

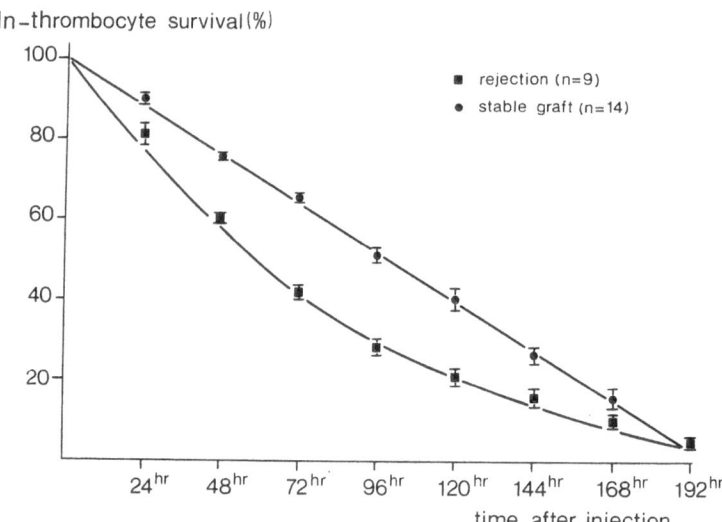

^{III} In-thrombocyte survival(%)

■ rejection (n=9)
● stable graft (n=14)

time after injection

Fig. 2

¹¹¹In-thrombocyte survival as found in patients after kidney transplan-
tation, demonstrating normal straight line kinetics (stable graft) or an
increased disappearance rate (rejection), concomitant with an increased
accumulation in the rejecting kidney (not shown). In vivo recovery: 60- 64%

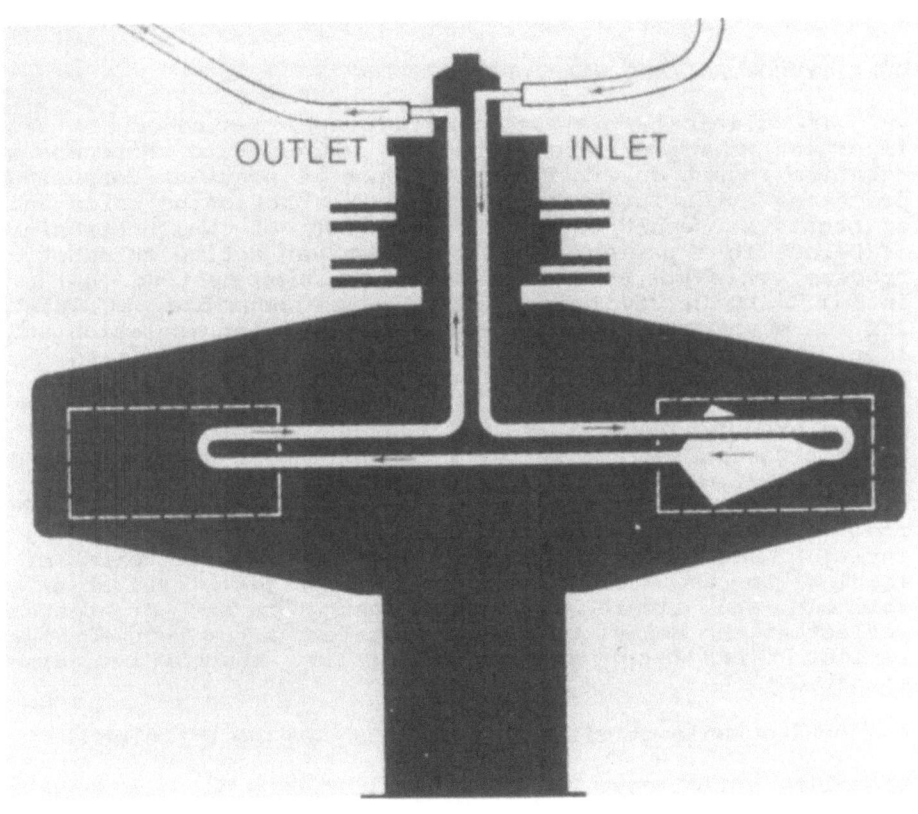

OUTLET   INLET

Fig. 3

Cross-section of the Elutriator-rotor (Beckman Instruments),
showing the separation chamber and centripetal flow pattern.

viability.

QUALITY CONTROL AND VIABILITY TESTING

In clinical platelet scintigraphic studies it is important that we are able to discriminate between a negative result due to a real absence of platelet consuming processes after injection of properly functioning cells and a negative result due to injection of malfunctioning platelets in a patient with or without an active thrombotic process. This means that platelet function testing [either in vitro or in vivo] is factually indispensible, at least for the evaluation and comparison of different isolation and labelling protocols, but it should, ideally, also be performed in parallel to each clinical study.

How can we predict the in vivo behaviour of such manipulated and possibly maltreated platelets? In this respect we can learn a lot from the extensive work performed by bloodtransfusion and other research centres dealing with the quality control of stored platelet concentrates. Apart from some specific aspects related to radioactivity, most interests of both groups of investigators go parallel, leading to the main question: do we have available a reliable and simple in vitro test [or set of tests] reflecting the behaviour of the platelets after reinjection? Besides this, other aspects of quality control are also involved.

Concerning Radioactivity	Concerning Platelets
Labelling efficiency	Sterility
Release of label	Visual inspection, cell count
	Platelet function
	Platelet viability

In contrast to the earlier mentioned transfusions of large amounts of platelets with the purpose to increase the number of circulating cells or to stop bleeding in the recipient, we have to deal usually with relatively small quantities of platelet concentrate with the consequence that there is also a small quantity of material available for in vitro testing. Therefore the tests should be performed as much as possible on a microscale. The labelling efficiency, for instance can easily be evaluated with the microhematocrit method [9].

The possible release of cell bound radioactivity could be checked occasionally [e.g. for comparison of different protocols] using a similar amount of cells as has been used for determination of the labelling efficiency, which could be incubated in a few ml of plasma for 24 hours at 37^0C.

Sterility testing should be performed at each occasion, but is usually resticted to evaluation of a new protocol only.

Visual inspection of the platelet suspension should reveal whether significant aggregation has taken place; in that case the suspension as such should not be injected.

Sometimes small aggregates are found which, after swirling the suspension mow and then slowly, will disappear after a while. Although [electronic] counting is needed in order to assess the number of platelets injected, visual appearance, especially the light density of the suspension, usually yields sufficient information about the platelet concentration.

PLATELET FUNCTION AND VIABILITY

Platelet viability can be defined as the capability of the cells to remain in the circulation with both a normal recovery or yield and life span; this term does not necessary include the capacity of the cells to function properly, and therefore a clear distinction between functionality and viability is indicated. There are indeed clinical situations in which malfunctioning cells circulate normally [e.g. thrombasthenia, use of aspirine,etc.]. As has been said before, it would be very appropriate if we had at our disposal simple and reliable in vitro tests for both functionality and viability. There are several possible candidates for such tests:

Regarding platelet function	Regarding platelet viability
Aggregation	Beta-Thromboglobulin release
Adhesion	Morphology
Chemotaxis	Serotonin uptake
	Hypotonic shock response

The best way to evaluate the relevance of a particular in vitro test is of course the direct comparison with the in vivo outcome. Because of ethical and practical considerations the probabilities for such an approach are scarce. We can use, however, the results of earlier in vivo experiments with respect to a.o. the optimal storage temperature for platelet suspensions, the effect of different anticoagulants, pH etc. and compare these with the in vitro test results performed under the same experimental conditions.

The major function of platelets is their hemostatic action and therefore, their capacity to adhere and aggregate in vitro have been evaluated as a quality control test for in vitro manipulated platelets. In 1962 the first publications by Born and O'Brien [21][22] about a nephelometric aggregation technique appeared in the literature and since then, this technique has been the basis of numerous publications. Although several modifications have been suggested, the same basic principles are still in use in many laboratories all over the world. A main reason for this popularity is undoubtedly its practical simplicity, however, there are also limitations: standardisation with respect to platelet number, environmental Ca^{2+} concentration, pH etc appeared to be necessary. Furthermore, a proper quantification of the obtained graphical results is cumbersome. Although the in vitro technique is simple, the physiological process behind is not and, in spite of a lot of research, the real mechanism of platelet aggregation has not been solved yet.

The test is useful for the assessment of intrinsic platelet defects and for the evaluation of the effect of endogenous or added plasma factors as well, but there are several reasons to assume that this in vitro test is not relevant at all as a predictor for in vivo function. In platelet storage experiments, the optimal storage temperature for maintenance of platelet aggregability is 4^0C [23] which is not the same as the temperature required for the best in vivo survival of the infused platelets, which appeared to be 22^0C [10].

Furthermore, it was demonstrated that platelets stored for 24 hours at 22^0C, having lost their aggregation response to ADP almost completely, were able to recover and aggregate in the same way as fresh platelets soon after transfusion [24][25]. Similar conclusions could be drawn from the work of Schmidt et al [26], dealing with both normal individuals and various patients undergoing platelet kinetic studies with 111-In labelled thrombocytes. Finally we were able to demonstrate that positive scintigraphic results can be obtained with autologous ^{111}In labelled platelets in a study of patients with left ventricular aneurisms, using platelets taken after intake of Aspirin and having a completely abolished in vitro aggregation ADP aggregation response [Fig 4]. On the other hand, it has been reported that, despite the fact that platelets displayed normal in vitro aggregation, "collection injury" was readily apparent from hepatic and blood pool activity curves [12]. Therefore, I want to emphasize again that in vitro platelet aggregometry is not relevant as an indicator for in vivo functioning of platelet suspensions and this test is thus not suitable for the comparison of various cell isolation and labelling techniques and may lead to an error of judgement [27][28].

Several in vitro tests are described dealing with the adhesion of platelets [29][30] or related biochemical markers like a decrease in membrane glycoproteins [31][32]. The same storage experiments as mentioned before have revealed that also with respect to the maintenance of platelet adhesiveness, a storage temperature of 4^0C is superior compared to 22^0C, in contrast to the experience regarding in vivo behaviour [23].

111-In labelled platelets are inherent to the procedure for the measurement of platelet chemotaxis [33] and could therefore be of use although comparison with fresh unlabelled cells is not possible. In our hands, however, the technique,including a 3 hour incubation, appeared to be cumbersome with considerable variation of the experimental results.

Beta thromboglobulin [BTG] is a platelet specific protein located inside the storage granules and prone to be ejected in the so called release reaction. Therefore, extracellular BTG has been investigated as a marker for platelet maltreatment. It has been shown, however, that platelets continue to circulate even though there is evidence of a reduction in their storage granules [34] and, again, results of storage experiments make it unlikely that the measurement of BTG can be of use as a quality control

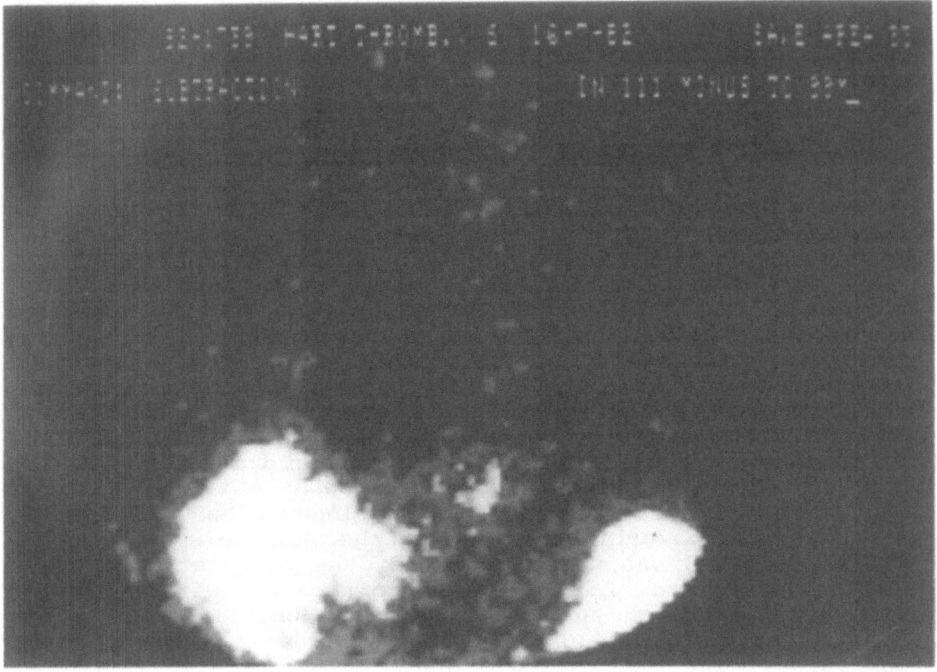

Fig. 4

Computer digitised scintigraph made 24 hours after re-injection of autologous 111In-thrombocytes in a patient with left ventricular aneurysm, and
after subtraction of 99mTc-erythrocyte bloodpool background activity. Due
to the use of aspirin several hours before blood withdrawal, the
111In-thrombocytes displayed a complete absence of secondary irreversible
aggregation, when tested before re-injection. Nevertheless, a clear hot
area can be distinguished in the region of the heart apex.

assay for monitoring the in vitro viability of platelets
[35].

Before platelets adhere and/or aggregate they become
activated, a state which is accompanied by a shape change
from disc to sphere, the latter generally considered as the
morphological marker for the activated state. Platelets,
however, belong to the contractory cells [like smooth muscle
cells] which means that they become "refractory" i.e.
temporarily inactive. It is not known how long this
refractory state will last and under which circumstances the
cells actually become irreversibly inactive, also
accompanied with distinct morphological changes. Therefore,
activation parameters are not suitable as platelet function
criterium, however, regarding its possible value as in vitro
viability indicator it should be mentioned here that
clinical situations where platelet survival is decreased
[e.g. Bernard-Soulier syndrome, Wiskott-Aldrich syndrome,
intravascular coagulation, thrombosis] are always associated
with changes in normal disc morphology [36]. Dealing with a
quantitative measurement of platelet shape change, a
practical and simple procedure has been suggested [37]. The
percentage of spherical platelets appear to correlate with
the ratio of extinction values measured at stirring rates of
700 and 200 rpm respectively and is independant of platelet
count and plasma extinction. Also other morphological scores
[38][39] as well as the capacity of the platelets for shape
change [39] are fairly well correlated with platelet
viability, although again the in vitro phenomenon of shape
change appears often reversible under physiological
conditions. That the discoid shape of a platelet is not an
absolute guarantee for normal survival is demonstrated by
the short survival after injection of neuraminidase treated,
discoid, platelets [40].

In 1982 the technical forum on the testing of platelet
function of the U.S. Bureau of Biologics suggested tests for
functional platelet integrity [41]. The top 3 tests were: 1]
Serotonin [5HT] uptake, 2] Hypotonic shock response [HSR],
3] Morphology.

Both 5HT uptake and HSR have been studied extensively
as potential viability criteria [42-48]. The relative
results with respect to the optimal storage temperature and
the effect of different anticoagulants on these parameters
were found to be in accordance with the in vivo results of
other investigators [20]. Direct correlation of changes in
these parameters with viability are, however, scarce
[43][46-49]. Further studies to prove their reliability in
different situations are necessary. There is no concensus
yet for a uniform interpretation of the HSR curves [Fig 5,
see also appendix 1].

EX VIVO TESTS.

As we have seen before, we should be very cautious with
the interpretation of in vitro test results in terms of in
vivo behaviour of platelets. Even if the measured
abnormalities are relevant, how sure can we be about their
irreversible character after transfusion?

Ex vivo experiments [i.e. study of a manipulated

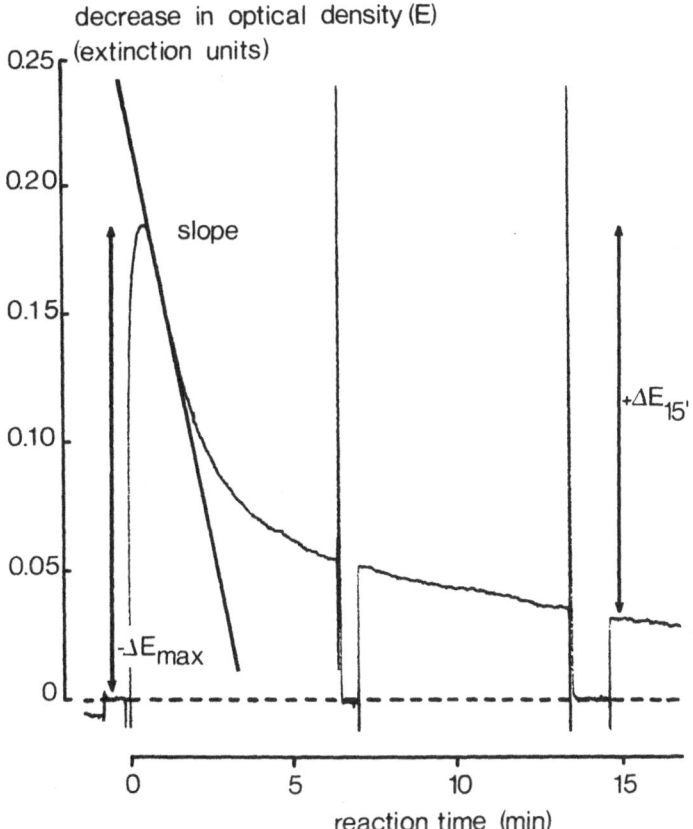

Fig. 5

Response of platelets to hypotonic shock.
The baseline was obtained by measuring the absorbance of 1.5 ml platelet-rich plasma mixed with 0.5 ml of a 0.154 M NaCl solution.
At time zero, 1.5 ml platelet-rich plasma was mixed with 0.5 ml of distilled water in a second cuvette and measured immediately thereafter. The maximal velocity of the return to the baseline was calculated by drawing the tangent along the steepest part of the curve. The vertical lines are due to reflection of the incident light beam by moving the cuvette holder and placing the other cuvette in position.

platelet population after transfusion and being in circulation for some time] may yield results that are far more conclusive. An almost classical example with respect to platelet function is te Borchgrevink retention test [50] based on comparison of platelet counts in blood obtained by venepuncture and in blood droplets that had oozed through a standard inscision of the skin. Shortening of a prolonged bleeding time has long been considered as the gold standard test for platelet function, however, it loks like everything is relative , since it has recently been shown [51] that platelet membrane vesicles [i.e. ^{111}In labelled platelet ghosts] can reduce microvascular bleeding time in thrombopenic rabbits. Schmidt et al [26] designed an ex vivo technique measuring simultaneous aggregation of unlabelled and labelled platelets after reinjection of the latter. In this way it could be confirmed that platelets manipulated in vitro can recover in vivo within a few minutes after reinjection.

We compared platelet retention with retention of radioactivity after reinjection of labelled platelets in blood taken with venepuncture and in drops of blood taken from standard inscisions in the forearm skin, like those in use for determination of the bleeding time [52]. In case the reinjected platelets are not functioning properly, they will not adhere on the inscision wound and the labelled platelet concentration in blood before and after passage of the fresh wound will hardly change although there is significant consumption of normal platelets.

Our clinical experience with the test is still limited. however, preliminary results demonstrated a refractory phase soon after transfusion of the labelled platelets, followed by normal function after one hour. The test is simple [see appendix 2]. We have the idea that this test can adequately reflect the function of the reinjected platelets and plan to perform it routinely now until a reliable preinjection test has definitely proven to be of value.

CONCLUSIONS.

Because of ethical considerations and for a proper interpretation of [negative] scintigraphic results it is important to obtain an indicator whether the injected platelets function well and remain sufficiently long in the circulation.

Platelet function defects demonstrated in vitro, after isolation and labelling of initially normal functioning platelets, are usually reversible in vivo. An in vitro protocol, describing conditions close to the physiological situation, enabling the platelets to recover before testing, is urgently needed. Ex vivo tests [i.e. after reinjection] may be useful and need further study.

Best candidates in vitro tests for platelet viability are:
- Serotonin uptake
- Hypotonic shock response
- Maintenance of disc shape.

Finally, I want to stress the need for a concensus about standard protocols for isolation, labelling and testing of platelets since these are the tools by which different laboratories can communicate about their results. Of course, such protocols will always have to be a compromise and probably not for everybody the optimal solution to a problem, however, to speak with Fratantoni [53]:

"although a camel may be the result of a committee attempting to design a horse, this provides, however, when one is in the desert, most satisfactory transportation".

REFERENCES

1. Weigert C. Fortschr Med. [1887] 5.193.
2. Page I.H. [1968] In: Serotonin. Yearbook Med Publ Inc. Chicago. 37
3. Dekhuyzen M.C. [1901] Anat Anz.19.529.
4. Tullis J.L. [1953] Blood cells and plasma protein. Acad Press Inc. N York.
5. Tocantins L.M. [1960] In: Blood Platelets. Ed: Johnson S.A. et al. Little Brown and Co. Boston pp3-6
6. Aster R.H. [1971] Effect of acidification in enhancing viability of platelet concentrates. Current status. Vox Sang.20.23-27.
7. Mourad N. [1968] A simple method for obtaining platelet concentrates free of aggregates. Transfusion.3.48
8. Wessels P. et al [1985] An improved method for the quantification of the in vivo kinetics of a representative population of ^{111}In labelled human platelets. Eur.J.Nucl.Med. 10.522-527.
9. Hardeman M.R. et al [1984] Labelling techniques of granulocytes and platelets with 111-In-Oxinate.In: Hardeman MT, Najean Y, eds. Blood cells in nuclear medicine. Part 1. The Haque: Nijhoff. 17-28
10. Murphy S, Gardner TH. Platelet preservation. Effect of storage temperature in maintenance of platelet viability - deleterious effect of refrigerated storage. New Eng.J.Med.1969:280: 1094-1098
11. Morrison TS, Baldini M. The favorable effect of ACD on the viability of fresh and stored human platelets. Vox Sang 1967:12:90-105
12. du P Heyns A, et al.Kinetics, distribution and sites of destruction of 111-Indium labelled human platelets. Br.J.Haematol,1980:44:269-280.
13. Peters AM et al.Intra hepatic kinetics of Indium 111-labelled platelets. Thromb and Haemostas 1985: 54: 5995-598
14. Hardeman MR et al.111-In-labelled platelets in the diagnosis of kidney transplant rejection. In: Hardeman MR Najean Y. eds. Blood cells in nuclear medicine Part 1. The Hague: N.Nijhoff. 1984:307-324
15. Adams SA. et al. Survival and recovery of human platelets stored for five days in a non-plasma medium. Blood 1986: 67:672-675

16. Mustard JF et al. Preparation of suspension of washed platelets from humans. Br.J.Haematol 1972. 22:193-204
17. Hytton RA et a;. Methods for the separation of platelets from plasma.Thromb Diath Haemorrh 1974.31:119-132
18. Zucker WH et al. Ultrastructural comparison of human platelets separated from blood by various means.AmJ.Pathol 1974; 77:255-267
19. Day HJ et al. Methods for separating platelets from blood and plasma. Thromb.Diath.Haemorrh. 1975:33:648-654
20. Hardeman MR. Cell Isolation Techniques: a critical review In: Thakur ML ed. Radiolabelled Cellular Blood Elements.New York, Plenum Publishing Corporation 1985: 51-66
21. Born GVR. Aggregation of blood platelets by adenosine diphosphate and its reversal. Nature 1962: 194. 927-929
22. O'Brien JR. Platelet aggregation. Some results from a new method of study.J.Clin.Pathol.19662:15:452-455
23. Shively JA et al.The effect of storage on adhesion and aggregation of platelets. Vox Sang 1970.18:204-210
24. Murphy S, Gardner FH. Platelet storage at 22°C: Metabolic morphologic and functional studies. J.Clin Invest.1971.50:370-377
25. Filip DJ, Aster RH. Relative hemostatic effectiveness of human platelets stored at 4°C and 22°C. J.Lab.Clin Med.1978.91:618-624
26. Schmidt KG et al. Function ex vivo of 111-In-labelled human platelets. Simultaneous aggregation of labelled and unlabelled platelets induced by collagen. Scand J Haemat 1982:29:51-56
27. Mortelmans L. et al Evaluation of three methods of platelet labelling. Nucl.Med.Commun.1986.7:519-529
28. Peters AM et al.Letter to the editor (comment on ref.27) Nucl Med.Commun.1987.8:183-184
29. Peters AM et al. A simple quantitative estimate of the function of radiolabelled platelets. Haemostasis 1984.14:333-336
30. McGill M, Brindley DC. Effects of storage on platelet reactivity to arterial subendothelium during blood flow. J.Lab Clin Med.1979.94:370-380
31. White GC et al. The effect of ambient storage on platelet membrane structure and response to thrombin transfusion 1979.19:411-419
32. George JN. Platelet membrane glycoproteins. Alteration during storage of human platelet concentrate. Thromb Res.1976.8:719-724
33. Lowenhaupt RW et al. A quantitative method to measure human platelet chemotaxis using Indium-111-Oxine labelled gel-filtered platelets. Blood 1982.60:1345-1352
34. Pareti FJ et al. Acquired storage pool disease in platelets during disseminated intravascular coagulation.. Blood 1976.48:511-515
35. Taylor MA. Release of ß-thromboglobulin during preparation, in vitro storage and cryopreservation of platelet concentrates. J.Clin Pathol.1983.36:811-813
36. McGill M. Correlations of platelet survivaland function

with the results of two in vitro tests.Vox Sang.1981.40 suppl.1.98-109

37. Holme S. Murphy S. Quantitative measurements of platelet shape by light transmission studies; application to storage of platelets for transfusion. J.Lab.Clin Med. 1978.92:53-64

38. Kunicki TJ et al. A study of variables affecting the quality of platelets stored at room temperature. Transfusion 1975.15:414-421

39. Hollme S et al. Effect of type of agitation on platelet morphology, vibability and function in vitro. Blood 1978.52:425-435

40. Greenberg J. et al.Effects on platelet function of removal of platelet sialic acid by neuraminidase. Lab.Invest 1975. 32:476-484

41. US Bureau of Biologics. Technical Forum. The testing of platelet function. Plasma Ther Transfus Technol. 1982.3:327-328

42. Hanin RJ et al. Platelet response to hypotonic stress after storage at $4^{O}C$ or $22^{O}C$. Transfusion 1970.10:305-309

43. Kim BK, Baldini MG. The platelet response to hypotonic shock. Its value as an indicator of platelet viability after storage. Transfusion 1974.14:130-138

44. Hardeman MR, Heynens CJ. Storage of human blood platelets; the rate of serotonin uptake and hypotonic shock response as in vitro viability test. Thromb Diath Haemorrh 1974.32:405-416

45. Mc Gill MR.Brindley DC. Effects of storage on platelet reactivity to arterial subendothelium during blood flow.J.Lab.Clin.Med 1979.94:370-380

46. Valeri CR et al. The relation between response to hypotonic stress and the 51-Cr recovery in vitro of preserved platelets. Transfusion 1974.14:331-337

47. Dayian G. et al.Improved procedure for platelet freezing.Vox Sang 1986.51:292-298

48. Lundberg A Murphy S. Survival in vivo of human blood platelets frozen without protective additives. Scand.H.Haemotol.1972.9:222-225

49. Synder EL. et al.In vitro characteristics and in vivo viability of platelets contained in granulocyte-platelet apheresis concentrate. Transfusion 91987.17:10-14

50. Borchgrevink CF. A method for measureing platelet adhesiveness in vivo. Acta Med.Scand.1960.168:157-164

51. Mc Gill et al.Platelet membrane vesicles reduced microvascular bleeding tine in thrombocytopenic rabbits. J.Lab.Clin.Med. 1987.109:127-133

52. Hardeman MR in preparation

53. Fratantooni JC. Comment on standardized procedures and the regulatory process. Transfusion 1986.26:36-37

APPENDIX 1

IN VITRO PLATELET VIABILITY TEST: RESPONSE TO HYPOTONIC SHOCK

The method described by Handin et al (1) was used with some modifications. Aa glass cuvette was filled at room temperature with either 0.2 ml of distilled water or 0.2 ml of 0.154 M saline (blank) and placed in a spectrophotometer (Hilger and Watts, Uvichem). To achieve immediate mixing 0.6 ml of PRP was brought to the bottom of the cuvette with a syringe. The change in absorbance (a) at 610 nm was recorded simultaneously on a Vitratron UR 400 recorder. The maximal deflection appeared to be dependent not only on the platelet concentration, but also on the final osmotic value, the latter, however, being standardized at 225 mOsm. For normal PRP, containing 300,000 - 450,000 platelets per ul, that magnification was chosen at which full scale deflection equaled 0.25 absorbance units. The response was followed, in duplicate, during 15 mins after the minimal absorbance had been reached (fig.5)

As a measure for the hypotonic shock response (HSR)-activity, the maximal slope of the return is usually taken, however, until a consensus has ben reached, it is advised to measure E_{max}, E_{15}, and platelet number as well. Further details regarding normal values, the influence of various experimental conditions and possible significance as in vitro viability test can be found in reference 2 and 3.

1.   Handin RI, Fortier NL, Valeri CR.
     Platelet response to hypotonic stress after storage at 4°C or 22°C. Transfusion 1970;10: 305.
2.   Hardeman MR, Heynens CJL.
     The active serotonin uptake and the hypotonic shock response of human blood platelets. Methods, normal values and the influence of various experimental conditions.
     Thromb Diath Haemorrh 1974;32:391
3.   Hardeman MR, Heymens CJL.
     Storage of human blood platelets; the rate of serotonin uptake and hypotonic shock response as in vitro viability test.
     Thromb Diath Haemorrh 1974;32:405.

APPENDIX 2

EX VIVO RADIO-LABELLED PLATELET-FUNCTION TEST (1)

The test is performed using EDTA-blood obtained from both a normal venepuncture and a few blood drops obtained after one or more standard incisions on the forearm at a cuff pressure of 40 mmHg.

The incision is made with the commercially available Simplate 11-device (General Diagnostics Inc.). The procedure, being essentially the same as in use for bleeding time determination, is almost painless, however, small scars will remain visible for a while.

Measure in both samples:

- cpm/ml
- platelet number/ml
- mmol Hb/l
  (The latter allows correction, if necessary, for either concentration due to evaporation or dilution due to tissue fluid)

  Calculate: % decrease in cpm/ % decrease in platelet number

(1) Hardeman et al (in preparation)

IMAGING THROMBUS WITH RADIOLABELLED MONOCLONAL ANTIBODY TO PLATELETS

Lavender J.P., Peters A.M., Stuttle A.W.J., Needham S.G., Loutfi I., Snook D., Epenetos A.A., Lumley P., Keery R.J., Hogg N.

Department of Diagnostic Radiology, Hammersmith Hospital, London

Glaxo Group Research Ltd., Ware Herts

Imperial Cancer Research Fund, London

INTRODUCTION

Indium-III labelled platelets introduced in the late 1970's as a new method of imaging thrombus have not gained widespread use and conventional radiographic techniques such as contrast phlebography for deep venous thrombosis remain as the favoured diagnostic approaches. The main drawback of Indium-III labelled platelets is the time and technical skill required for cell separation and labelling and this has resulted in only a few regional centres making use of this technique. Oster et al have demonstrated the possibility of labelling platelets by the use of a radiolabelled monoclonal antibody in the dog and we have recently explored this technique in man.

MATERIAL AND METHODS

MONOCLONAL ANTIBODY - P256

P256 is a IgG1 mouse monoclonal antibody which reacts with the platelet membrane glycoprotein complex 11b/111a.

EFFECTS OF ANTIBODY ON PLATELET FUNCTION

The effects of P256 on platelet function at different levels of receptor occupancy were studied in vitro by measuring aggregation in citrated platelet rich plasma induced by proaggregants.

RADIOLABELLING OF P256

P256 was labelled with indium-III using the bifunctional chelating agent DTPA. One to two molecules of DTPA were complexed giving a specific activity of 5 mCi/mg

26

Ch. Kessler et al. (eds.), Clinical Application of Radiolabelled Platelets, 26–27.
© 1990 Kluwer Academic Publishers.

antibody. At this activity no impairment of antibody immunoreactivity could be detected.

PLATELET LABELLING

Platelet labelling using the monoclonal antibody has been performed both in vitro and in vivo. In vitro labelling was performed using platelet rich plasma incubated with the monoclonal antibody with a calculated receptor occupancy of 6%. In vivo labelling was performed by injecting 100 ug of radiolabelled antibody intravenously labelled with 100-200 uCi of indium-III.

RESULTS

FUNCTION OF PLATELETS CARRYING P256

Platelets carrying P256 underwent spontaneous aggregation to an extent that was proportional to the percentage of receptors occupied. At or below an occupancy of 3%, however, no difference in spontaneous aggregation could be detected between platelets carrying the antibody and control platelets.

IN VIVO PLATELET KINETICS

In vitro labelled platelets showed some evidence of activation with a rising activity over the liver, but splenic pooling was regarded as similar to that seen with conventional labelling platelets. With in vivo labelling platelet behaviour was more normal showing no evidence of activation.

IMAGING

Total body distribution showed platelet pooling in the spleen where the distribution was similar to that of conventional labelled indium-III platelets. There was clear localisation of activity in thrombus.

REFERENCES

1. Oster Z.M., Srivastava S.C., Som P. et al. (1985) Thrombus radioimmuno-scintigraphy: an approach using monoclonal anti platelet antibody. Proc. Natl. Acad. Sci. U.S.A. 82: 3465-8.
2. Peters A.M., Lavender J.P., Needham S.G. et al. (1986) Imaging thrombus with radiolabelled monoclonal antibody to platelets. Br. Med. J. 293: 1525-27.

HAEMODILUTION IMPROVES III-IN-PLATELET LABELLING EFFICIENCY

Galvin D.A.J., Meek A.C., Harper R.A., McCollum C.N.

Department of Surgery, Charing Cross Hospital, Fulham Palace Road, London SW6 8RF

INTRODUCTION

Since the original description of radiolabelling of platelets with III-Indium Oxine by Thakur in 1976 (9), the applications of this technique have widened. Radiolabelled platelets have been used to assess platelet uptake on atheromatous tissue (2), in prosthetic grafts (3, 4, 7), models of surgical shock (8), transplanted organs (1), platelet vessel wall interaction following arterial surgery (6) and platelet inhibitory therapy (5). However, the preparation of platelets for radiolabelling requires an adequate platelet harvest from anticoagulated blood and at times this has been impaired by a high haematocrit. It has been suggested that haemodilution may improve platelet harvest and we have applied this to our platelet labelling technique in a canine model measuring thrombogenicity in prosthetic grafts in greyhounds.

MATERIALS AND METHODS

Greyhounds were used to investigate platelet deposition on prosthetic grafts and to assess the effect of platelet inhibitory therapy. Initially to obtain platelets for labelling venous blood, anticoagulated with sodium acid citrate, was spun for 10 mins at 200G to obtain platelet rich plasma (PRP. However, this frequently produced insufficient quantities of PRP to proceed to labelling. In 15 subsequent procedures 10 mls. of normal saline was added to the 20 mls. of anticoagulated venous blood and although this improved platelet separation, platelet harvesting was not yet optimal. Finally, anticoagulated blood was diluted with 20 mls. of calcium free Tyrode's solution containing 280 ng of PGE1, and in all subsequent cell separation procedures, satisfactory platelet harvesting was achieved.

Platelets were labelled using a method similar to that described by Wilkinson et al. (10). Seventeen mls. of venous blood was anticoagulated with 3 mls. of 3.4% sodium acid citrate and used undiluted for cell separation or diluted with either 10 mls. of 0.9% saline or 20 mls. of calcium

Ch. Kessler et al. (eds.), Clinical Application of Radiolabelled Platelets, 28–32.
© 1990 *Kluwer Academic Publishers.*

free Tyrode's solution with PGE_1. Blood was then spun at 200 G for 10 minutes to obtain a sample of platelet rich plasma (PR). This was separated using a Pasteur pipette and diluted to twice its volume with calcium free Tyrode's solution with PGE1 and then spun again at 640 G for a further 10 minutes producing a platelet pellet. The supernatant was retained and the platelets were first washed and then resuspended in 2.5 mls. of Tyrode's solution. Following the addition of 220 uCi III-Indium oxine the platelet suspension was incubated at room temperature for 10 minutes. Supernatant plasma was added to stop the labelling reaction and a further spin at 640 G isolated a pellet of radiolabelled platelets. This was then resuspended in platelet poor plasma and the labelling efficiency calculated before reinjection into each animal. Platelet aggregometry was performed at the end of each labelling procedure to assess the total aggregating response of labelled platelets to ADP. This was performed on a Payton 300B light transmittance aggregometer by adding 10 ul of a 10 ug/ml solution of ADP to 100 ul of PRP and following the aggregation response on a chart recorder (Fig. 1).

The labelling efficiency was calculated using a well crystal by measuring radioactivity from the labelled platelets and expressing it as a percentage of the total activity in platelet suspension and supernatant from the final spin.

RESULTS

Mean (-/+ sem) haematocrit in all blood samples used for labelling was 50.7 -/+ 0.66 percent. In only 8 out of 14 attempts was sufficient volume of PRP obtained from undiluted blood to proceed to platelet labelling. Saline dilution attempted in 15 animals successfully harvested platelets in 13 cases while all 40 procedures with Tyrode's dilution were successful. Mean (-/+ sem) labelling efficiency was 94.7 -/+ 0.34 percent in the Tyrode's dilution group and this was significantly higher than with saline at 86.6 -/+ 2.2 percent (p<0.0001) or the successful undiluted samples at 90.1 -/+ 1.8 percent (p<0.001) (Fig. 2). The total platelet aggregating response was unaffected by dilution at 95.2 -/+ 1.4% in whole blood, 94.2 -/+ 0.63% with saline and 93.6 -/+ 0.76% in the Tyrode's/PGE1 dilution group.

DISCUSSION

This study has demonstrated that haemodilution improves platelet harvesting in blood taken from greyhounds. The figure 1 method has yielded improved labelling efficiencies without adversely affecting platelet function as measured by platelet aggregometry to ADP. Although this method is especially applicable to greyhounds which have a mean haematocrit of approximately 51%, it may be indicated in any radiolabelling procedure where cell separation is impeded by high haematocrit and may be used if difficulties are encountered in obtaining a satisfactory cell separation.

REFERENCES

1. Buckels J.A.C., Chandler S., Hawker J.A., Smith N., Barnes A.D., McCollum C.N. (1983) Indium labelled platelet uptake in rejecting renal transplants. Surg. Gyaen. Obstet. 157: 242-246.
2. Davis H.H., Siegel B.A., Sherman L.A., Heaton W.A., NaidichT.P., Joist J.H., Welch M.J. (1980) Scintigraphic Detection of Carotid Atherosclerosis with Indium-III-labelled Autologous Platelets. Circulation 61: 982-988.
3. Goldman M., Norcott H.C., Hawker R.J., Drolc. Z., McCollum C.N. *1982) Platelet accumulation on mature Dacron grafts in man. Br. J. Surg. 69: 538-540.
4. Goldman M., Norcott H.C., Hawker R.J., Hail C., Drolc Z., McCollum C.N. (1982) Femoro-popliteal Bypass Grafts - an Isotope Technique allowing in vivo Comparison of Thrombogenicity. Br. J. Surg. 69(7): 380-382.
5. Lane I.F., Irwin J.T.C., Jennings S.A., Postkitt K.R., Meek A.C., McCollum C.N. (1986) The effect of the cyclo-oxygenase inhibitor Indobufen on platelet accumulation in prosthetic vascular grafts. Br. J. Surg. 73: 563-565.
6. Meek A.C., Lane I.F., Harper R.A., McCollum C.N., Greenhalgh R.M. (1986) Radiolabelled platelets in the evaluation of platelet inhibitory therapy following carotid endarterectomy. Nucl. Med. 25: 85.
7. Mergerman J., Christenson J.T., Hanel D.C., Strauss H.W., Abbott W.M. (1983) Imaging vascular grafts in vivo with Indium-III-labelled platelets. Ann. Surg. 198: 178-184.
8. Poskitt K.R., Irwin J.T.C., Abbondati G.G., Kox W., McCollum C.N. (1985) Pulmonary failure in surgical shock: the role of platelet aggregates studied in pigs. Br. J. Surg. 72: 399-400.
9. Thakur M.L., Welch M.J., Joist J.H., Coleman R.E. (1976) Indium-III labelled platelets: studies on preparation and evaluation of in vitro and in vivo functions. Thromb. Res. 9: 345-357.
10. Wilkinson A.R., Hawker R.J., Hawker L.M. (1978) III-Indium labelled canine platelets. Thromb. Res. 13: 175-182.

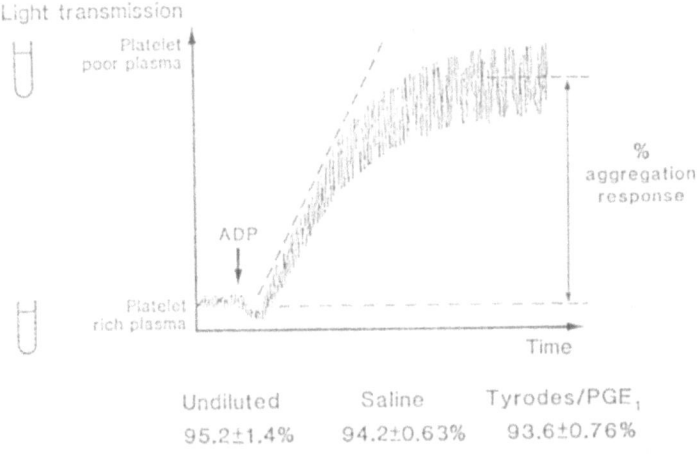

Fig 1

Total platelet aggregometry responses to ADP measured by light transmission aggregometry

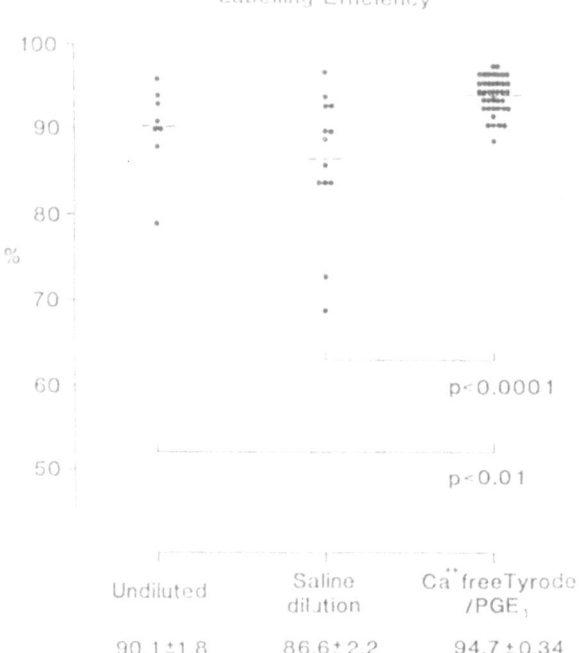

Labelling Efficiency

Undiluted	Saline dilution	Ca⁺⁺freeTyrode /PGE₁
90.1±1.8	86.6⁺2.2	94.7±0.34

p<0.0001

p<0.01

Fig 2

Comparison of platelet labelling efficiency following headmodilation of anticoagulated blood

TC-99m HMPAO AS A POTENTIAL PLATELET LABELLING COMPOUND: FIRST IN VIVO AND IN VITRO RESULTS

W. Becker (1) U. Borst, M. Weppler, (1) E.P. Kromer, W.Burner.

SUMMARY

First results of platelet labelling with Tc-99m hexamethylproplene-amineoxime (HMPAO) in-vitro (n=7) and in-vivo (n=3) are described. After platelet isolation the best incubation time is 20 min (37°C). The in-vitro Tc-99m elution out of platelets amounts to about 7%/60 min. After reinjection of the labelled cells, the organ distribution of Tc-99m is comparable to activity distribution patterns after In-111-oxin labelling with a maximum in the spleen, minor activity in the liver and total visualisation of the blood pool. Already after reinjection of the cells a kidney and bladder activity can be seen as a consequence of tracer excretion. The localisation of bowel activity after 2h p.i. also is a consequence of a Tc-99m complex elution through the intestine. A positive demonstration of Tc-99m HMPAO labelled platelets uptake in a fresh thrombus can be demonstrated.

INTRODUCTION

First results of labelling leukocytes with a new lipophilic Tc-99m complex, Tc-99m Hexamethylpropylene-amineoxime (HMPAO), primarily introduced for brain imaging, were published (6,8,10).

The advantage of a Tc-99m labelled compound over In-111 labelled compounds are comparable for the labelling of leukocytes and of platelets. These advantages are higher convenience, lower radiation dose, better image quality and the 24h availability in every nuclear medicine department. So, although first results with monoclonal platelet antibodies are reported, (9,11) the possibility of labelling platelets with Tc-99m HMPAO is an interesting question. (2).

2 METHODS AND PATIENTS
Platelet isolation and labelling

All procedures of cell separation and Tc-99m labelling were carried out aseptically in a laminar flow cabinet using sterile one way material. All centrifugation steps were completed without use of the centrifuge brake.

Thirty-four milliliters of venous blood were drawn into

33

Ch. Kessler et al. (eds.), Clinical Application of Radiolabelled Platelets, 33–44.
© 1990 Kluwer Academic Publishers.

one sterile 50ml polystyrene syringe, containing 8ml of NIH (ACD formula A; Biostabil^R) and were gently mixed. Platelet rich plasma (PRP) was obtained by centrifugation of the blood at 180 g for 15 min. Red cells trapped in the PRP were separated by another centrifugation (180g: 15 min) of the supernatant of the first centrifugation step (PRP)(7). After acidifying to pH 6. 2-6. 5 with ACD the platelets were sedimented by centrifuging the PRP at 800g for 15 min. The supernatant (PPP = platelet poor plasma) was withdrawn and stored separately in a 20ml syringe at 37°C. The platelet pellet was resuspended in 1 - 2ml of physiological saline (37°C). 555 MBq of Tc-99m HMPAO was added and incubated alternatively at 22° or 37°C for 5,10, 20 or 25 min. The labelled platelets were washed with physiologic saline (800g; 10 min), the supernatant was discharged and the platelet pellet was resuspended in the stored autologous platelet-poor plasma. 250 NBq-350 MBq labelled platelets were reinjected or used for in-vitro studies.

Tc-99m HMPAO preparation

The procedure of Tc-99m IMPAO labelling was in accordance with the instructions of **AMERSHAM-BUCHLER**
For this reason a vial was placed in a shielding container and 5ml (555MBq) of a sterile elute from a Tc-99m generator was injected. Before withdrawing the syringe from the vial 5ml of gas were withdrawn from the space above the solution to normalise the pressure in the vial. The shielded vial was shaken for 10 seconds to ensure a complete dissolution of the powder.

IN-VITRO STUDIES

To examine the best incubation time of the isolated platelets with Tc-99m HMPAO different incubation times were used (5,10,20 and 25 min). Additionally the incubation temperature was varied (22°C and 37°C).
The Tc-99m elution out of the platelets in vitro was tested by incubating the labelled cells for 70 mins. in autologous platelet poor plasma. The platelet suspension then was centrifuged (800g; 15 min) and the Tc99m activity was determined after a decay correction in the supernatant and in the sedimented pellet.
In another assay the labelled platelets were centrifuged every 20 min. to determine the Tc-99m elution in-vitro after a short incubation period (10 min, 50,min 70 min).

IN-VIVO STUDIES

After injection of the labelled cells every 30 min over a period of 270 min 5ml of venous blood was taken to determine the Tc-99m plasma activity.

CAMERA IMAGES

After reinjection of the labelled platelets gamma camera (GE 400 T) images were acquired 30 min, 1h, 2h and 20h p.i. with a parallel hole, low energy, general purpose collimator on-line to a computer (DEC GAMMA 11) using the 140 KeV peak +/-20%.

PATIENTS

Subjects included 3 patients with suspected thrombus, two endomyocardial thrombi (one female, 59 years; one male 71 years, and one suspected venous thrombo-embolus, female 53 years).

Following i.v. bolus injection the kinetic pattern of the Tc-99m labelled platelets were dynamically registered by a dynamic flow study over 30 min. Time activity curves of heart, liver and spleen were reconstructed taking regions of interest over these organs. The percentile distribution of Tc-99m activity was calculated between the heart, the liver and the spleen.

RESULTS
Labelling efficiency and stability of the label in-vitro

The purity of the isolated cell pellet was high. The number of contaminating red cells and leukocytes was less than 1%.

The labelling efficiency was dependant on the incubation temperature and incubation time (Fig 1). The note physiologic room temperature showed a slightly lower labelling efficiency than the incubation at 37°C. the longer the incubation period, the better was the labelling efficiency. The longest incubation period tested was 25 min, because according to the instructions of the producer of HMPAO the complex should be used within 30 minutes after reconstitution of the complex.

After an in-vitro incubation the tested Tc-99m elution amounted to about 11% during 70 min p.i. A regular centrifugation every 20 min resulted in a Tc-99m elution of about 7% of the activity per centrifugation-step (Fig 2).

IN-VIVO TC-99M ACTIVITY CURVES

The measured in-vivo activity showed a nearly linear decline of the curve after a single decrease of activity 60-min after reinjection of the cells.

Patients

The time activity curves recorded over the lungs, the cardiac blood pool and the spleen by dynamic imaging over 30-min after platelet reinjection were similar to those seen

fig.1

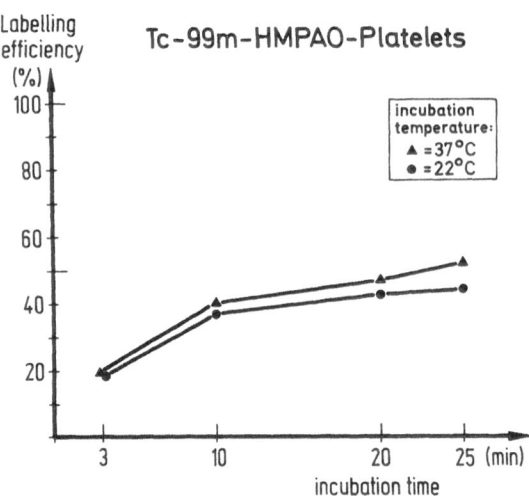

Influence of temperature and incubation
time on the labelling efficiency of Tc-99m-HMPAO
labelled platelets

fig.2

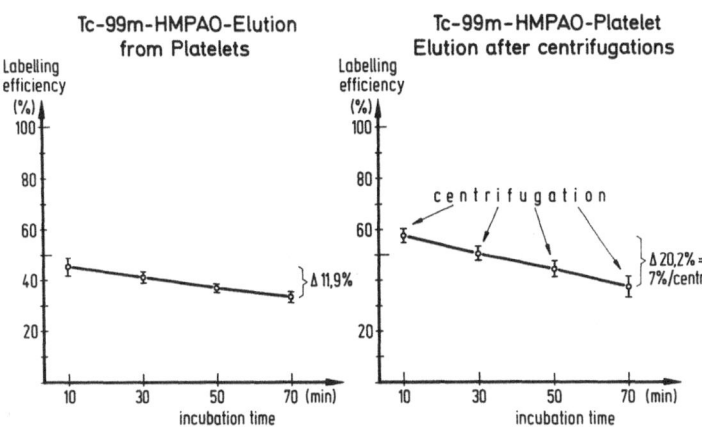

In-vitro-stability of Tc-99m-HMPAO of
platelets after permanent incubation
(37°C) (left) and repeated centrifugation (37°C)
every 20 min after labelling (right)

after reinjection of In-111 oxine labelled platelets. The whole body distribution was identical to the distribution known after injection of platelets labelled with in-111 oxine. There was an intensive splenic activity (1h: 22,4 + 1, 0%/2h: 20, 8 + 0, 6%), and blood pool imaging (heart 1h: 23,1 + 3, 8%/2h: 22, 3 + 0, 6%).

Immediately after renal perfusion of the labelled platelets a Tc-99m complex excretion by the kidneys leads to an increase of the bladder activity (Fig 3a, b). 1,5 to 2 hours after reinjection of the labelled cells, no gallbladder visualisation could be recognised, but later on the small bowel and also large bowel could be seen (Fig 4a, b).

The examined 71-year old male with a pathologic platelet uptake admitted to the hospital after a myocardial infarction, showed echocardiographically a suspicious left ventricular mass. Scintigraphically 1h and 2h after injection of the labelled platelets a pathologic uptake could be clearly delineated in projection to the left ventricular mass (Fig 5). The activity of the thrombus was comparable to the spleen activity and could be clearly delineated from the blood pool activity (Fig 5).

The other two examined patients both were treated by anti-coagulants over at least 48-hours. One female showed echocardiographically an endomyocardial thrombus, the other female showed a scintigraphically diagnosed lung embolism without pathologic platelet uptake in the deep vein or the lung (figure 3a,b).

DISCUSSION

The 'golden standard' of platelet labelling is the In-111-oxine method (4,12). This disadvantages of this method are the physical characteristics of this isotope and the time and technical skill required for the platelet isolation procedure (3,5). The last problem seems to be theoretically solved by the possibility of thrombus imaging with In-111-labelled monoclonal antibodies in man (9,11). The first problem, physical characteristics, is present up to now. Tc-99m would be an ideal isotope for labelling, because of its 24-hour availability in every nuclear medicine department, the better imaging quality and the lower radiation exposure to the patient. But the desired shorter physical half- life of Tc-99m makes it impossible to use Tc-99m labelled platelets for platelet kinetic studies; so only thrombus localisation would be possible. For this reason the stability of the label and kinetic dates of the Tc-99m-HMPAO-labelled platelets or the elution of a Tc-99m-complex out of the cells has to be known.

The tested labelling efficiency is best at 37°C after 25 min. incubation period in vitro (Fig 1). The elution rate of the isotope in-vitro amounts to about 10% over 70-min. The character of the eluted isotope is completely

fig.3a

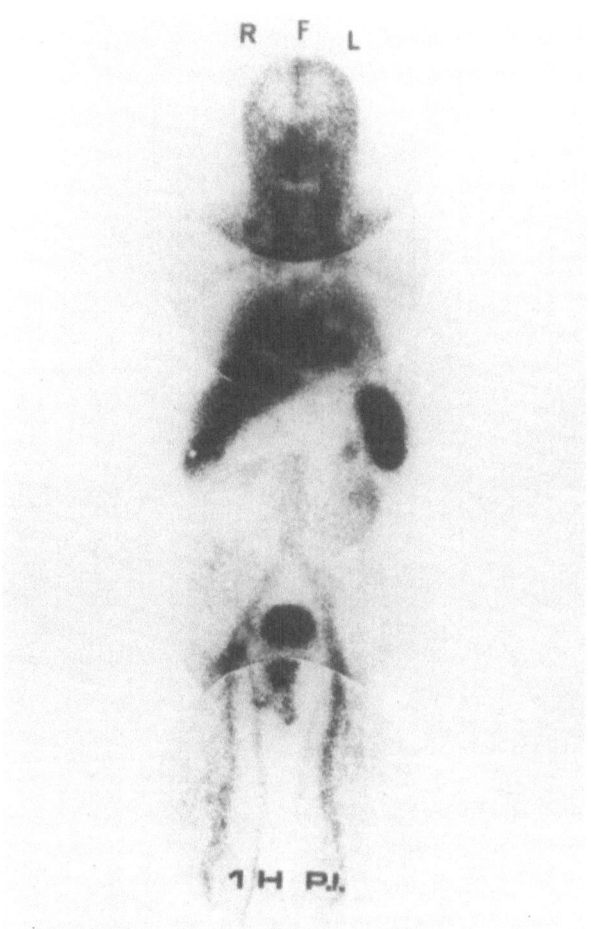

Whole body distribution of Tc-99m-HMPAO- labelled
platelets 1 hour (a) and 2 hour (b) after
reinjection. The maximum of activity is
concentrated in the spleen and minor in the liver.
The blood pool is clearly delineated. Note the
missing thyroid and brain uptake, the renal and
bladder activity as a consequence of Tc-99m
complex elution (53 year old female)

fig.3b

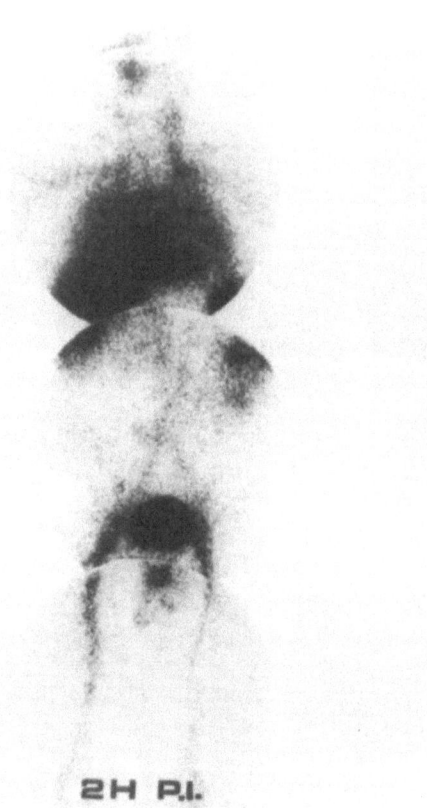

Fig 4.

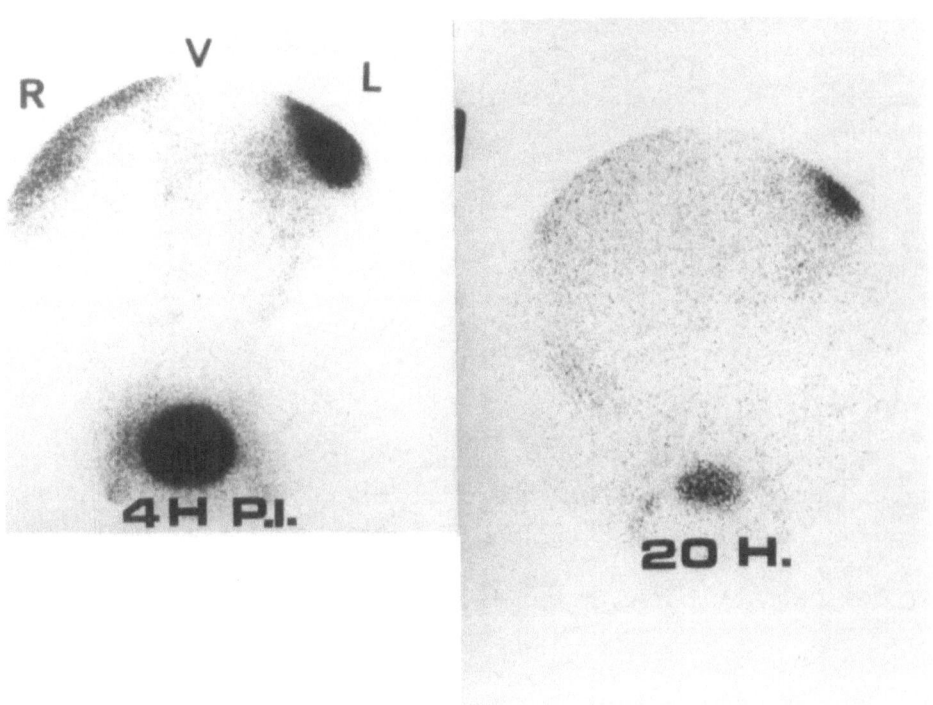

Normal platelet distribution in spleen and liver
with additional kidney and bladder activity and
delineated bowel activity 4 hours and 20 hours
p.i.

fig.5

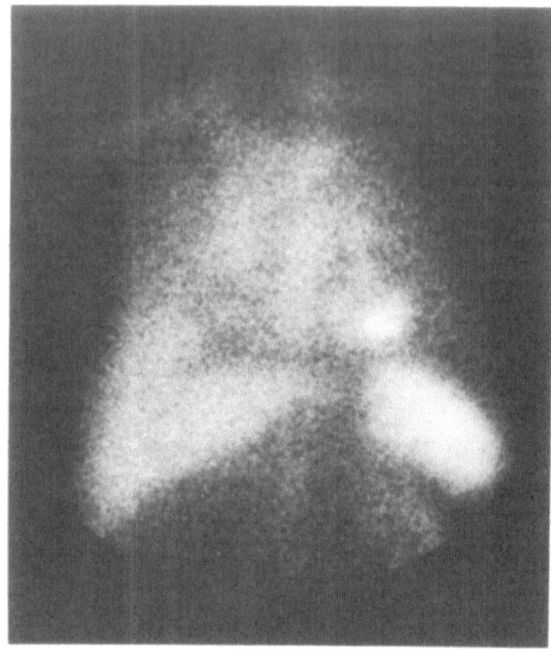

Intensive Tc-99m-HMPAO platelet uptake in a
ventricular thrombus in a 71-year old male 2 hours
after reinjection of the labelled platelets (2)

unknown, this may be the isotope or a Tc-99m-complex. Because the percentage of contaminating red cells and leukocytes is lower than 1%, it seems reasonable that the eluted label derives from the platelets themselves. As a consequence immediately after renal perfusion the kidneys are visualised and shortly after bladder activity increases. The eluted complex also is intestinally excreted.

Incidently to the behaviour of Tc-99m-HMPAO as a leukocyte label in all our examined patients a Tc-99m-complex elution could be seen (1.8). This seems not to be TcO_4^- because in none of the examined patients a thyroid uptake could be seen. The excreted Tc-99m-complex seems to be similar to that in leukocyte labelling studies. because a renal and intestinal excretion could be identified. The intestinal pathway leads to a bowel activity, that could be seen about 1,5 to 2-hours after reinjection of the labelled platelets. Deriving from these Tc-99m-complex elutions diagnostic problems arise concerning abdominal thrombus localisation. The eluted complex also is not the label Tc-99m-HMPAO itself, because no brain imaging results.

The percentage of Tc-99m-distribution over the heart, liver and spleen in the first hour p.i. is comparable to In-111-oxine platelet studies (4) and allows to suppose a high Tc-99m-stability in the labelled platelets.

The stability of this label and the reproducability of our results still has to be proven in future patient studies. So Tc-99m-HMPAO seems to be a promising platelet labelling compound for clinical studies in imaging thrombosis, although diagnostic problems are present in the abdomen; of course platelet survival studies are not possible due to the short physical half-life of Tc-99m.

REFERENCES

1   W.Becker, E Schomann, W.Fischbach, W.Börner, K.G.Gruner. Comparison of Tc-99m-HMPAO and In-111-Oxine-labelled granulocytes in man: First clinical results (in preparation)

2   W.Becker, W.Borner, U.Borst, E.P.Kromer, K.R.Gruner. Tc-99m-HMPAO: A new platelet labelling compound? Eur.J.Nucl.Med. (in press)

3   M.R.Dewanjee, S.A.Rao, P.Didisheim. Indium-111 Tropolone, a new high-affinity platelet label: Preparation and evaluation of labelling parameters J.Nucl.Med. 22 (1981) 981-987

4   A.duP.Heyns, M.G.Lötter, P.N.Bradenhorst, O.R.van Reenen, H.Pieters, P.C.Minaar, F.P.Retief. Kinetics, distribution and sites of destruction of 111-Indium-labelled human platelets. Brit.J.Haemat. 44 (1980) 269-280

5   R.L.Hill-Zobel, S.Gannon, B.McCandless, M.F.Tsan Effects of chelates and incubation media on platelet

labelling with Indium- 111.J.Nucl.Med. 28 (1987) 223-228

6   K.Joseph, V.Damann, G.Engeroff, K.R.Gruner. Markierung von leukozyten mit Technetium-99m-HMPAO: Erste klinische Ergebnisse. Nuc Compact 17 (1986) 277-283

7   A.Moisan, J.le Cloirec, J.Y.Herry. Marquage des plaquettes et des granulocytes par l'oxine-indium-111. J.biophys.et med.nucl.7 (1983) 113-115

8   A.M.Peters, H.J.Danpure, S.Osman, R.J.Hawker, B.L.Henderson, H.J.Hodgson, J.D.Kelly, R.D.Neirinck, J.P.Lavender. Clinical experience with Tc-99m hexamethylpropyleneaminoxime for labelling leukocytes and imaging inflammation lancet 11 (1986) 946-949

9)   A.M.Peters, J.P.Lavender, S.G.Needham, T.Loufti, D.Snook, A.A.Epenetos, P.Lumley, R.J.Keery, N.Hogg. Imaging thrombus with radiolabelled monoclonal antibody to platelets. Brit.Med.J. 293 (1986) 1525-1527

10   C.Schumichen, J.Schölmerich. Tc-99m-HMPAO labelling of leukocytes for detection of inflammatory bowel diseases. Nuc Compact 17 (1986) 274-276

11   P.Som, Z.H.Oster, P.O.Zamora, K.Yamamoto,D.F.Sacker, A.B.Brill, K.D.Newell, B.A.Rhodes. Radioimmunoimaging of experimental thrombi in dogs using technetium-99m-labelled monoclonal antibody fragments reactive with human platelets. J.Nucl.Med.27 (1986) 1315-1320

12   M.L.Thakur, M.J.Welch, H.J.Hoist, E.R.Coleman. Indium-111 labelled platelets: studies on preparation and evaluation of in vitro and in vivo functions. Thromb.Res.9. (1976) 345-357

PLATELET LABELLING WITH III-IN-TROPOLONATE

Louwes H. and Schuur J.J.

Department of Nuclear Medicine, R.K. Ziekenhuis, Groningen,
The Netherlands.

INTRODUCTION

Thrombocytopenia may be caused by production
disturbance, by abnormal distribution or by an increased use
or destruction. There is no simple laboratory method
available to determine the cause of a thrombocytopenia. One
method could be the determination of platelet survival time.
Until the end of the seventies ^{51}Cr was used as a
label, when it was replaced by III-In complexes. These
complexes like tropolonate, oxinate, 2-mercapto pyridine-N-
oxide (MERC) and actylacetonate are not cell-specific. That
means that a blood sample with erythrocytes, granulocytes,
lymphocytes, monocytes and platelets will have to be
separated from the rest in order to obtain a specific cell
suspension for labelling. Separating cells from whole blood
requires skill, which may be obtained with some
perseverance. The most important rule is to separate the
cells in such a way that normal function is retained after
labelling and re-injection into the patient.
In 1981/1982 4 independent reports were published in
which the use of tropolonate was described (Dewanjee 1981;
Burke 1982; Danpure 1982; Dewanjee 1982).
The important advantage of III-In-tropolonate over III-
In-oxinate and III-In-acetylacetonate is that the platelets
may be labelled in a plasma environment (Danpure 1982). In
plasma the cell viability will be better maintained. III-
In-tropolonate is a lipophilic substance and diffuses
relatively easy through the platelet membrane. Within the
cell III-In-tropolonate falls apart and III-In will
irreversibly bind to the cytoplasma (Thakur 1977). Next to
the determination of the Mean Platelet Life, III-In labelled
platelets may be used to follow platelet Kinetics. Peters
and Lavender (1983, 1984) have described platelet kinetics
in a number of publications.
In our hospital, III-In labelled platelets have been
used since 1977, first with III-In-oxinate and since 1984
with III-In-tropolonate, also with excellent results.

45

Ch. Kessler et al. (eds.), Clinical Application of Radiolabelled Platelets, 45–60.
© 1990 *Kluwer Academic Publishers.*

LABELLING PROTOCOL

- fill 60 ml syringe, fitted with an 186 needle, with 7,5 ml of ACD
- withdraw 42.5 ml of blood, without pressure.
- mix contents of syringe well, avoid foaming.
- divide contents of syringe over 2 sterile conical tubes.
- spin tubes for 15 min. at 200 x g.
- remove Platelet Rich Plasma (PRP) as much as possible.
- transfer PRP into a sterile polystyrene tube.
- determine the PRP volume.
- adjust the pH of the PRP to 6.0-6.5 (0.1 ml ACD per ml PRP).
- mix carefully, avoid foam formation.
- spin PRP 15 min. at 650 x g.
- removed Platelet Poor Plasma (PPP).
- store PPP in a sterile tube.
- transfer 0.5 ml PPP onto the platelet pellet.
- resuspend cell pellet carefully, avoid aggregates.
- add 18,5 Mbq (0.5 mCi) of III-In-tropolonate to the platelet suspension.
- incubate 20 min. at room temperature.
- after incubation add 5 ml. of PPP to the platelet suspension.
- measure the tube in the dose calibrator.
- spin PRP 15 min. at 650 x g.
- remove the radioactive supernatant PPP.
- add 1 ml non-radioactive PPP and gently resuspend the cells.
- add another 5 ml. of PPP.
- mix carefully and measure tube again in the dose calibrator.
- the labelling efficiency may now be calculated.
- fill a syringe with 5 ml. of cell suspension for reinjection into the patient.
- 1 ml. of cell suspension is retained for quality control testing.

QUALITY CONTROL

The following parameters are determined
- a) labelling efficiency
- b) activity bound to   -erythrocytes
                         -plasma
- c) platelet viability

ad a) labelling efficiency is determined as follows :

$$\text{Labelling Efficiency} = \frac{P}{P + W}$$

P: activity in platelet suspension
W: activity in washing solution (=supernatant PPP)

ad b 1) activity bound to erythrocytes

0.1 ml platelet suspension is mixed with 1.9 ml ammonium oxalate. After 25 min. incubation this mixture is centrifuged for 20 min. at 300 x g. The activity is measured before and after centrifugation. Labelling percentage to erythrocytes may be calculated according to the same formula.

ad b 2) activity bound to plasma

0.1 ml of platelet suspension is mixed with 1.9 ml saline. After 25 min. incubation this mixture is centrifuged for 20 min. at 300 x g. The activity is measured before and after centrifugation. Labelling percentage to plasma may thus be calculated.

PLATELET VIABILITY

- visual check by holding the suspension against the light. Platelets have a typical shine.
- microscopic check of platelet in ACD plasma shows them as flat, oblong to circular discs.
- microscopic check on aggregates.
- ability to aggregate by means of ADP and an aggregometer.
- hypotonic shock response. (Hardeman 1974,1990) The addition of water to the platelet suspension causes hypotonicity. The platelets will increase in size because of osmosis. Water taken up by the platelets, is actively removed. Thereafter the increase in size of the platelets and its return may be measured with an aggregometer.

IN-VITRO INVESTIGATION

0.1 ml of the injected labelled platelet suspension is used for a standard solution, diluted in 250 ml HCl 4N.
After administration blood is sampled at the following points in time: 0, 15, 30, 45, 60, 90, 105, 180 and 240 min. and during 5 - 7 days twice a day. The blood samples are centrifuged for 10 min. at 200 x g. One ml of plasma supernatant is transferred into a counting tube. All samples are counted (at the same time) for 1 min.
The Mean Platelet Life is calculated according to a linear, exponential, gamma function, mean and weighted mean arithmatic model. Calculations were performed following the recommendations of the International Panel of Diagnostic Applications of Radioisotopes in Haematology (ICSH) (1977).

INITIAL PLATELET RECOVERY

The initial Platelet Recovery (IPR) was calculated from the total blood activity extrapolated to zero time as a fraction of the injected radioactivity. The Patient blood volume (BV) in liters needed for this calculation was estimated from the subjects height (H) and weight (W) using the following formula (Bowring 1981):

-   males $BV = 0.417 H^3 + 0.0450 W - 0.03$

-   females $BV = 0.414 H^3 + 0.0328 W - 0.03$

where H is in m. W in kg and BV in 1.

PLATELET PRODUCTION RATE

Assuming that platelet destruction is a random process the survival curve will be mono-exponential. The Fractional Platelet Production Rate (FPPR) is equal to the reciprocal of the Platelet Survival (PS), in formula :

$$FPPR = \frac{1}{PS} \ (d^{-1})$$

If the number of platelets per litre (NPF) is known the platelet production rate per litre (PPRL) may be calculated:

$$PPRL - NPL \cdot FPPR = \frac{NPL}{PS} \ (1^{-1} \cdot d^{-1})$$

After correction for the initial platelet recovery and for splenic pooling (factor 0.90, Harker et al. 1969) the PPRL is calculated using the formula:

$$PPRL = \frac{NPL \cdot 0.90}{PS \cdot IPR} \ (1^{-1} \cdot d^{-1})$$

By multiplication with the patient Blood Volume, the Total Platelet Production Rate (TPPR) is found:

$$TPPR = \frac{BV \cdot NPL \cdot 0.90}{PR \cdot IPR} \ (d^{-1})$$

ORGAN UPTAKE

The hepatic and splenic uptake were measured with a

large-field-of-view gamma camera interfaced with a computer
(A^2 Medical Data System). The gamma camera visualised the
heart, lungs, spleen and liver simultaneously. Before
injection the patients were positioned by marking the
xiphoid and anterior iliac spines as points of reference. In
posterior position 60 one minute digital frames were
recorded. Recording of a 60 min. time activity curve over
the spleen enables the determination of the wash-in curve
and calculation of the T 1/2. If it is assumed that the
first hour represents pooling only, kinetics may be
described as a two compartmental model. The relation between
the activity in compartment 1 (blood) and 2 (spleen) may be
represented as described in appendix 1. Also the calculation
of the Splenic Blood Flow (SBF) and the Transit Time (TT) is
described in appendix 1. Following the dynamic investigation
static acquisition is started for 5 minutes in anterior and
posterior position. Twice daily these views are repeated
along with blood sampling for the determination of platelet
half life. Using standardised regions of interest techniques
the geometric mean counts of liver and spleen were
calculated as a percentage of the amount of radioactivity
injected (Fleming 1979).

RADIATION DOSE

In order to obtain insight into the radiation dose of
III-In-platelets the absorbed dose and the effective dose
equivalent were calculated in normals (n=11). Cumulative
activity was calculated by integration of the time curves.
The organ dose was calculated with the aid of the S-values
for III-In as used in the MIRD Tables. The effective dose
equivalent was calculated following the instructions of ICRP
26.

STATISTICS

All values are expressed as mean with one standard
deviation. Significance was taken as p <0.005.

RESULTS

In normals (n=11), having an average number of
platelets of 237 -/+ 37 x 10 9/1 a labelling efficiency of
87 -/+ 8% was found. In patients (n=58) with an average
platelet number of 56 -/+ 32 x 10 9/1 this value was 79 -/+
12%,

QUALITY CONTROL

Next to the labelling efficiency, the percentage
labelling to contaminating erythrocytes and to plasma were
determined. For normals 0.2 -/+ 0.4% and 0.9 -/+ 0.7%
respectively. In patients these values were: 0.9 -/+ 1.2%
and 1.2 -/+ 0.9%.

Under the microscope no aggregates were seen.
The relative percentage of aggregation in order to check the platelet viability in normals as well as patients after addition of ADP was 95 -/+ 7%. The relative hypotonic shock response was 92 -/+ 5%.

IN-VITRO

The results of the calculations of the mean platelet life, initial recovery, total platelet production, transport constant (k12), transit time and splenic blood flow are stated in Table 1.

IN-VIVO

The uptake in the liver and the spleen is displayed in Table 2 (normals and patients).

DOSIMETRY

The absorbed dose and the body effective dose equivalent are to be found in table 3.

DISCUSSION

The tropolonate concentration in the final cell suspension (5×10^{-5} M) was lower than stated in literature: Danpure and Osmone (1981) ; Dewanjee (1986) and Vallabhajosula (1986).
As the labelling efficiencies in normals as well as in patients were higher than 75% and III-tropolonate is readily available in this form as a radiopharmaceutical there was no reason for us to increase the tropolonate concentration.
The labelling efficiency lies within the same range as reported by other authors: Dewanjee 1986 ; Goldsmit 1986 and Vallabhajosula 1986.
The plasma bound activity was significantly lower (0-1.7%) than found by Dewanjee (1986) (3 - 5%). This percentage increased in the course of 5 days to approx. 20%, while in our hands the value remained stable throughout the investigation.
Results of the Mean Platelet Life (in normals) and initial recovery compare well with those found in literature (Table 4). In all patients the value of mean platelet life was shorter than in normals (p <0.005). MPL in patients with a thrombocytopenia due to decreased production was longer than the MPL found in patients.
The initial recovery in patients does not differ significantly from the value for normals, except for patients with hypersplenism, whose initial recovery is lower.
Total Platelet Production Rate is compared to the

able 1: results of the mean platelet life(MPL),initial recovery(IR),platelet production rate(TPPR), splenic blood flow(SBF),transittime(TT),transportconsant (k12),half time($T_{1/2}$) wash-in curve spleen.

est	units	normals	thrombocytopenia immune	thrombocytopenia decreased production	thrombocytopenia hypersplenism	thrombocytopenia recurrent
r platelets	$10^9 l^{-1}$	237 ± 37	55 ± 32	60 ± 40	87 ± 28	53 ± 22
PL (l)	d	9.5 ± 1.4	3.0 ± 1.8	6.2 ± 2.6	5.7 ± 2.2	2.9 ± 1.7
PL(e)	d	7.3 ± 1.5	1.3 ± 1.3	4.7 ± 2.3	4.2 ± 1.8	1.6 ± 1.2
PL(g)	d	9.2 ± 1.5	1.9 ± 1.6	5.1 ± 2.3	4.6 ± 1.8	1.9 ± 2.0
PL(m)	d	8.3 ± 1.3	2.4 ± 1.5	5.4 ± 2.6	4.9 ± 2.0	2.3 ± 1.5
IPL(wm)	d	9.4 ± 1.3	2.9 ± 1.7	6.1 ± 2.5	5.6 ± 2.0	2.9 ± 1.7
ecovery(l)	%	59 ± 12	45 ± 20	55 ± 14	33 ± 13	63 ± 17
ecovery(e)	%	60 ± 12	47 ± 20	56 ± 14	34 ± 13	66 ± 18
ecovery(g)	%	60 ± 12	48 ± 20	55 ± 14	34 ± 13	65 ± 18
PPR(l)	$10^9\ d^{-1}$	214 ± 55	267 ± 287	73 ± 38	320 ± 370	135 ± 70
PPR(e)	$10^9\ d^{-1}$	275 ± 70	692 ±1560	90 ± 49	480 ± 628	311 ± 200
TPR(g)	$10^9\ d^{-1}$	220 ± 69	692 ± 226	94 ± 80	470 ± 635	264 ± 189
T1/2	min	4.3 ± 0.5	4.8 ± 2.2	5.1 ± 2.0	3.7 ± 1.3	9.3 ± 0.8
(12	$1000.min^1$	53 ± 7	67 ± 55	52 ± 40	117 ± 56	2 ± 1
TT	min	10.7 ± 1.2	11.0 ± 6.2	10.1 ± 4.0	13.8 ± 7.6	13.9 ± 0.8
SBF	ml/min	287 ± 83	308 ± 270	187 ± 120	587 ± 387	7 ± 5

l = linear;e = exponential;g = gammafunction; w = mean;gw = weighted mean

<u>table 2</u>:organ uptake in normals and patients with thrombocytopenic disorders.

time after injection (h)	Organuptake (%)				
	normals	thrombocytopenia immune	thrombocytopenia decreased production	thrombocytopenia hypersplenism	thrombocytopenia recurrent
spleen					
1	38 ± 2	29 ± 9	33 ± 13	54 ± 15	4 ± 2
4 - 5	35 ± 2	29 ± 8	35 ± 16	52 ± 12	6 ± 3
21 - 28	37 ± 2	30 ± 8	39 ± 19	52 ± 12	14 ± 6
48 - 54	36 ± 2	31 ± 9	40 ± 20	52 ± 12	17 ± 11
72 - 80	36 ± 2	30 ± 9	41 ± 20	52 ± 12	19 ± 9
liver					
1	10 ± 1	10 ± 3	13 ± 4	6 ± 2	36 ± 25
4 - 5	11 ± 1	10 ± 2	14 ± 5	5 ± 2	43 ± 24
21 - 28	10 ± 2	12 ± 4	17 ± 6	5 ± 2	57 ± 23
48 - 54	10 ± 2	13 ± 4	20 ± 9	5 ± 2	60 ± 20
72 - 80	10 ± 2	14 ± 4	18 ± 9	5 ± 2	60 ± 22

table 3:Absorbed Dose and Effective Dose Equivalent

[111]In-labeled platelets in normals(n=11)

target organ	SOURCE ORGAN			
	spleen mGy/MBq	liver mGy/MBq	total body mGy/MBq	total mGy/MBq
spleen	8.63 ± 0.82	0.008 ± 0.003	0.09 ± 0.01	8.73 ± 0.75
liver	0.030 ± 0.001	0.36 ± 0.06	0.089 ± 0.008	0.48 ± 0.06
muscles	0.043 ± 0.005	0.011 ± 0.002	0.076 ± 0.005	0.13 ± 0.01
lungs	0.064 ± 0.005	0.021 ± 0.003	0.081 ± 0.001	0.16 ± 0.01
marrow	0.041 ± 0.003	0.011 ± 0.003	0.105 ± 0.001	0.16 ± 0.01
thyroid	0.0032 ± 0.0001	0.002 ± 0.0003	0.070 ± 0.005	0.08 ± 0.01
bone	0.027 ± 0.003	0.011 ± 0.003	0.095 ± 0.008	0.13 ± 0.01
pancreas	0.58 ± 0.06	0.032 ± 0.005	0.105 ± 0.008	0.71 ± 0.05
stomach	0.28 ± 0.03	0.027 ± 0.011	0.097 ± 0.008	0.40 ± 0.02
kidneys	0.26 ± 0.02	0.032 ± 0.001	0.089 ± 0.008	0.39 ± 0.02
testes	0.002 ± 0.003	0.001 ± 0.0003	0.068 ± 0.005	0.07 ± 0.01
ovaries	0.016 ± 0.001	0.004 ± 0.001	0.094 ± 0.001	0.12 ± 0.01

The effective dose equivalent(mSv): men: 0.62 ± 0.04

women: 0.63 ± 0.04

table 4: initial recovery(IR), mean platelet life(MPL):comparison with other authors

Author	IR %	MPL linear (d)	MPL exponential (d)	MPL gammafu. (d)
Heyns*(1980)	72 ± 16	9.0 ± 0.7		
Robertson*(1981)	74 ± 10	8.3 ± 0.25	7.4 ± 1.4	7.5 ± 0.5
Heaton*(1979)	71 ± 4	8.8 ± 0.25	6.8 ± 0.4	7.3 ± 0.5
Heaton***(1979)	47 ± 7	9.8 ± 0.3	8.0 ± 0.4	7.7 ± 0.6
Schmidt*(1983)	58 ± 3	8.7 ± 0.25	2.5 ± 0.4	6.2 ± 1.9
Bolin* (1982)	38 ± 11	8.8 ± 2.2	4.6 ± 2.2	10.4 ± 1.0
Scheffel*(1982)	57 ± 11	9.9 ± 0.8	3.5 ± 0.6	8.7 ± 1.0
Dewanjee**(1986)	56 ± 10	10.0 ± 0.9	6.9 ± 1.0	8.8 ± 1.6
Dewanjee***(1986)	56 ± 10	9.0 ± 0.6	5.8 ± 0.6	8.2 ± 0.8
Dewanjee**(1986)	56 ± 10	10.6 ± 0.8	6.8 ± 0.9	10.4 ± 1.0
Heyns*(1986)	61 ± 12			9.4 ± 1.0
Heyns***(1986)	68 ± 13			9.2 ± 1.0
Lotter*(1986)		9.7 ± 0.6	4.1 ± 0.7	9.3 ± 0.7
Vallabhajosula*(1986)	57 ± 11	9.5 ± 0.8	6.3 ± 0.9	9.3 ± 1.2
Vallabhajosula**(1986)	66 ± 17	10.7 ± 1.5	7.3 ± 1.5	9.3 ± 1.4
present study** (1987)	60 ± 12	9.5 ± 1.5	7.3 ± 1.4	9.2 ± 1.4

* ^{111}In-oxinate ;** ^{111}In-tropolonate;***[51]Cr used as label.

table 5:Uptake in liver and spleen spleen: comparison with other authors

	liver (% uptake) (after 1 hour)***	spleen (% uptake) (after 1 hour)***
Heyns(1980)	15.8 ± 0.7	25.9 ± 4.1
Robertson(1982)	8.6 ± 0.8	42.3 ± 3.2
Scheffel(1982)	12.5 ± 1.6	36.8 ± 2.8
Klonizakis(1980)	7.0 ± 1.0	25.9 ± 4.1
Heyns(1986)	9.6 ± 1.2	31.1 ± 6.1
Dewanjee*(1986)	5.8 ± 3.4	35 ± 10
RKZ*(1987)	10.1 ± 2.6	36 ± 2

***author dependant

values found by Heyns (1986), Branehog (1977) and Harker
(1969) are within the same range as our results with III-In-
tropolonate.

Platelet production in patients with thrombocytopenia
due to decreased production is indeed lower than in normals
(p <0.005). The range was very wide in patients with an ITP,
but none had lower than normal values.

Liver and spleen uptake after one hour in normals
correlates well with the values found in literature (Table
5). Also, the absolute uptake in spleen and liver does not
differ from values published by other authors. However, in
the course of our investigation Dewanjee (1986) and duP.
Heyns (1980) published significantly increased values of
absolute uptake in liver as well as spleen. Scheffel (1982)
did not find a significant increase in the course of the
investigational procedure.

In patients with ITP, the one hour splenic uptake
varied from 9 - 58%. In 18 (= 62%) of these patients the
splenic uptake increased with time. The one hour hepatic
uptake ranged from 5 - 24%. In 24 % of those the uptake
increased with time.

The patients with thrombocytopenia Due to decreased
production showed a one hour splenic uptake from 12 - 43%.
In one patient the uptake increased during the consecutive
days. The one hour hepatic uptake carried from 8 - 14%. In 7
(= 44%) of these patients the hepatic uptake increased with
time.

The group of patients with hypersplenism had a one hour
splenic uptake with a higher value (43 - 83%) than in
normals. In none of them the value increased in the course
of time.

Uptake of activity over the spleen during the first
hour after administration of III-In-labelled platelets may
be looked upon as pooling. An increase in activity over the
liver or the spleen during the consecutive days should be
considered as increased destruction. As absolute uptake in
normals is relatively constant, this might indicate that
destruction and pooling is a continuous process and that
they run parallel. The rate of destruction is sometimes
called destruction-pooling ratio (D/P). It might be more
adequate to replace the D/P ratio by dt/da ratio in which dt
is a function of time and da a function of the absolute
increase of activity in one of both organs.

One of the possible causes of increased liver uptake
could be degree of damage to platelets, caused by the
separation process. In our hands, microscopic checking and
viability testing did not show any changes in platelet
aspect or function.

It is assumed that in patients with ITP two processes
occur: lysis and phagocytosis. Lysis takes place within the
circulating blood, phagocytosis happens by the macrophages
in liver and or spleen. Hirsch (1983) assumes that platelets
with a lot of platelets antibodies are phagocytosed by liver

macrophages and platelets with a few antibodies by those of the spleen. It would be interesting to compare organ uptake with titrated platelet antibodies. In our investigation this comparison was not included.

In 2 patients with recurrent thrombocytopenia after splenectomy, accessory spleen was found. The one hour uptake in the splenic tissue was 2 and 5% respectively, and increased to 12% in the one patient (after 24 hrs) and to 22% in the other (after 48 hrs). The 1 hour hepatic uptake varied from 12 - 60%. In all patients the hepatic uptake increased with time.

Comparison of the calculated results of the transport constant (k12), transit time and splenic blood flow, with those of Peters (1980), shows a very good correlation. In nearly all patient groups k12, transit time and splenic blood flow are more or less comparable. Only splenic blood flow in patients with hypersplenism was -obviously-increased.

In platelets within the splenic blood flow are in (dynamic) equilibrium with circulating platelets, it may be concluded that splenic blood flow dependant upon 2 factors: size of the spleen and the transit time. In patients with thrombocytopenia no correlation has been found between splenic blood flow and the absolute splenic uptake.

Neither could be a correlation be established between Initial Recovery and the absolute splenic uptake. It may be possible that the absolute splenic uptake is not the right parameter to determine splenic size. It might be better to correlate the data obtained with the splenic volume instead of uptake.

CONCLUSION

In general, one might say that the method of separating and labelling platelets with III-In-tropolonate can easily be performed (technically). Mean platelet life, initial recovery, total platelet production and the uptake in time of the liver and the spleen are clinically relevant parameters. The value of the other data as calculated with the two compartmental model still remains to be established in further studies.

REFERENCES

1. Bolin R.B., Greene J.R. (1986) Stored platelet survival data analysis by a gamma model. Transfusion 26: 28-30.
2. Bowring C.S. (ed.) : Radionuclide tracer techniques in haematology. Butterworths, London, Boston, Sydney, Wellington, Durban and Toronto. (1981) ; 40-41.
3. Branehog H.I., Ridell B. and Weinfeld (1977) On the Analysis of Platelet survival curves and the Calculation of Platelet Production and Destruction. Scand. J. Haemtol. 19: 230-231.

4. Burke J.E.T., Roath S., Ackery D., Wyeth P. (1982) The comparison of 8-hydroxyquinoline, tropolone and acetylacetone as mediators in the labelling of polymorphonuclear leucocytes with Indium-III: a function study. Eur. J. Nucl. Med. 7: 73-76.

5. Danpure H.J., Osman S., Brady F. (1982) The labelling of blood cells in plasma with III-In-tropolonate. Br. J. Radiol. 55: 247-249.

6. Dewanjee M.K. Rao S.A., Didisheim P. *1981) Indium-III-tropolone a new high-affinity platelet label: preparation and evaluation of labelling parameters. J. Nucl. Med. 22: 981-987.

7. Dewanjee M.K., Wahner H.W., Dum W.L., Robertson J.S., Offord K.P., Fuster V.P. Chesebro J.H. (1986) Comparison of tree Platelet Survival Time in Healthy Volunteers. Mayo Clin. Proc. 61: 327-336.

8. Dewanjee M.K., Rao S.A., Rosemark J.A., Chowakwry S., Didisheim P. (1982) Indium-III Tropolone, A new Tracer for Platelet Labelling. Radiology 145: 149-153.

9. Fleming J.S. (1979) A technique for the measurement of activity using a gamma camera and computer. Phys. Med. Biol. 24: 176-180.

10. GoldsmithS.J., Vallabhajosula S., Machac J., Lipszyc H., Brown C., Badimon L., Fuster V (1985) III-In-labelled Platelets for Kinetic Studies and Thrombus Imaging: Tropolone vs Oxine. Eur. Nucl. Med. Congress, London, September 3-6, 1985.

11 Hardeman M.R Heynes C.J.L.(1974) The Active serotonin uptake and the hypotonic shock response of human blood platelets. Thromb.Diath Haemorrh. 32:391-404

12 Hardeman M.R. (1990) Platelet isolation technique and viability testing. This volume.

13 Harker L.A. and Finch C.A. (1969) Thrombokinetics in man. J. Clin. Invest. 48: 963-974.

14. Heaton A.W.A., Davis H.H., Welch M.J. Mathias C.J., Joist J.H., Sherman L.A., Siegel B.A. (1979) Indium-III: A new radionuclide label for studying human platelet kinetics. Br. J. Haem. 42: 613-622.

15. Heyns duP. A., Badenhorst P.N., Pieters H., Lotter M.G., Minnaar P.C., Duyvene de Wit C.J., Reenen O.R. van, Retief E.P. (1980) Preparation of a viable population of Indium-III labelled human platelets. Thromb. Haemost 42: 1473-1482.

16. Heyns duP. A., Lotter M.G., Badenhorst P.N., Reenen van O.R., Pieters H., Minaar P.C., Retief F.P. (1980) Kinetics, Distribution and Sites of Destruction of III-Indium-labelled Human Platelets. Br. J. of Haemtol. 44: 269-280.

17. Heyns duP. A., Badenhorst P.N., Pieters H., Lotter M.G., Wessels P., Kotze H.F. Platelet Turnover and Kinetics in Immune Thrombocytopenic Purpura: Results with Autologous III-In-labelled Platelet Differ. Blood 1096: 69: 86-92.

18. Hirsch J., Brain E.A., (1983) Hemostatis and

Thrombosis. Churchill Livingstone New York, Edinburgh, London, and Melbourne : 54-65.

19. Kloniozakis I., Peters A.M., Fitzpatrick M.L., Kensett M.J., Lewis S.M., Lavender J.P. (1980) Radionuclide distribution following injection III-Indium-labelled platelets. Br. J. Haemotol 46: 595-602.

20. Lotter M.G., Heyns duP. A., Badenhorst P.N., Wessels P., Zyl van J.M., Kotze H.F., Minnaar P.C. (1986) Evaluation of Mathematic Models to Assess Platelet Kinetics. J. Nucl. Med. 27: 1192-1201.

21. Peters A.M., Kolnizakis Y. (1980) Dynamic studies with Indium-III labelled platelets. Br. J. Radiol. 53: 923.

22. Peters A.M., (1983) Platelet Kinetics In: Thakur M.L. (ed.) Radiolabelled Cellular Blood elements, Plenum Press, New York and London. pp 111-133.

23. Peters A.M., Walport M.J., Well R.N., Lavender P.J. (1984) Methods of Measuring Splenic Blood Flow and Platelets Transit Time with Indium-III-Labelled Platelets. J. Nucl. Med 25: 86-90.

24. Peters A.M., Lavender J.P. (1982) Factors controlling the intrasplenic transit of platelets. Eur. J. Clin. Invest. 12: 191-195.

25. Peters A.M., Lavender J.P. (1983) Platelet kinetics with Indium-III platelets: comparison with Chromium-51 platelets. Semin. Thromb. Hemost. 9: 100-114.

26. Peters dA.M., Saverymuttu S.H., Wonke B., Lewis S.M., Lavender J.P. (1984) The interpretation of platelet kinetic studies for the identification of sites of abnormal platelet destruction. Br. J. Haemtol. 57: 637-649.

27. Ries C.dA. and Price C.D. (1974) [51]Cr Platelet Kinetics in Thrombocytopenia. Ann. Inter. Med. 80: 702-707.

28. Robertson J.S., Dewanjee M.K., Brown M.L., Fuster V., Chesebro J.H. (1981) Distribution and dosimetry of III-In-labelled platelets. Radiology 140: 169-176.

29. Scheffel U., Tsan M., Mitchel T.G., Camargo E.E., Braine H., Ezekowitz M.D., Nickoloff E.L., Hill-Zobel R., Murphy E., McIntyre P.A. (1982) Human Platelets labelled with In-8-hydroxyquinoline: kinetics, Distribution and Estimates of Radiation Dose. J. Nucl. Med. 23: 149-156.

30. Schmidt K.G., Rasmussen J.W., Arendrup H. (1983) Comparative studies of the in vitro kinetics of simultaneously injected III-In- and ^{51}Cr-labelled human platelets. Scand. J. Haematol. 30: 485-488.

31. Thakur M.L., Welch M.J., Joist J.H. and Coleman R.E. (1976) Indium-III labelled platelets. Studies on preparation and evaluation of in-vitro and in-vivo functions. Thromb. Research 9: 345-357.

32. Vallabhjosula S., Machac J., Goldsmit S.J., Lipszyc H., Badimon L., Rand J., Fuster V. (1986) Indium-III Platelet Kinetics in Normal Human Subjects: Tropolone versus Oxine Methods. J. Nucl. Med. 27: 1669-1674.

33. I.C.S.H.panel on Diagnostic Application of

radioisotopes in Haematology: Recommended methods for radioisotope platelet survival studies. Blood (1977) 50: 1137-1144.

appendix 1

$$X_1 = A_1 + A_2 e^{-mt} \tag{1}$$

$$X_2 = B \, (1 - e^{mt}) \tag{2}$$

$$A_1 = \frac{k_{12}D}{(k_{12} + k_{21}) \, V_1} \tag{3}$$

$$A_2 = \frac{k_{12}D}{(k_{12} + k_{21}) \, V_1} \tag{4}$$

$$m = k_{12} + k_{21} \tag{5}$$

$$B = \frac{k_{12}D}{(k_{12} + k_{21}) \, V_2} \tag{6}$$

After 1 hour a stable situation is reached:

$$X_1 V_1 = \frac{k_{12}D}{(k_{12} + k_{21})} \tag{7}$$

$$X_2 V_2 = \frac{k_{12}D}{(k_{12} + k_{21})} \tag{8}$$

$$\frac{X_1 V_1}{X_2 V_2} = \frac{k_{12}}{k_{12}} \tag{9}$$

$$\frac{A_2}{D} = \frac{X_2 V_2}{D} = \frac{k_{12}}{(k_{12} + k_{21})} \tag{10}$$

$\dfrac{A_2}{D}$ is equals absolute splenic uptake (S) after 1 hour.

(10) gives :

$$k_{12} = S \ (k_{12} + k_{21}) \qquad (11)$$

$$k_{12} + k_{21} = \dfrac{0.693}{T_{1/2}} \qquad (12)$$

$T_{1/2}$ may be calculated from the splenic wash-in curve

$$SBF = k_{12} \ V_1 = S(k_{12} + k_{21})V_1 \qquad (13)$$

Splenic blood flow in conclusion is dependent on the following parameters: Absolute splenic uptake, transport constants K12 and K21 and the total blood volume.
Transit time equals according to the compartmental model, the inverse of K21.

RADIOLABELLED PLATELETS IN CARDIOVASCULAR DISEASES

Mrinal K. Dewanjee
Director, Radiopharmaceutical Laboratory
Professor Radiology
Mayo Medical School
Rochester, MN   55905

INTRODUCTION

The recognition of the various factors controlling platelets vessel wall interaction in normal hemostasis and the role of platelets, clotting factors, and prostaglandins, in thromboembolic disease, atherosclerosis and post-prostheses implantation have stimulated interest in the evaluation of in vivo thrombus formation, embolization, and the evaluation of various prophylactic and therapeutic interventions. In vitro studies of platelets adhesion to deendothelialized vessel or biomaterials (catheters, synthetic vascular grafts, arterio-venous shunts, conduits, mechanical valves, ventricular assist devices and artificial heart) involve the use of light or electron microscopy and/or 51-Cr or III-In-platelets and Iodine-labelled clotting factors, mainly fibrinogen (1-6). In vivo consumption of platelets has been measured with several tracers including 51-Cr and III-In-labelled platelets (7-9). Chromium-51 appears to be a marker of platelet activation and III-Indium appears to be a marker of platelet consumption. Although platelets had been labelled with Technetium-99m, the radionuclide washes off from the platelets with time after administration. Recently. lipid soluble 99m-Tc-complex (99m-Tc-hexamethylene propyleneamine oxine) had been used for granulocyte and platelet labelling. This tracer may be useful for repeated measurements of platelets thrombosis and surface passivation.

Platelet survival study representing global platelet consumption is not a sensitive technique, whereas imaging study allows estimation of regional platelet consumption. Currently 123-I⁻ 131-I-labelled and III-In-DTPA coupled antibodies against platelet glycoproteins (IIb, IIIa) and fibrin are being evaluated in the experimental animal models (5,6). Due to faster blood clearance of these antibodies, early imaging could be carried out with these agents. The sensitivity of these latter techniques for detecting the sites of chronic low-grade thrombosis has not been tested.

The present techniques of diagnosis of thrombosis and atherosclerosis resulting in partial or total stenosis of

Ch. Kessler et al. (eds.), Clinical Application of Radiolabelled Platelets, 61–110.
© 1990 *Kluwer Academic Publishers.*

vessels are based on the measurement of projected lumen diameter at the affected site or the resultant hemodynamic abnormalities. These techniques include impedance plethysmography, Doppler ultrasonography, phonoangiography, nuclear magnetic resonance, digital subtraction, and III-In-platelet scintigraphy (10-52). The neutral complexes of III-Indium, i.e. III-In-oxine, III-In-acetylacetone, III-In-tropolone, and III-In-mercaptopurine-N-oxide, penetrate cell membrane due to high lipid solubility. These tracers after intracellular dissociation bind mainly to soluble proteins, organelles, and membrane proteins (1-2). The more stable complexes of III-In-tropolone and III-In-mercaptopurine-Oxide also permit cell labelling in plasma media, III-In-oxine permits cell-labelling only in plasma-free media. Commercial preparation of III-In-oxine also contains a surface-active agent (100 μg of Tween-80 per mCi of III-In) to prevent adhesion of III-In-oxine to the vial. III-Indium, unlike 51-Cr, is released after membrane lysis, and a major fraction of the III-Indium then binds to transferin present in plasma. Only a small percentage of the III-Indium (less than one percent) is excreted in the urine in clinical evaluations. In addition, III-In-labelled granulocytes or monocytes (where PMN granulocytes are separated by Ficoll-Hypaque or elutriation technique) and III-In-lymphocytes might be ideal markers for quantification of granulocyte infiltration in inflammation, foreign body response, infection, abscess, and transplant rejection (16).

Imaging thrombus was possible in the case of large thrombus in the acute phase for vessels with deep injury or thrombogenic surface of prostheses. In the chronic phase where a small number of single layers of adherent platelets is formed, the deposition of the labelled platelets on the wall is relatively small with respect to the circulating radioactivity in the blood. In this situation, the imaging is not possible. Despite these limitations, the dynamic process of platelet deposition in most of the denuded atherosclerosed vessels and thrombogenic surfaces of the prosthesis in the circulatory system can be recorded. This ongoing thrombosis and embolization had been observed in one to fifteen-year-old vascular grafts of Teflon and Dacron biomaterials. These studies also permitted the evaluation of platelet-inhibitor drugs; for example aspirin, persantin, sulfanpyrazone, motrin, several thromboxane inhibitors, anagrelide, prostacyclin, ticlopidine and calcium channel blockers. Decrease (minimal to moderate) in platelet deposition on prosthetic surface due to medical intervention had been observed by noninvasive imaging with III-In-platelets in animal models and patients. Subtraction of blood pool radioactivity with 99m-Technetium-labelled autologous red blood cell (99m-Tc-RBC) and determination of thrombus-bound III-Indium radioactivity on the wall of the prostheses have been made. The nature of the platelet deposition depends on thrombogenicity of the surface, the amount of blood flow, the diameter and configuration of the prosthesis, and the time-interval after prosthesis implantation. In the vascular prosthesis, platelet deposition as measured from III-In-radioactivity in the midsection of the graft is equal to, less than, or higher than the anastomotic site giving rise to three types of platelet distribution, flat curved, concaved or convexed. The nature of this platelet deposition also changes with time post-implantation. At least in two types of prostheses, we had the opportunity of quantifying platelet thrombosis in the acute and chronic phases. For valvular prosthesis, similar techniques could be used for the quantification of the total number of adherent platelet deposition over a period of several hours. In addition, the effects of other medications were evaluated in the tissue valve and mechanical valve implanted in calves, dogs and patients.

It has been suggested that in platelet adhesion, the initial attachment and spreading occurs because of platelet glycoproteins (Ia and Ib) and in the latter phase of platelet aggregation and continuation of the thrombus formation, other glycoprotein complexes (IIb and IIIa) participate along with plasma proteins present in blood. The concentration of fibrinogen is about 3,000 μg/m and that of fibronectin about 300 μg/ml, Von Willebrand (vWd) factor 7 μg/ml and thrombospondin 0.02 μg/ml. Both the vWd factor and fibronectin are synthesized by vascular endothelial cells and appear as glue between circulating platelets and vessel-wall-collagen. The nature of the binding of vWd factor and fibronectin to platelet glycoproteins might be dependent on the shear rates, the type of surfaces, and the concentration of these adhesive proteins present at the site of interaction. With labelled platelets and proteins, we were able to identify the molecular and cellular composition of thrombi in the arterial and venous system. Although the extent of activation of platelet and thrombus formation may be different, the platelet-fibrin organization in adherent thrombus on the de-endothelialized surface and prosthetic surface of grafts and valves implanted in calves and dogs at different sites appear similar; it is interesting to note that the composition of the thrombus calculated with the radioisotopic technique appears to be very similar for thrombi in the acute and chronic phases. in the in vitro model, because of the precipitation of some fibrinogen along with fibrin, the number of fibrin per platelet tends to be higher. In addition, we have also evaluated the type of platelet damage, platelet consumption, and platelet release during open-heart surgery with bubble and membrane oxygenator. The labelled platelets and clotting factors thus provide very important markers for quantitative studies in animal models, and semi-quantitative studies by imaging in animal models and patients.

III-In-platelets provide a direct technique for quantification of regional platelet thrombus formation; in addition it can provide indirect information about the process of embolization. The embolization is usually indicated by the increase in the tissue/blood radioactivity ratio in the distal bed. In general, it has been thought that if the amount of thrombus formation is higher, the sequential event of embolization from prosthesis also should be higher, and the data of platelet thrombosis suggests that on most of the prostheses, thrombus formation decreases with time post-implantation as the surface of the prostheses undergoes organizational changes leading to passivation.

Numerous studies in our laboratory and others demonstrate that mild injury resulting in endothelial injury results in the adherence of a single layer of platelets which is difficult to image. On the other hand, in case of complex and deep injury, the large platelet aggregates which are formed at the site of injury, could be imaged successfully with III-In-platelets.

Calcium ion (59) plays a key role in platelet activation (Fig 2a). The mechanism of platelet thrombosis on denuded vessel and synthetic surface is shown in Fig. 2b. The list of drugs affecting platelet thrombosis is shown in Fig. 2c.

Several cyclooxygenase and thromboxane synthetase inhibitors (56, 58) are also found to decrease the platelet deposition on denuded vessel and synthetic graft (Fig 2d). The potent platelet-disaggregating agent, prostacyclin, and the platelet aggregating agent,thromboxane, are produced by endothelial cell and platelet, respectively. The poststenotic vortices trap aggregated platelets and their releasate (Fig 2f).

Coronary Artery Disease is a continually repeating cycle of endothelial damage and repair which manifests specific symptoms of angina pectoris and ischemic damage to myocardium. The first cycle is stable atheroma - endothelial ulceration - platelet adhesion - ulcer healing by endothelial cell repair and coverage. When an atheroma develops endothelial ulceration, platelet aggregates form on the ulceration site, thrombus formation and embolization result in sudden death or ischemic cardiomyopathy. When the ulcer heals due to incorporation of thrombus and lipid, there is rapid progression of luminal stenosis at the ulceration site. The second cycle is endothelial ulceration - partial thrombosis, thrombus evolution-thrombus incorporation, and stable atheroma. When the thrombus results in complete occlusion, myocardial infarction results. The thrombi may undergo lysis or may be incorporated in the vessel wall. This cycle of ulceration and thrombus in coronary artery is shown in Fig 2e.

SCINTIGRAPHY WITH III-INDIUM -LABELLED PLATELETS

The half-life of 2.8 days, physical decay by electron capture process and high photon abundance of III-Indium radionuclide (90 percent of 171 keV and 96 percent of 245 keV) make this radionuclide ideal for noninvasive imaging. The gamma camera head used for scintigraphic studies consist of a disk of thallium doped sodium iodide crystal (25-54 cm in diameter, 6,4-12.7 mm in thickness) fitted with several photomultiplier tubes. The thinner disc (6,4 mm) in the portable gamma camera can be fitted with a specially designed collimator for bedside studies, although the detection efficiency is lower. In general, for most of the scintigraphic studies a large field of view gamma camera with a 12.7 thick crystal fitted with a medium energy parallel hole collimator are used. The spectrometer windows (20% of photopeak energy) are adjusted to i8nclude the 171 and 245 keV peaks. Gamma rays of 320, 140, 159 and 364 keV are used for in vitro radioactivity measurements of 51-Cr-, 99m-Tc-, 123-I- and 131-I-radionuclides with a gamma counter respectively. Attenuation and scatter of III-Indium from platelet pool in the spleen and liver degrade the spatial resolution of the gamma camera images. The intrinsic spatial resolution of the gamma camera is 2-4 mm, but in practice is much higher. In spite of this limitation, the validation of in vivo distribution studies in animal models, the use of test objects with computerized gamma cameras, and in vitro measurements of isolated organs and components with gamma counters provide acceptable quantitative information of III-In-platelet distribution by scintigraphy. Since only a small percentage of labelled platelets participate in thrombosis on the wall of the injured vessel or prostheses, and platelet survival time is relatively long, a high blood background radioactivity is always present in the early phase. Ideal imaging time is usually two to five days post-injection of III-In-platelet. Several methods of measurement of thrombogenicity indices with III-In-platelets are shown in Table 1. The schematics of platelet labelling with III-In-tropolone and radioiodination of fibrinogen with Iodogen-transfer technique are shown in Fig 1A and 1B, respectively.

Platelet survival times with 51-Cr- and III-In-labelled autologous platelets in healthy volunteers obtained in our laboratory (7) are shown in Table 2. Platelet clearance from blood was analysed with linear, exponential, and multi-hit models. No significant difference in platelet survival values due to labelling in ACD-plasma and ACD-saline media was observed with III-In-tropolone and III-In-oxine. The linear platelet survival time in different species are as follows: Human (10-11d) > Baboon, dog (5-7d) > Calf (5-6d) . pig, rabbit, rat (3-4d). The reactivity of platelets to proaggregating agents from human, calf and pig is lower than that of the dog.

The estimated radiation dose for 500 microcuries of III-In-platelet administration is 1.13 rad to liver, 0.70 rad to lung, 16.75 rad to spleen, 1.16 rad to kidneys, 0.27 rad to red marrow, 0.17 rad to ovaries, 0.07 rad to testes, and 0.30 rad to the whole body. Adequate platelet survival studies can be performed with 100-150 microcuries of III-In-labelled platelets. The experimental and clinical studies carried out with III-In-platelet are summarized in Table 3. Due to high radiation dose to the spleen, most of the clinical studies with III-In-labelled platelets were performed with 500 microcuries requiring longer imaging times (5-15 minutes per view of approximately 100,000 counts). During imaging, the motion of the patient or experimental animal should be reduced to a minimum. This is essential for blood pool subtraction with 99m-Tc-RBCs (2 mCi of 99m-Tc for 0.5 mCi of III-In). III-In-excess (%) had been determined for thrombus on atherosclerosed carotid and aortic plaque in primate. Gore-Tex grafts in dogs in acute and chronic phase, Gore-Tex grafts in patients, thrombus in coronary artery and left ventricle; graft undergoing thrombotic occlusion had 2-3 times more III-In-excess than patent graft. III-In-excess values ranged from (3-80)%; in experimental study a good correlation was obtained between III-In-excess and thrombus weight and platelet-content. Blood-pool radioactivity in reference region is chosen at similar depth of that of region of interest; frequently blood-pool in heart is used. By in vitro measurement, we also determined the RBC/platelet ratio in thrombus. Several images in both anterior and posterior views are necessary for quantitative distribution of III-In-labelled platelets in the whole body. From the geometric mean of the radioactivity in the anterior and posterior views, the percentage distribution of radioactivity in the liver, spleen, lungs and the site of platelet thrombosis could be quantified more accurately. For most of the platelet deposition studies on injured vessel wall and cardiovascular prostheses, the peak time of III-In-platelet deposition had been obtained in experimental and clinical studies. The time course of platelet deposition depends on the diameter of the vessel lumen, texture of surface, blood flow, shear rate, types of biomaterials used in prostheses, presence of drugs, and platelet reactivity (Fig 3a-3e)

The site of platelet thrombus formation could be imaged only for reasonably large thrombi in valvular prostheses, vascular grafts, ventricular assist devices, artificial heart, aneurysm, and ulcerating atherosclerosed plaque. An imaging technique is successful most of the time in the acute phase post-injury or after prostheses implantation. Noninvasive imaging without background subtraction is not always a very sensitive technique for detection of platelet deposition in patients. We attempted to image platelet deposition on aorta coronary saphenous vein bypass grafts in ten patients (control) immediately post-surgery. The site of sternotomy incision only was visualized, but not the coronary bypass graft. In five patients (control) with carotid artery disease, platelet deposition could not be imaged, although platelet deposition at the sites of endarterectomy was imaged. Six patients with bacterial endocarditis were scanned for the evaluation of platelet deposition without success. Three of these patients were treated with antibiotics. Platelet deposition on the sewing ring of mechanical and tissue valve prostheses could not be imaged in several patients at one to five years post-valve prostheses implantation; at this period the sewing ring is covered with fibroblasts and most of the platelet thrombosis occurs on the disc of the leaflets. Our experimental study also indicates that the platelet thrombus provide a nucleation site for calcification in the tissue valve. Treatment with aspirin-persantin reduces both platelet thrombosis and calcification. The subtraction of blood-pool radioactivity with 99m-Tc-RBC and calculation of III-In-excess factor (13) for the site of platelet thrombus formation increases the sensitivity of the diagnostic technique. The following sections will describe the applications of III-In-labelled platelets for noninvasive imaging and quantification of platelet deposition on ulcerating plaque, aneurysm, venous thrombus, coronary bypass graft, (29) artery undergoing angioplasty (43), synthetic vascular grafts, valvular prostheses, conduits, and artificial heart.

SEMIQUANTITATIVE ESTIMATION OF PLATELET DEPOSITION ON VASCULAR GRAFTS WITH III-IN-PLATELET SCINTIGRAPHY.

Platelet labelling with III-In-oxine and III-In-tropolone permits quantification of platelet thrombosis in atherosclerosis and thrombosis in the acute and chronic phase. About 6000,000-700,000 vascular grafts are implanted annually in the United States; of these, 200,000-250,000 are autogenous vein grafts. 70,000-90,000 are vein bypass grafts, 200,000-225,000 are aorta coronary bypass grafts, and the rest are synthetic vascular grafts (greater than 5 mm in diameter). Most of the grafts in high blood flow and low resistance region of the aorta, iliac and proximal femoral artery perform quite satisfactorily. The scheme of bilateral femoral graft implantation and the pattern of platelet and fibrin deposition and possibility of scintigraphy is shown in Fig 4-6, respectively. The change in the nature and extent of regional platelet deposition and effect of treatment on coronary bypass graft is shown in Fig 7. The amount of thrombus formation, embolization, and platelet survival time could be measured simultaneously with III-In-labelled platelets. For determination of platelet survival times, it is essential to subtract the plasma-bound III-Indium-activity from total radioactivity in blood. Several approaches have been made for measurement of platelet deposition on different types of prostheses, vascular grafts, and evaluation of the effect of drugs (Fig. 8-20). Qualitative estimation of platelet thrombosis was made with a gamma camera at 12-120 hours after administration of III-In-platelets, and 5-10 days after graft implantation. Subsequent follow up of platelet consumption included measurement of platelet survival time and platelet deposition on the graft. Unlike animal models, endothelial coverage occurs only at proximal and distal anastomosis in patients, the rest of the area is covered with fibrin-collagen matrix with a few fibroblasts scattered on the graft. This surface is thrombogenic and platelet deposition can be observed at 5 to 15 years post graft-implantation (Fig 11). High platelet deposition in the acute phase might lead to graft occlusion. Within one to two hours of perfusion, a dumb-bell shape of platelet deposition is observed, more deposition at anastomoses and less in the middle. The decline in III-In-platelet-activity in the graft may be due to embolization of platelet aggregates. In the chronic phase, platelet deposition is observed in the midsection of the graft. In some studies, Indium-excess in graft was calculated after administration of III-In-platelets and 99m-Tc-RBC. In corporation of red cell in thrombus, presence of plasma-bound III-Indium, proximity of vein, presence of III-Indium in bone marrow, and motion artifacts make proper background subtraction difficult for III-In-excess calculation.

In some studies, platelet deposition in the graft was compared with that in the contralateral femoral popliteal vessel. Atherosclerosis, phlebosclerosis, varicosity in the contralateral vessel along with blood pool and marrow activity also lead to error in estimating the radioactivity ratios. Stratton et al. (32) evaluated graft thrombogenicity by measurement of graft III-Indium activity with a gamma camera and blood radioactivity with a gamma counter. The graft/blood ratio is higher in more thrombogenic surface. Due to continuous platelet sequestration, this graft/blood ratio increases in both normal vessel, more so in the grafts and other thrombogenic surfaces. In our studies, (30) we have determined the number of III-Indium counts/pixel/microcurie on the graft surface. A smaller number of counts per pixel necessitates longer imaging time. We have also evaluated platelet thrombosis in Dacron grafts and effect of medication (30). Like other synthetic vascular grafts, higher platelet deposition occurs at two to three days post administration of labelled platelets.

QUANTITATION OF PLATELET DENSITY ON VASCULAR GRAFTS IN ANIMALS WITH III-IN-LABELLED PLATELETS.

Thrombosis is a surface reaction. In quantitative studies, the most important parameters of thrombosis are to obtain the number of adherent platelets per unit area of atherosclerosed vessel or vascular graft and the analysis of the components of thrombus (e.g. fibrin-monomer/platelet). This is only possible in experimental animal studies on harvested grafts and tissue valves. In spite of meticulous tracer and surgical techniques in measurement of platelet deposition, we observed a great deal of variation in platelet density (47, 48). This variation might be due to fibrinolysis, embolization, heretogenous degree of platelet activation due to differential synthesis of thromboxane by platelet and prostacylin by endothelial cell, and other rheological factors of blood flow. The equations describing the calculation of platelet and fibrin density and fibrin per platelet on the graft surface are shown in Table 4.

To understand the mechanism of occlusion in aorto coronary bypass (ACB) graft in patients, we have used a canine model and developed a treatment protocol with aspirin and persantin (Figs 4-7) to increase ACB graft patency in dogs (29). This has also been shown to be useful in clinical studies in patients. In vitro studies of the interaction of platelet and coagulation factors with biomaterial surfaces provide incomplete information in that individual parts of this complex synergistic process can be studied at one time. In our laboratory, the in vivo deposition of platelets and the formation of thrombus on ACB graft and cardiovascular prostheses have been imaged and quantified with the use of III-Indium-labelled platelets in several animal models and humans. We have also evaluated the effect of several platelet-inhibitor drugs in reducing platelet thrombosis. The comparison of platelet inhibiting drugs after myocardial infarction is summarized by Fuster et al. (58) (Table 4). Presently aspirin persantin combination appears as one of the best mode of therapy for platelet thrombosis on bypass graft and other prostheses.

The dynamic process of build-up of platelet thrombus and embolization on the ulcerating atherosclerosed plaque, as well as thrombogenic surface, had been imaged non invasively in animal models and human patients. The platelet activation due to higher shear rate, loss of endothelial cells, or ulceration of the plaque results in platelet thrombosis at this site. Powers et al. (13) evaluated platelet deposition on atherosclerosed plaque of aorta in cholesterol-fed primates after balloon injury. They have calculated III-In-excess factor for platelet deposition in plaques. The platelet uptake correlates with the severity of atherosclerotic lesion. The scintigraphic evidence of platelet deposition on arteriographically confirmed plaques in several series was quite variable and has ranged from 0-78 percent. Powers et al. (17) recently reported results from 100 patients with suspected severe vascular diseases; scintigrams of platelet deposition on ulcerated carotid plaques are shown in Fig 9. Platelet deposition was observed at 41 percent of lesions shown in angiography and 13 percent in arteriography at the normal sites. The detection sensitivity as measured by test objects suggest that a carotid thrombus must contained at least 0.11 percent of injected dose of III-In-platelet for scintigraphic detection, and the same order of magnitude is required for successful imaging of venous thrombosis. Plaque could be imaged only when the plaque to blood radioactivity ratio is about 4.0-5.0. Due to the dynamic process of thrombus formation and embolization in the high flow region of small diameter carotid artery, more frequent imaging might be necessary.

EVALUATION OF PLATELET THROMBOSIS IN ANEURYSMS

The turbulence of blood flow and stagnation in these cavities (53-56) give rise to formation of thrombus of platelet, fibrin and red cell, and continuous incorporation of platelet and fibrin on the upper-most layer of thrombus. III-In-platelet was used successfully for imaging these thrombus formations. The optimum time for imaging was 96-120 hours post-injection of III-In-platelets (Fig 10). Surgical repair of aneurysms and scintigrams of platelet deposition on Dacron grafts are shown in Fig 10. Patients with abdominal aortic aneurysms and bilateral femoral artery aneurysms had higher III-In-platelet activity at the site of aneurysm. No significant difference of platelet deposition was observed when the patients were medicated with aspirin and persantin, and sulfinpyrazone. Heyns et al. (24) observed (4.7 -/+ 3.6) percent of total administered III-In-radio-activity at 8-10 days post-injection in the aortic aneurysm.

III-INDIUM PLATELET SCINTIGRAPHY IN THE DISEASES OF THE VENOUS SYSTEM

Thakur et al. (1) first imaged venous thrombi in the canine jugular veins induced by electric current injury. Knight et al. (3) studied the effect of aging of venous thrombi on platelet incorporation in dogs. All thrombi could be visualized two hours after III-In-platelet injection. The optimum time of imaging was 12 to 15 hours post injection. The thrombus to blood radioactivity ratio decreases from greater than 20 at 1-12 hours, 2-25 at 12-24 hours, and 1-5 at 24-48 hours. Similar effects of aging and anticoagulant on III-In-platelet incorporation and pulmonary embolus was also observed in the canine models by several investigators. Several clinical studies using venography, plethysmography, and III-In-platelet scintigraphy were utilized for diagnosis of venous thrombosis. In general, the thrombus could be visualized at three to six hours after injection of III-In-platelet (Fig 13); therapy with anticoagulant, i.e. heparin, decreases platelet incorporation in the thrombus and decreases the sensitivity of this test.

As Ezekowitz et al. (22) used III-In-platelets for imaging hematologically active thrombi in the left ventricle; in comparison with two-dimensional echocardiography, thrombus imaging was far more specific, although the former was more sensitive. False positive studies were quite common. The thrombus radioactivity measured at autopsy was 10-15 times higher than blood. Fig 14 demonstrates platelet deposition in ventricular thrombi obtained in our laboratory. No significant effect of anticoagulant and platelet inhibitor drug was observed in this study. The optimum time for imaging was three to four days post injection of III-In-platelets.

EVALUATION OF MICROVASCULAR INJURY AND PLATELET THROMBOSIS
IN TRANSPLANTED ORGANS AND VESSELS.

The activation of T-lymphocytes is the predominant
factor for allograft rejection resulting in the loss of
endothelial cells. Humoral antibodies also may dominate the
rejection process resulting in membrane damage (cytolysis by
complement activation). The loss of endothelial cells to
smaller vessels of transplanted organs (kidneys, heart,
liver, heterologous blood vessels and lungs) due to
lymphocytes might lead to platelet thrombus formation on
subendothelial collagen and occlusion of vessel causing foci
of microinfarcts. This platelet deposition could be imaged
in the acute phase with III-In-labelled platelets. Platelet
deposition in the infarcted tissue is three to five times
less than that in the normally perfused organ. However,
French et al. (25) observed one to two times higher platelet
deposition in the rejected kidney than normal kidney.

Prostacyclin infusion resulted in decrease of platelet
incorporation and prolonged platelet survival time.
Medication with aspirin, persantin and sulfinpyrazone tends
to increase renal graft viability. Platelet deposition at
the anastomosis would not be observed in liver transplant
patients in the acute phase; although both the survival and
recovery were drastically reduced. Platelet deposition in
transplanted dog heart was found twice as high as that of
normal heart at four to five days post transplantation.

QUANTITATION OF PLATELET THROMBOSIS IN VALVULAR PROSTHESES
IN ANIMALS.

A variety of mechanical and tissue prosthetic valves
are used in patients with diseases of cardiac valves (38).
The major limitation of the former is propensity of thrombus
formation, embolization, and that of the latter is
calcification. With III-In-labelled platelets we have been
able to image platelet deposition in the acute phase on both
the mechanical and tissue valve prostheses implanted in dogs
and calves (39-42). These valves were implanted in the
mitral annulus and platelet deposition was followed for a
one to three month period. In addition, in vitro studies
with gamma counter permitted quantitation of the number of
adherent platelets on the components of the mitral valve
prostheses. In addition, higher tissue to blood
radioactivity ratio in skeletal muscle and kidneys was
observed due to embolization. Fig 16 shows the dynamic
process of platelet incorporation in the mitral annulus of
bovine pericardial tissue valve prostheses in calves. The 24
hour platelet deposition showed a consistent decrease on all
components of the tissue valve prostheses at 1, 14, 30 and
90 days post implantation. These results of quantitative
studies of platelet density and total platelet deposition
are shown in Figs 17-19, respectively. Our studies also
indicate that platelet vesicles provide a nucleation site

for calcification in collagenous valvular prostheses and synthetic polymers (42).

PLATELET DEPOSITION ON EXTRACARDIAC CONDUITS IN CLINICAL STUDIES.

The use of porcine valved extracardiac conduits (Dacron tube 10-20 cm long, 1.2-2.6 cm external diameter, with or without porcine valve) in several congenital cardiac lesions, e.g. pulmonary atresia, has permitted corrective surgery. We have measured platelet deposition on conduits (six with valves and three without) with III-In-labelled platelets in nine young patients (37), In this study, III-In-platelets (290-483 microcuries) were administered either immediately or on the fifth to eighth post operative day and imaging was performed between one and six days. Highest platelet deposition on conduit was observed at three to four days post injection (Fig 20). Treatment with aspirin (75 to 325 milligrams) administered orally three times a day caused no recognizable changes. Three patterns of platelet deposition (no uptake, diffuse uptake and focal uptakes at anastomoses and valves) were observed.

PLATELET DEPOSITION IN VESSELS UNDERGOING ANGIOPLASTY

Angioplasty of the occluded artery by balloon dilation causes endothelial cell loss, cracking of internal elastic lamina, hemorrhage under the plaque, medial damage followed by necrosis and exposure of blood to subendothelial thrombogenic contents of plaque (42). Platelet deposition at the site of deep injury could be imaged with III-In-platelets. Occasionally platelet deposition could also be observed in the embolus of cerebral artery and femoral artery. The site of arterial puncture for catheterization, hematoma at the site of biopsy and site of inflammation and infection also accumulate platelets. As the vessel undergoes partial re endothelization, the platelet density (Platelet/cm2 for 1- and 24- hour deposition) decreases from 45×10^6 at one day, to 1.2×10^6 at one week to 0.1×10^5 at two months post angioplasty (43).

PLATELET DEPOSITION ON CATHETERS IN ANIMAL AND CLINICAL STUDIES.

Lipton at al. (44) studied platelet deposition on polyethylene catheters placed in the carotid artery of dogs and goes for a period of 30 minutes to 24 hours. III-In-platelets were injected before and after catheter insertion. Direct correlation was obtained between thrombus weight on catheter and III-Indium radioactivity. Highest activity in dogs was found at 40 minutes post injection. At later periods due to fibrinolysis, thrombus disaggregation and embolization, the III-Indium activity decreased. Heparin-bonded catheters accumulated fewer platelets than control

catheters. Similar studies were carried out by O'Connell
(46) in patients undergoing angiography; as catheters were
pulled out, the adherent thrombus embolized and this site of
catheter insertion and embolus could be shown in the
scintiphoto (Fig 12). The full width at half of maximum
(FWHM) of the time for increase, peaking and decrease of
platelet deposition is much broader in a larger orifice or
lumen than for a smaller lumen. This is particularly high in
the case of a catheter study; due to substantial decrease in
lumen diameter due to catheter insertion the higher shear
rate might increase platelet deposition on the catheter.
Fortunately a lot of these platelet aggregates in acute
adherent thrombi are not well organized, they may embolize
or disintegrate because of fibrinolytic activity in the
circulatory system, and thus may cause less complications
after angiography. For a smaller lumen, the FWHM is almost a
spike function, either the lumen is patent (nonthrombogenic
surface) or occluded (thrombogenic surface); for a large
diameter graft, the rate of embolization of small-size
platelet aggregates may be higher; patency might be
maintained with the underlying risk of embolization.

In spite of limited clinical applications, we believe
that tracer techniques will be essential for evaluation of
platelet-active drugs in cardiovascular diseases, bypass
grafts vessels undergoing angioplasty, and development of
biocompatible prostheses, small vessel (< 4mm) grafts,
valves and ventricular pumps.

REFERENCES

1. Thakur M.L., Welch M.J., Joist J.H., Coleman R.E.
    (1976) Indium-III balled platelets: studies on
    preparation and evaluation of in vitro and in vivo
    functions. Thromb. Res. 9: 345-357.
2. Dewanjee M.K., Rao S.A., P. Didisheim P. (1981) Indium-
    III troplone, a new high-affinity platelet label:
    preparation and evaluation of labelling parameters. J.
    Nucl. Med. 22: 921-987.
3. Knight L.C., Primeau J.L., Siegel B.A., Welch W.J.
    (1978) Comparison of In-III-labelled platelets and
    iodinated fibrinogen for the detection of deep vein
    thrombosis. J. Nucl. Med. 19: 891-894.
4. Dewanjee M.K. (1987) Radioiodinated Tracers. CRC Press.
    Boca Raton, Florida.
5. Oster Z.H., Srivastava S.C., Som P., Meinken G.E.,
    Scudder L.E., Yamamoto K., Atkins H.L., Brill A.B.,
    Coller B.S. (1985) Thrombus radioimmunoscintigraphy: an
    approach using monoclonal antiplatelet antibody. Proc.
    Natl. Acad. Sci. 82:3465-3468.
6. Rosebrough S.F., Kudryk B., Grossman Z.D., McAfee J.G.,
    Subramanian G., Ritter-Hrncirik C.A., Witanowski L.S.,
    Tillapaugh-Fay G. (1985) Radioimmunoimaging of venous
    thrombi using iodine-131 monoclonal antibody. Radiology

156: 515-517.

7. Dewanjee M.K., Wahner H.W., Dunn W.L., Robertson J.S., Fuster V.D., Chesebro J.H. (1986) Comparison of three platelet markers for measurment of platelet survival time in healthy volunteers. Mayo Clinic. Proc. 61: 327-336.

8. Mustard J.F., Packham M.A., Kinlough-Rathbone R.L. (1981) Platelets, atherosclerosis and clinical complications in vascular injury and atheroscleroris, in Biochemistry of Disease. S. Moore (ed.) Vol. 9:79. M. Dekker, Inc. New York.

9. Harker L.A. (1986) Antiplatelet drugs in the management of patients with thrombotic disorders. Sem. Thromb. Hemostasis 12: 134-155.

10. Schefel U., Tasan M.F., Mitchell T.G., Camargo E.E., Braine H., Ezekowitz Mk.D. Nickloff E.L., Hill-Zobel R., Murphy E., McIntyre P.A. (1982) Human platelets labelled with IN-III 8-hydroxyquinoline: kinetics, distribution, and estimates of radiation dose. J. Nucl. Med. 23: 149-156.

11. Robertson J.S., Dewanjee M.K., Brown M.L., Fuster V., Chesebro J.H. (1982) Distribution and dosimetry of III-In-labelled platelets. Radiology 140: 169-176.

12. Peters A.M. (1982) Splenic blood flow and blood cell kinetics. (1983) Clin. Haematol. 12: 421-447.

13. Powers W.J., Mathias C.J., Welch M.J., et al. (1982) Scintigraphic detection of platelet deposition in atherosclerotic macques: a new technique for investigation of antithrombotic drugs. Thromb. Res. 25: 137-143.

14. Evaluation of cardiovascular devices and prostheses during in vivo function. Chapter 10. In Guidelines for blood-material interactions. Report of the NHLBI Working Group. NIH Publication No. 85-2185. U.S. Dept. of Health and Human Services.

15. Dewanjee M.K. (1985) III-In-platelets in bypass grafts: experimental and clinical applications. NATO Symposium "Radiolabelled Cellular Elements of Blood", Thakur M.L., Hardeman M., Ezekowitz M.D. (eds.) Plenum Press, N.Y., 229-263.

16. Dewanjee M.K. (1984) Cardiac and vascular imaging with labelled platelets and leukocytes. Semin. Nucl. Med. 14(3): 154-187.

17. Powers W.J., Siegel B.A., Davis H.H., Mathias C.J., Clark H.B., Welch M.J. (1982) Indium-III platelets scintigraphy in cerebrovascular disease. Neurology 32: 938-943.

18. Fedullo P.F., Moser K.M., Moser K.S., Konopka R., Hartman M.T. (1982) Indium-III labelled platelets: effect of heparin on uptake by venous thrombi and relationship to the activated partial thromboplastin time. Circulation 66: 632-637.

19. Sostman H.D., Neumann R.D., Zoghbi S.S., Lord P.F., Thakur M.L., Carbo P., Greenspan R.H., Gottschalk A.

(1982) Experimental studies with III-Indium labelled platelets in pulmonary embolism. Invest. Radiol. 17: 367-374.

20. Davis H.H., Heaton W.A., Siegal B.A., Mathias C.J., Joist J.H., Sherman L.A., Welch J.J. (1978) Scintigraphic detection of atherosclerotic lesions and venous thrombi in man by Indium-III autologous platelets. Lancet 1: 1185-1187.

21. Penech A., Hussey J.K., Smit F.W., Dendy P.P., Bennett B., Douglas A.S. (1981) Diagnosis of deep vein thrombosis using autologous indium-III-labelled platelets. Br. Med. J. 282-1020-1022.

22. Ezekowitz M.D., Wilson D.A., Smith E.O., Burow R.D., Harrison L.H., Parker D.E., Elkins R.C., Peyton M., Taylor F.B. (1982) Comparison of indium-III-platelet scintigraphy and two-dimensional echocardiography in the diagnosis of left ventricular thrombi. N. Eng. J. Med. 306: 1509-1513.

23. Ezekowitz M.D, Pope C.F., Sostman H.D., Smith E.O., Glickman M., Rapoport S., Sniderman K.W., Friedlaender G., Pelker R.R., Taylor F.B., Zaret B.L. (1986) Indium-III platelet scintigraphy for the diagnosis of acute venous thrombosis. Circulation 73: 668-674.

24. Heyns A., Lotter M.G., Badenhorst P.N., Pieters W., Nel C.J.C., Minnaar P.C. Kinetics and fate of Indium-III labelled platelets in patients with aortic aneurysms. Arch. Surg. 117: 1170-1174.

25. French A., Nicholls A., Smith F.W. (1981) Indium (iii-In)-labelled platelets in the diagnosis of renal transplant rejection: preliminary findings. Br. J. Radiol. 54: 325-327.

26. Dewanjee M.K., Pumphrey C.W., Murphy K.P., Josa M. (1978) Imaging platelet deposition with III-In-labelled platelets in coronary artery bypass grafts in dogs. Mayo Clinic. Proc. 53: 327-331.

27. Hanson S.R., Harker L.A., Ratner B.D. (1980) In vivo evaluation of artificial surfaces with a nonhuman primate model of arterial thrombosis. J. Lab. Clin. Med. 95: 289-304.

28. Dewanjee M.K., Pjmphrey C.W., Murphy K.P., Fuster V.D., Kaye M.P., Rosemark J.A., Chesebro J.H. (1982) Evaluation of platelet-inhibitor drugs in a canine bilateral femoral graft implant model. Trans. Am. Soc. Artif. Intern. Organs 28: 504-509.

29. Dewanjee M.K., Tago M., Josa M., Fuster V., Kaye M.P. (1984) Quantification of platelet retention in aortocoronary femoral vein bypass graft in dogs treated with dipyridamole and aspirin. Circulation 69: 350-356.

30. Pumphrey C.W., Chesebro J.H., Dewanjee M.K., Wahner H.W., Hollier L.H., Pairolero P.C., Fuster V. (1983) In vivo quantititation of platelet deposition on human peripheral arterial bypass grafts using Indium-III-labelled platelets. Effect of dipyridamole and aspirin. Am. J. Cardiol. 51: 796-801.

31. Callow A.D., Connolly R., O'Donnel T.F., Gembarowicz R., Keough E., Ramberg-Laskaris K., Valeri R. (1982) Platelet-arterial synthetic graft interaction and its modification. Arch. Surg. 117: 1447-1455.

32. Stratton J.R., Ritchie J.L. (1986) Reduction of indium-III platelet deposition on Dacron vascular grafts in humans by aspirin plus dipyridamole. Circulation 73: 325-330.

33. Goldman M.D., Simpson D., Hawker R.J., Norcott H.C., McCollum C.N. (1983) Aspirin and dipyridamole reduce platelet deposition on prosthetic femoropoliteal grafts in man. Ann. Surg. 198: 713-716.

34. Gloviczki P., Dewanjee M.K., Trastek V.F., Hoffman E.A., Kaye M.P. (1984) Experimental replacement of the inferior vena cava: factors affecting patency. Surgery 63: 657-666.

35. Christenson J.T., Mergerman J., Hanel K.C., L'Italian G.J., Strauss H.W., Abbot W.M. (1981) The effect of blood flow rates on platelet deposition in PTFE arterial bypass grafts. Trans. ASAIO 27: 188-191.

36. Didisheim P., Dewanjee M.K., Frisk C.S., Kaye M.P. (1984) Animal models for preducting clinical performance of biomaterials for cardiovascular use. In: Contemporary Biomaterials. Material and Host Response. Clinical Applications, New Technology and Legal Aspects. J.W. Boretos (ed.) M. Eden Noyse Publications. Park Ridge N.J. pp. 132-179.

37. Agarwal K.C., Wahner H.W., Dewanjee M.K., Fuster V., Puga F.J., Danielson G.K., Chesebro J.H., Feldt R.H. (1982) Imaging of platelets in right-sided extracardiac conduits in humans. J. Nucl. Med. 23: 342-347.

38. Harker L.A., Slichter S.J. (1970) Studies of platelet and fibrinogen kinetics in patients with prosthetic heart valves. N. Engl. J. Med. 283: 1302-1305.

39. Dewanjee M.K., Trastek V.F., Tago M., Torianni M., Kaye M.P. (1983) Noninvasive radioisotope technique for detection of platelet deposition on bovine pericardial mitral valve prosthesis and in vitro quantification of visceral microemboli in dogs. Trans. Am. Soc. Artif. Intern. Organ 29: 188-193.

40. Dewanjee M.K., Fuster V., Rao S.A., Forshaw P.L., Kaye M.P. (1983) Noninvasive radioisotope technique for detection of platelet deposition in mitral valve prostheses and quantitation of visceral microembolism in dogs. Mayo Clinic. Proc. 58: 307-314.

41. Dewanjee M.K., Didisheim P., Kaye M.P., Solis E., Zollman P.E., Francis M.D., Torianni M., Trastek V.S., Tago M., Edwards W.D. (1984) Platelet deposition on and calcification of bovine pericardial valve. Eur. Heart J. 5 (Suppl. D): 1-5.

42. Dewanjee M.K., Solis E., Mackey S.T., Lenker J., Didisheim P., Chesebro J.H., Zollman P.E., Kaye M.P. (1986) Quantification of regional platelet and calcium deposition on pericardial tissue valve prosthesis in

calves and effect of hydroxyethylene diphosphonate. J. Thorac. Cardiovas. Surg. 92: 337-348.

43. Steele P.M., Chesebro J.H., Stanson A.W., Holmes D.R. Jr., Dewanjee M.K., Badimon L., Fuster V. (1985) Balloon angioplasty. Natural history of the pathophysiological response to injury in a pig model. Cir. Res. 57: 105-112.

44. Lipton M.J., Doherty P.W., Goodwin D.A., Bushberg G.T., Prager R., Meares C.F. (1980) Evaluation of catheter thrombogenicity in vivo with indium-labelled platelets. Radiology 135: 191-194.

45. Rodvien R., Robinson R., Mitchell R.R., Litwak P., Price D.C. (1982) A new model for in vivo platelet and thrombus kinetics, in Cooper S.L., Peppas N.A., Hoffman A.S. and Ratner B.D. (eds.): Biomaterials, Artifacial Phenomena and Applications. Washington D.C., American Chem. Society, Chapter 3: 25-34.

46. O/Connor M.K., Brennan S.S., Shanik (1986) Indium-III-labelled platelet deposition following transfemoral angiography. Radiology 158: 191-194.

47. Dewanjee M.K., Solis E., Mackey S.T., Gonzales G., Chesebro J.H. (1986) Quantification of platelet and fibrinogen deposition on PTFE and vein grafts in dogs and the effect of vitamin E on graft thrombosis in the acute phase. Trans. ASAIO 32: 187-192.

48. Dewanjee M.K., Solis E., Lenker J., Tidwell C., Mackey S.T., Didisheim P., Kaye M.P. (1986) Quantification of platelet and fibrinogenfibrin deposition on components of tissue valves (Ionescu-Shiley) in calves. Trans. ASAIO 32: 591-596.

49. Badimon L., Fuster V., Dewanjee M.K., Romero J.C. (1982) A sensitive new method of ex vivo platelet deposition. Thromb. Res. 28: 237-250.

50. Hope A.F., Heyns A., Lotter M.G., v. Teenen O.R., Kock F.D., Badenhorst P.N., Pieters H., Kotze H., Meyer J.M. Minnaar P.C. (1981) Kinetics and sites of sequestration of Indium-III-labelled human platelets during cardiopulmonary bypass. J. Thorac. Cardiovas. Surg. 81: 880-886.

51. Peterson K.A., Dewanjee M.K., Kaye M.P. (1982) Fate of indium-III-labelled platelets during cardiopulmonary bypass performed with membrane and bubble oxygenators. J. Thorac. Cardiovas. Surg. 84: 39-43.

52. Heyns A.D.P., Badenhorst P.N., Lotter M.G. (1985) Platelet kinetics and imaging. Vol. 1. Techniques and Normal Platelet Kinetics. Vol. 2. Clinical Applications. CRC Press, Boca Raton, Florida.

53. Roach M.R. (1978) A model study of why some intracranial aneurysms thrombose but others rupture. Stroke 9: 583-387.

54. Dewanjee M.K. (1986) Methods of assessment of thrombosis in vivo. New York Acad. Sci. (In press).

55. Nurden A.T., George J.N., Phillips D.R. (1986) Platelet membrane plycoproteins: their structure, function and

modification in disease. Chapter 4 in Biochemistry of Platelets. Eds. Phillips D.R. Shuman M.A. Academic Press, New York, pp. 159-212.

56. Harker L.A. (1986) Antiplatelet drugs in the management of patients with thrombotic disorders. Sem. Thromb. Hemos. 12: 134-155.

57. Goldsmith H.L., Karino T. (1981) Flow patterns and localization of thrombus formation. Theologic contribution to thrombosis and hemotasis. N.I.H. Conf., June 4-5, 1981, Bethesda, MD.

58. Fuster V., Adams P.C., Badimon J.J., Chesebro J.H. (1987) Platelet-inhibotor drugs' role in coronary artery disease. Prof. Cardiovasc. Disc. 29: 325-348.

59. Majerus P.W., Connolly T.M., Deckmyn H., Ross T.S., Bross T.E., Ishii H., Bansal V.S., Wilson D.B. (1986) The metabolism of phosphoinostide-derived messenger molecules. Science 234: 1519-1526.

60. Houslay M.D. (1987) Egg activiation unscrambles a potential role for IP4-Trends in Biochemical Sciences 12: 376-377.

61. Feinstein M.B., Zavoico G.B., Halenda S.P. (1985) Calcium and cyclic AMJP: Antagonistic modulators of platelet function. Chapter 10, The Platelets, Physiology and Pharmacology Ed. G.L. Longnecker, Academic Press, Orlando, Florida pp. 237-270.

Table 1: THROMBOGENICITY INDICES FROM MEASURMENT OF ^{111}IN-PLATELET
RADIOACTIVITY IN ORGANS AND PROSTHESES

1. Relative graft radioactivity
    (Equal No. of pixels on graft $= \dfrac{^{111}\text{In-CPM on graft}}{^{111}\text{In-CPM on normal vessel (contralateral)}}$
    and vessel)

2. Relative thrombogenicity
    (Equal No. of pixels on $= \dfrac{^{111}\text{In-CPM on graft-}^{111}\text{In-CPM in soft tissue}}{^{111}\text{In-activity (μCi) X No. of pixels}}$
    graft and soft tissue)

3. Geometric Mean Method
    a) Geometric mean ^{111}In-CPM= (Anterior ^{111}In-CPM X Posterior ^{111}In-CPM)$^{\frac{1}{2}}$

    b) Corrected organ ^{111}In-CPM =

    $\dfrac{\text{Transmission Coefficient}}{\text{Sensitivity (}^{111}\text{In-CPM/μCi)}}$ X   Geometric mean ^{111}In-CPM

    where transmission coefficient and sensitivity of gamma camera are
    determined by measuring a known amount of ^{111}In-radioactivity in a
    test object (phantom).

4. Determination of focal wall-adherent ^{111}In-platelet radioactivity at region
    of interest (ROI) by subtraction of circulating ^{111}In-platelet radioactivity
    in blood-pool (ROI).

a. [^{111}In-CPM at focal thrombus]$_{\text{Excess}}$=Total ^{111}In-CPM(ROI)-^{111}In-CPM(Blood-pool)

    Assuming all counts from ^{99m}Tc-RBC are in blood pool and only small ^{111}In-CPM
    from wall-adherent thrombus,

b. ^{111}In-CPM(Blood-pool of ROI) = ^{99m}Tc-CPM (ROI)$\times\dfrac{^{111}\text{In-CPM(Reference Region)}}{^{99m}\text{Tc-CPM(Reference Region)}}$

    Where reference region refers to a regio of blood pool with no thrombus.

c. $\left[\begin{array}{c} ^{111}\text{In-CPM} \\ \text{of focal thrombus} \end{array}\right]_{\text{Excess}}^{\%}$ = $\dfrac{[^{111}\text{In-CPM}]_{\text{Excess}}}{^{111}\text{In-CPM(Blood-pool of ROI)}}$ X   100

Table 2: Platelet Survival Time in Days (Mean+Standard Deviation) of
^{111}In- and ^{51}Cr-Labeled Autologous Platelets in Human Volunteers:
Data Were Analysed With Three Model Calculations

	^{51}Cr-Platelets	^{111}In-Platelets (Oxine-ACD-Saline)	^{111}In-Platelets (Tropolone-Plasma)
Linear	10.1 ± 0.9	8.8 ± 0.6	10.2 ± 0.7
Exponential	6.8 ± 0.9	5.1 ± 0.6	5.4 ± 0.7
Multiple Hit	9.1 ± 1.1 (men) 9.8 ± 1.6 (women)	7.7 ± 0.9 (men) 8.1 ± 1.2 (women)	8.9 ± 1.4 (men)

Table 3: Qualitative and Quantitative Studies of Platelet Incorporation
in Thrombus and Embolization With ^{111}In-Platelets in
in Experimental and Clinical Studies

A. Arterial Diseases
1. Arterial grafts (internal mammary artery)
   Vein grafts (saphenous vein graft)
   Gore-Tex grafts
   Dacron grafts
   Polyurethane grafts (experimental)
   Endothelial cell seeded graft (experimental)
   Platelet inhibitors, prostacyclin and other drugs
2. Aneurysms
   Thoracic aorta
   Abdominal aorta
   Dissecting aneurysm
   Intracranial aneurysm
3. Atherosclerosis (deendothelialization and cholesterol feeding of
   animals), thrombosis and embolization
   Carotid artery (Ulcerating plaques)
4. Endothelial damage
   Balloon angioplasty (rabbit, pig, human)
   Vein graft denudation (Coronary and peripheral bypass)
   Renal artery thrombosis
   Coronary thrombosis and thrombolysis
   Homocystinuria, smoking, hypertension, hyperlipidemia
   Catheter damage during angioplasty
   Endarterectomy
5. Vasculitis (temporal arteritis)

B. Venous Diseases
1. Venous thrombosis
2. Renal vein thrombosis
3. Sagittal sinus thrombosis
4. Vena cava graft
5. Pulmonary embolism
6. Role of anticoagulants and thrombocytic agents

C. Cardiac Diseases
1. Atrial thrombosis
2. Ventricular thrombosis
3. Bacterial endocarditis
4. Valvular prostheses and vascular conduits
   (Acquired and congenital defects)
5. Myocardial hemorrhage

D. Microvascular Injury (Organ transplantation)
1. Kidney
2. Heart

E. Miscellaneous Prosthesis (temporary and semipermanent)
   Blood-biomaterial interactions
   Catheter induced thrombosis and embolization
   Cardiopulmonary bypass (bubble and membrane oxygenator)
   Artery-vein shunts and other ex vivo circuits
   Left ventricular assist devices
   Artificial heart (4 mechanical valves, two pumps; most thrombogenic
   device)

Table 4 **Comparison of Platelet-Inhibiting Drugs After Myocardial Infarction in Eight Prospective Randomized, Double-Blind Placebo-Controlled Trials**

Trial	Time Between MI and Entry (Mean Mo)	Duration of Follow-up (Mean Mo)	Drug	Dosage (mg/d)	Total No. Patients	Results of Therapy	End Point(s)
Elwood et al[121]	2½	12	ASA	300	1,239	Favorable trend	Total mortality
Coronary drug project[122]	3	22	ASA	972	1,529	Favorable trend	Total and CAD mortality, MI and other CV events
Breddin et al[123]	1½	24	ASA + Phen	1,500	946	Favorable trend	SD, MI (fatal and nonfatal)
Elwood and, Sweetnam[124]	¼	12	ASA	900	1,682	Favorable trend	Total mortality
AMIS[125]	25	38	ASA	1,000	4,524	No benefit	Total and CAD mortality, MI, stroke
PARIS[126]	20	41	ASA	972	2,026	Favorable trend	Total and CAD mortality, CAD incidence
			ASA + D	972 + 225		Favorable trend	Total and CAD mortality, CAD incidence
ART[127]	1	16	Sulf	800	1,558	Decreased SD only	Total and CAD mortality, CAD incidence
ARIS[128]	⅔	19	Sulf	800	727	Decreased MI only	MI, SD, CAD, total mortality
PARIS[129]	2	23	ASA + D	972 + 225	3,128	Decreased all end points	Total and CAD mortality, MI, CAD incidence

Abbreviations: ASA, aspirin; CAD, coronary artery disease; MI, myocardial infarction; CV, cardiovascular; SD, sudden death; Phen, phenprocoumon (Liquamar); AMIS, Aspirin Myocardial Infarction Study Research Group; PARIS, Persantine-Aspirin Reinfaction Study Research Group; D, dipyridamole (Persantine); ART, The Anturane Reinfarction Trial Research Group; Sulf, sulfinpyrazone (Anturane); ARIS, Anturane Reinfarction Italian Study.

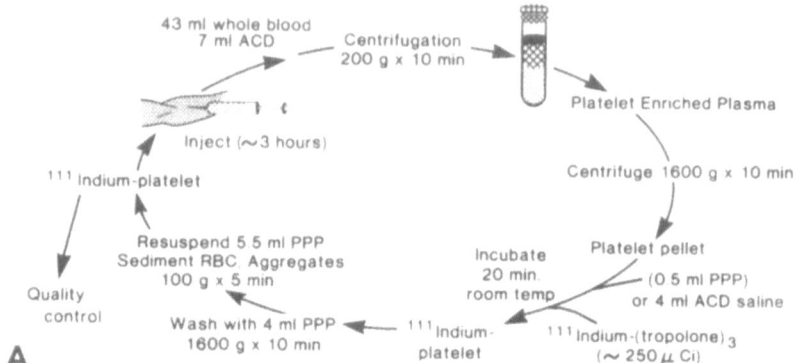

RADIOIODINATION OF FIBRINOGEN (Iodogen)

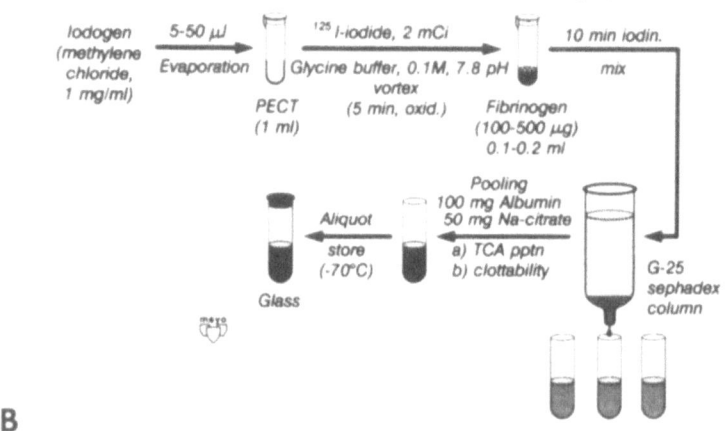

B

Fig 1a
Autologous platelet labelling with III-In-tropolone. Harvested platelets resuspended in 0.5 ml of plasma was incubated with iII-In-tropone. After removing unbound III-In, labelled platelets are injected into the subject.

Fig 1b
Radioiodination of fibrinogen with Iodogen-transfer technique. In this method only oxidized radioiodide comes in contact with protein, thus reducing the probability of protein oxidation. After intravenous administration, denatured labelled fibrinogen is usually removed by liver.

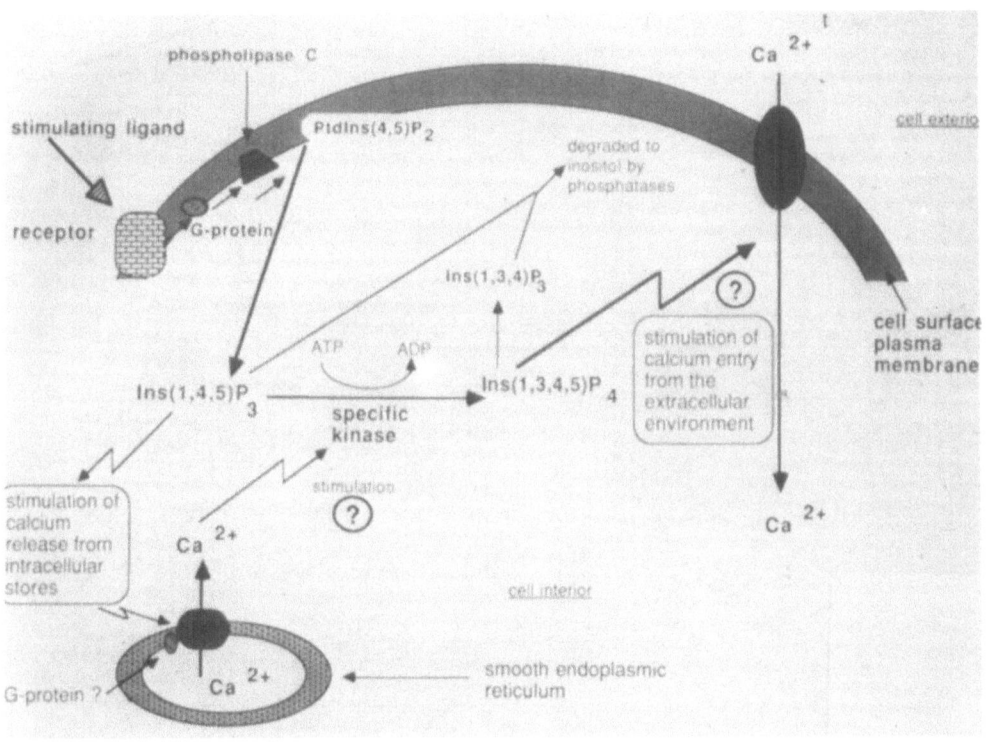

Fig 2a

The second messenger system in platelet and contractile cells involves both cyclic AMP and phosphatidyl inositols. The increase in cytosolic calcium and its association with calmodulin activate both contraction of actomyosin in microfilament and polymerization of microtubules. The contraction of microfilament propels the granules along the pathways determined by the microtubules. Thus cytosolic increase in free calcium plays an important role in the secretory process of aggregatory substances from alpha and dense granules from activated platelets. The precise mode of action of cylic AMp is uncertain; it is suggested to increase cytosolic calcium from intracellular pools and phosphorylation of microtubular proteins. The stimulation of inositol phospholipid metabolism causes the hydrolysis of phosphatidylinositol 4,5-bisphosphate Ptd Ins (4,5) P_2 produce two intracellular messengers, diacylglycerol (DAG) and inositol 1,4,5-triphosphate Ins (1,4,5) P_3, referred to here as IP_3. Diacylglycerol inter reacts with protein kinase C causing its activation, possible translocation to the plasma membrane, and the phosphorylation of various intracellular proteins. IP_3 binds to a membrane-bound intracellular receptor which is believed to reside in the smooth endoplasmic recticulum in muscle cells. Occupancy of this receptor by IP_3 releases Ca^{2+} ion into the cytosol, probably by a guanine nucleotide regulatory protein. (Courtesy of Houslay M.D. Ref. 60).

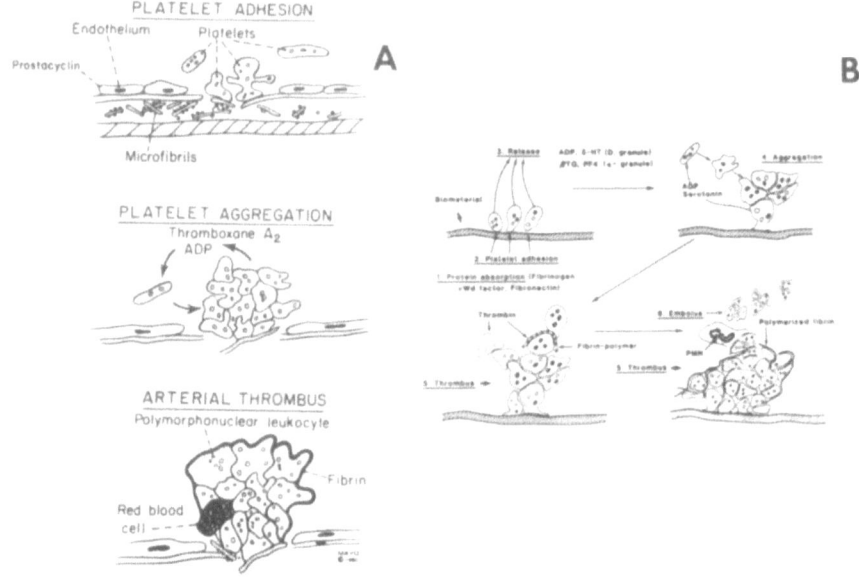

Fig 2b

Platelet thrombosis in denuded vessel wall (Left): several types
(I, III, V) of collagen fibers activate the platelets leading to
secretion from dense and alpha-granules, further platelet
aggregation and thrombosis on denuded vessel wall. Small injury
is repaired within 1-3 weeks. Occasionally, some thrombus is
incorporated in the plaque which is covered by a layer of
endothelial cells. The platelet thrombosis on the surface of
synthetic (Right) vascular graft (Dacron, Teflon and other
polymer surface); absorbed fibrinogen in the acute phase, a mixed
matrix of fibrinogen-fibrin-collagen and von Willebrand factor in
the chronic phase activate platelets leading to the continuous
process of thrombus formation and embolization. The fibroblast in
the pseudo-neointima, media and anastomoses result in collagen
build-up on synthetic graft surface.

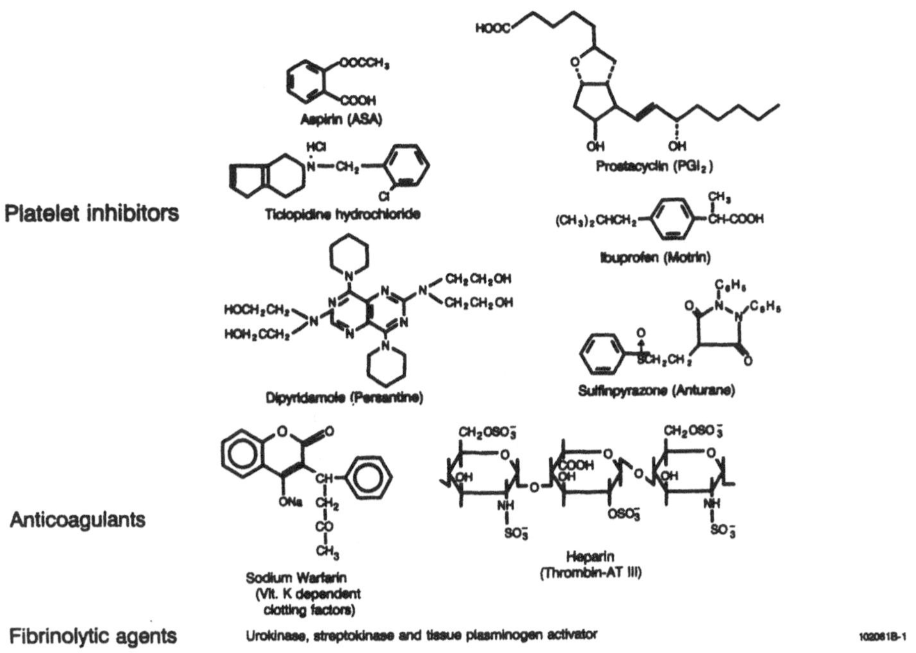

Fig 2c
Several drugs in the category of platelet inhibitors, anticoagulants and thrombolytic agents decrease the rate of thrombus formation, embolization and fibrinolysis.

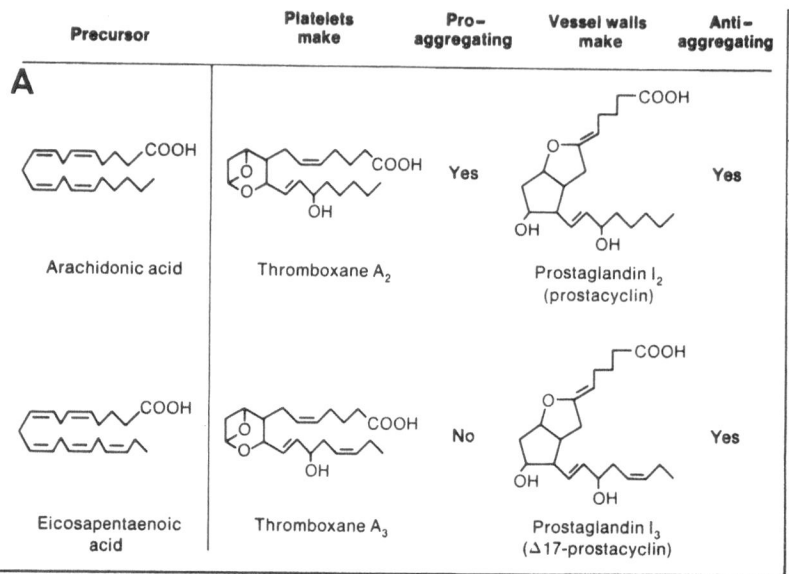

A

Precursor	Platelets make	Pro-aggregating	Vessel walls make	Anti-aggregating
Arachidonic acid	Thromboxane A₂	Yes	Prostaglandin I₂ (prostacyclin)	Yes
Eicosapentaenoic acid	Thromboxane A₃	No	Prostaglandin I₃ (Δ17-prostacyclin)	Yes

B

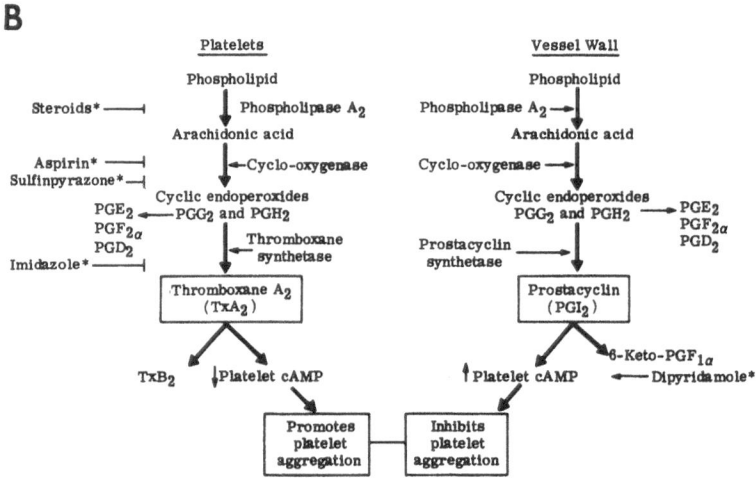

Fig 2d

Generation of prostaglandin derivatives by endothelial cells, smooth muscle cells and fibroblasts in vessel wall. Arrows indicate probably sites of action of platelet inhibitor drugs on platelet enzymes. (Reproduced with permission from Fuster V. Ref. 58)

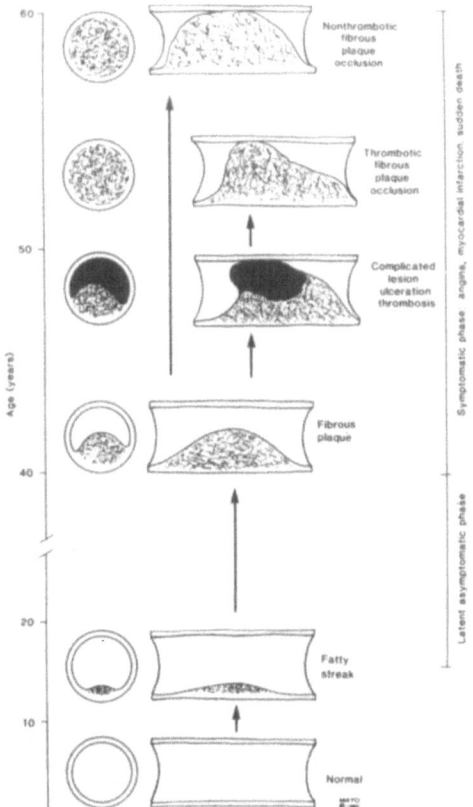

Fig ₂ₑ

Schematics of evolution of atherosclerosis and occlusion of lumen
by intimal proliferation are relatively slow, thrombus formation
at partially occluded lumen may lead to total luminal occlusion.
(Reproduced with permission form Fuster V. Ref. 58).

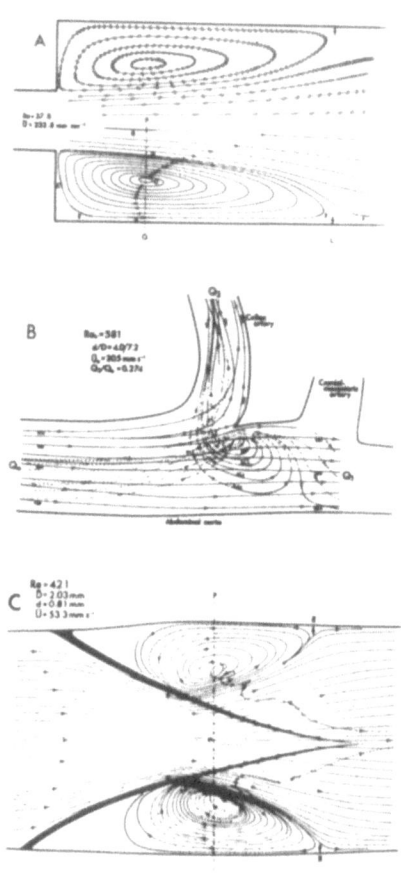

Fig. 2f
Theology of blood flow at stenosis, valve and bifurcation of blood vessels, vortices in these nonlinear systems are shown by turbulence. (Courtesy of Goldsmith H.L. Ref. 57)

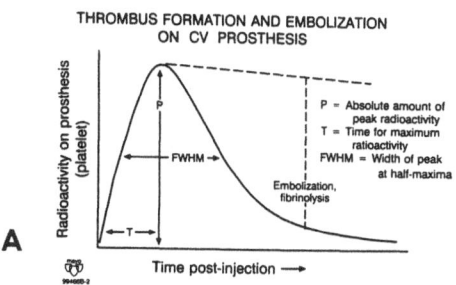

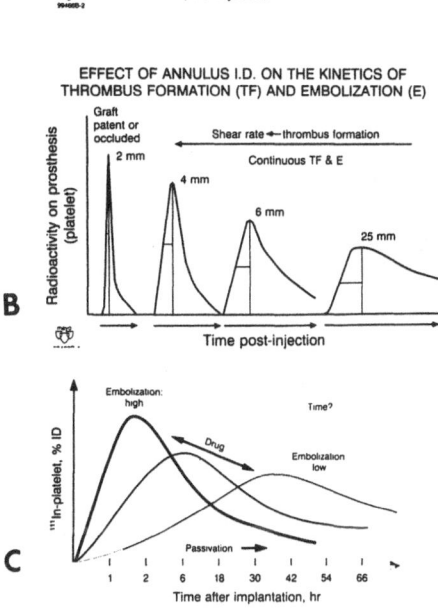

Fig. 3a(A)
The dynamics of the process of thrombus formation and embolization on cardiovascular prostheses could be followed by imaging of III-Indium-platelet deposition with a gamma camera.

Fig: 3a(B)
The processes of thrombus formation and embolization depend on the annulus I.D. and the shear rate. The smaller the vessel diameter, the higher the shear rate. In addition, the peak time for highest platelet deposition also increases with the increase in the diameter of the prosthesis.

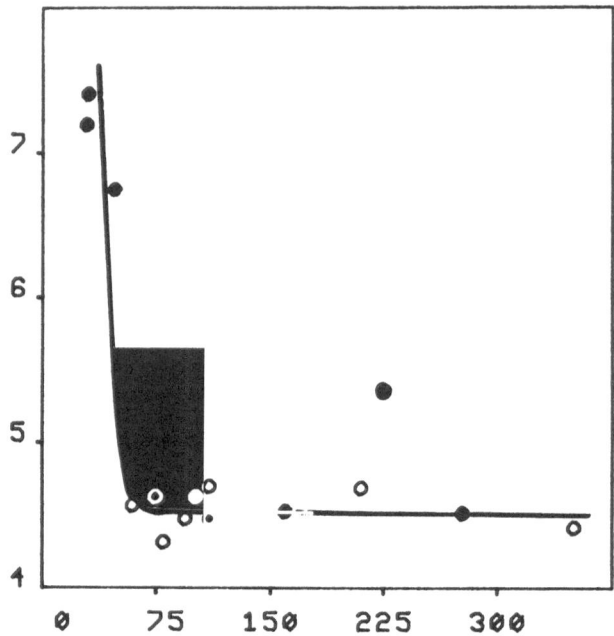

Fig 3b
The dependence of velocity of blood flow rates on platelet deposition. Platelet deposition drastically decreases after a cut-off value of 75 milliliter per minute of blood flow. In this study, the ipsilateral femoral vein was either open (o) or ligated to reduce blood flow through the graft (o).

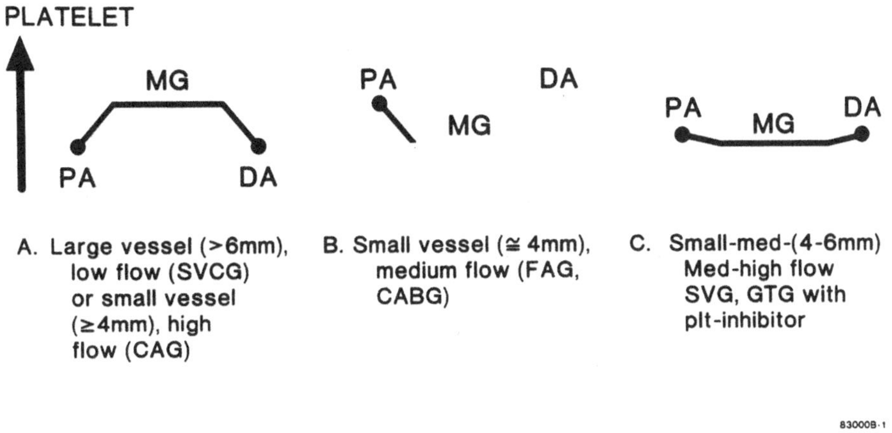

Fig 3c
Summary of regional platelet-deposition on segments of Gore-Tex grafts in the dog model. The three shapes of platelet deposition depend on hemodynamic parameters implanted in the arterial and venous system.

TRIAD OF IDEAL PROSTHESIS

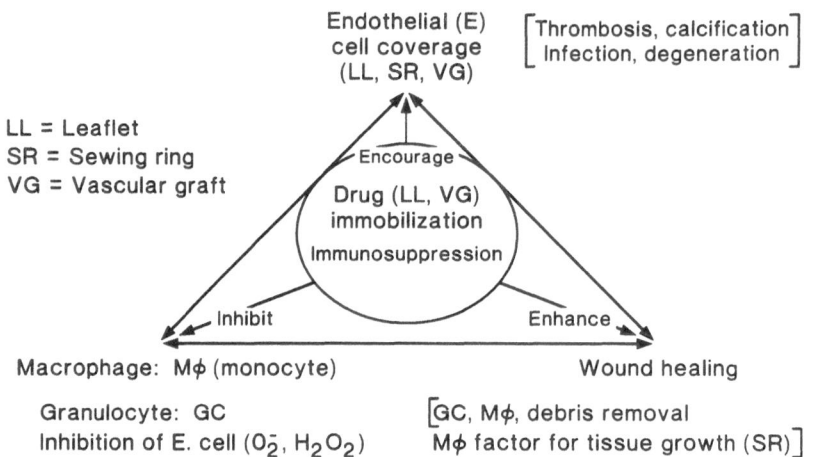

LL = Leaflet
SR = Sewing ring
VG = Vascular graft

Endothelial (E)
cell coverage
(LL, SR, VG)

[Thrombosis, calcification
Infection, degeneration]

Encourage

Drug (LL, VG)
immobilization

Immunosuppression

Inhibit

Enhance

Macrophage: Mφ (monocyte)

Wound healing

Granulocyte: GC
Inhibition of E. cell (O_2^-, H_2O_2)

[GC, Mφ, debris removal
Mφ factor for tissue growth (SR)]

84880B 2A

Fig 3d

The triad of endothelial cell coverage, macrophage and monocyte
infiltration and would healing depends on a variety of factors
leading either to the pathological changes, e.g. thrombosis,
calcification, infection, degeneration, or endothelial cell
coverage. The role of macrophage in wound healing in the early
phase is important, but in the later phase foreign body response
prevents endothelial cell coverage.

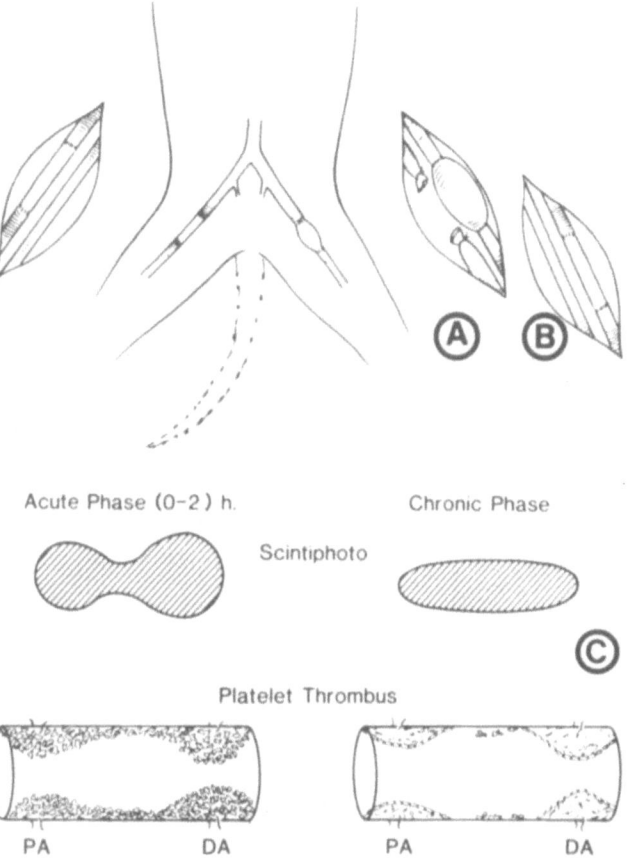

Fig 4a

Scheme of bilateral femoral graft implantation in dogs. (A) EPTFE-bein graft, (B) EPTFE-EPTFE graft at one and three hours perfusion. (C) III-In-platelets in vascular grafts. Schematics of platelet deposition in the acute and chronic phase; in the acute phase more platelets are deposited at the proximal and distal anastomoses; less in the middle and converse is true for chronic phase. Scintiphoto indicates similar platelet distribution on vascular grafts in patients. Occasionally hot spots for focal thrombi were found in the mid region of the graft. The dynamics of the difference of platelet deposition at anastomosis and mid-section of the small diameter (4 mm I.D.) graft. The platelet deposition is higher always at the anastomosis than at the mid-section. In addition, in the occluding small vessel prosthesis, higher platelet deposition occurs in the mid-section at later hours. Dewanjee M.K. (16). Reproduced with permission from the publisher.

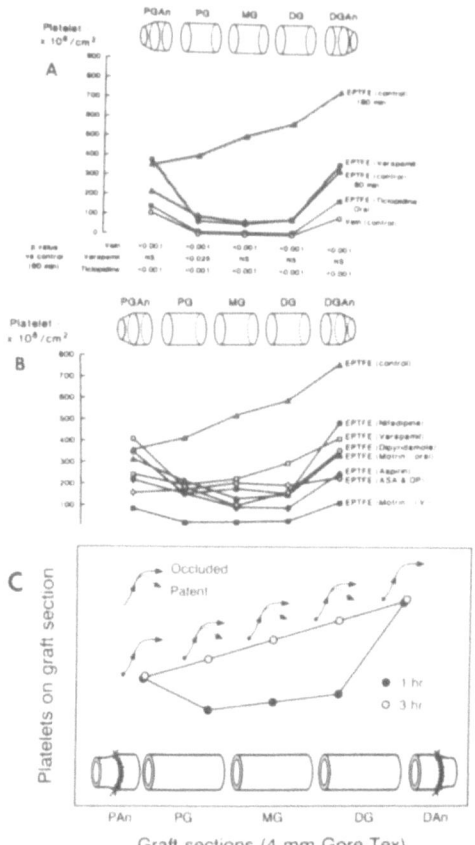

Fig 5a

Platelet deposition on vein- and EPTFE-graft at 60 minutes of perfusion in control and treated dogs. The shaded area represents different rate of regional platelet deposition during the two-hour interval from 60 to 180 minutes of perfusion; platelet deposition rate is higher at distal anastomosis.

Fig 5b

Platelet deposition on vein- and EPTFE-graft at 180 minutes of perfusion in control and treated dogs. Intravenous motrin reduces thrombogenicity of EPTFE graft to that of femoral vein graft; aspirin, aspirin-persantin, and motrin are more effective than calcium-channel blockers in reducing platelet deposition. Dewanjee et al. (28) Reproduced with permission from the publisher.

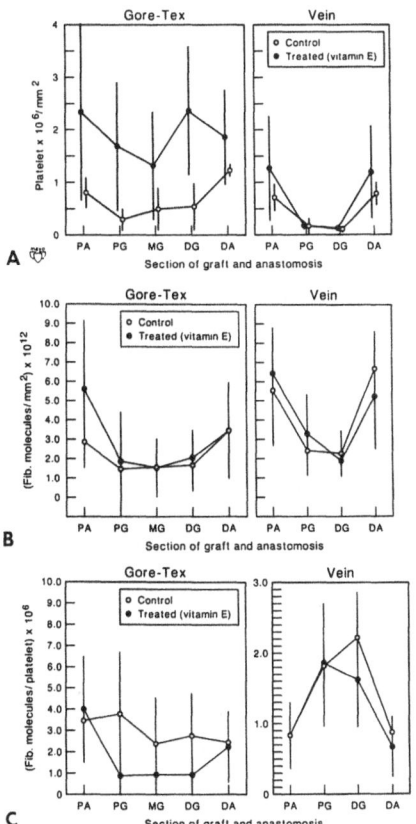

Fig. 6a
Platelet density on anastomosis and midsections of Gore-Tex and vein grafts after one hour of perfusion in control and vitamin E treated dogs.

Fig 6b
Density of fibrin on sections of the same grafts.

Fig 6c
Fibrin/platelet ratio on sections of the same grafts Dewanjee et al. (47). Reproduced with permission from the publisher

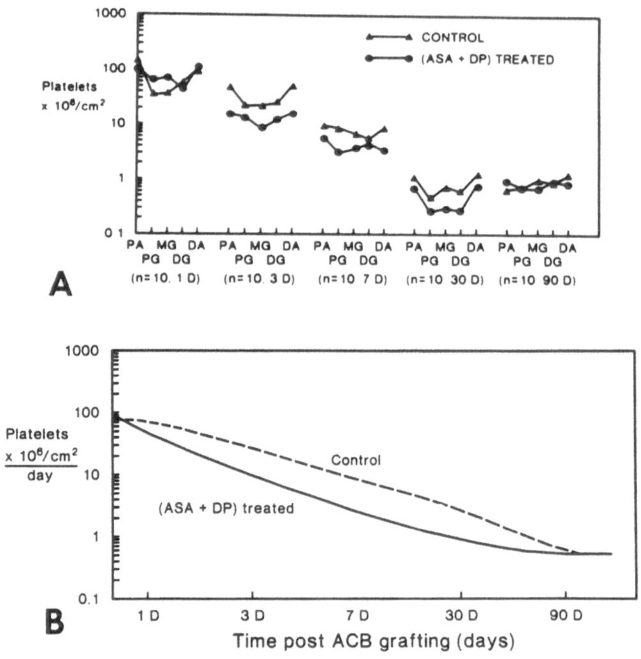

96

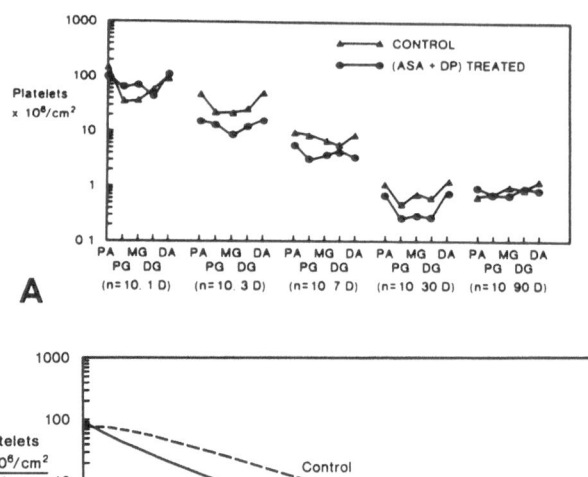

A

B

Time post ACB grafting (days)

Fig 7a
Time course of change in regional platelet deposition as
represented by surface density of platelets on aorto coronary
bypass graft in control and treated dogs. Platelets/cm^2 on graft
surface (24 hours post injection) of untreated ("control") dogs
and dogs treated orally with dipyridamole and aspirin, were
determined with III-In-platelets. Persantin (2.5 mg/kg/day) was
administered two days prior to surgery and aspirin (15 mg/kg/day)
immediately post-operation. Five dogs in each group were
sacrificed at 1, 3, 7, 30 and 90 days after grafting. In each
group of five joined points, the points, left to right, represent
mean values from proximal anastomosis (PA), proximal graft
segment (PG), mid-graft segment (MG), distal graft segment (DG),
and distal anastomosis (DA). Note lower platelet density in the
treated group at 3,7 and 30 days. Twenty-four hour platelet
deposition is similar at day 1 and day 90. Dewanjee M.K. (29)
Reproduced with permission from the publisher.

Fig 7b
Continuous level of higher platelet deposition leads to faster
occlusion at the narrower distal anastomosis.

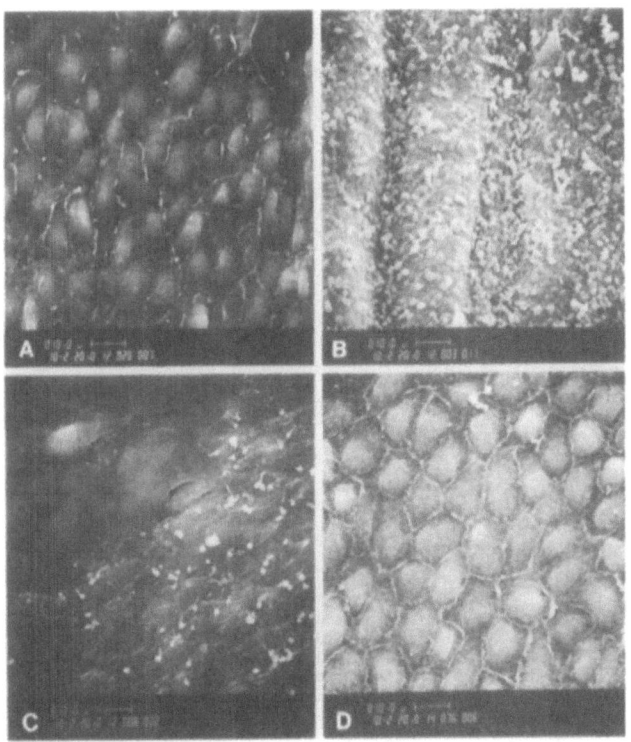

Fig 8

Scanning electron micrograph of vessels undergoing angioplasty.
Residual endothelial cells cover the intima by proliferation.

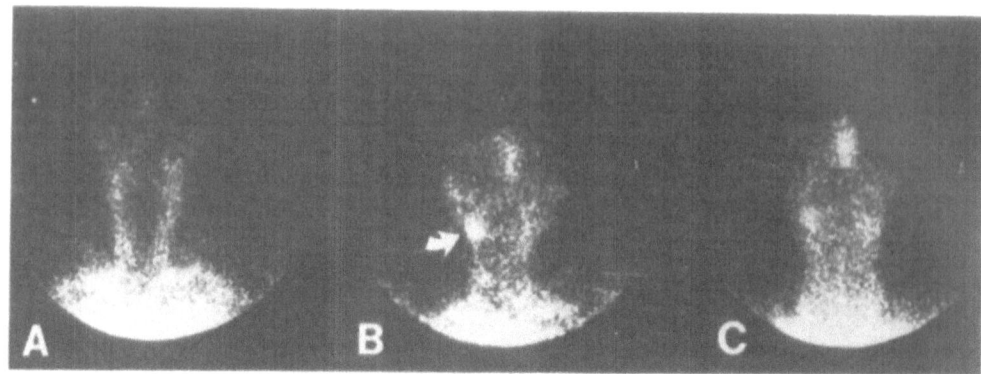

Fig 9

III-In-platelet scintigrams of the head and neck (anterior view of a 37-year-old woman). (A) Normal scintigram, III-In-platelets in major vessels of carotid artery and jugular vein and nasopharyngeal blood pool are clearly outlined (8). A well-defined focus (white arrow) of increased III-In-platelets at the right carotid bifurcation of a 42-year-old man who had an infarction of the ipsilateral cerebral hemisphere five days earlier. (C) A typical scintigram showing diffuse uptake at the carotid bifurcation of a 59-year-old man with right-sided amaurosis fugax. Due to the transient nature of thrombosis and embolization, these thrombi could be followed by imaging with a gamma camera. Powers et al. (17)

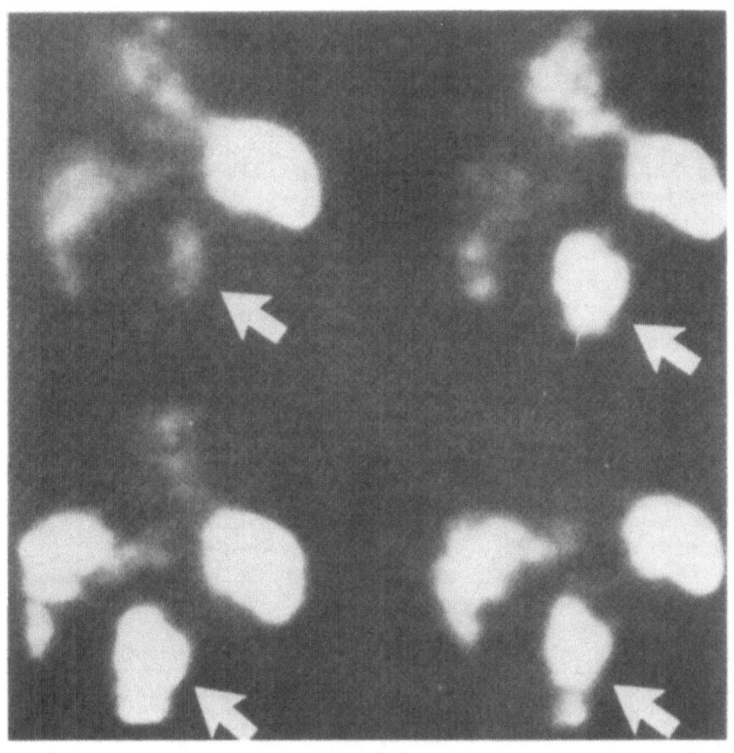

Fig 10

Scintigrams of a patient with abdominal aortic aneurysm (arrow) at 90 minutes (top left), 24 hours (top right), 48 hours (bottom left), and 144 hours (bottom right) post injection of III-In-platelets. Optimum imaging time of accumulation of III-In-platelet in aneurysm is approximately 72-96 hours; note the dynamic nature of platelet incorporation in the aneurysm. Splenic pooling and hepatic sequestration are visible in the anterior view image. Heyns et al. (24). Reproduced with permission from the publisher.

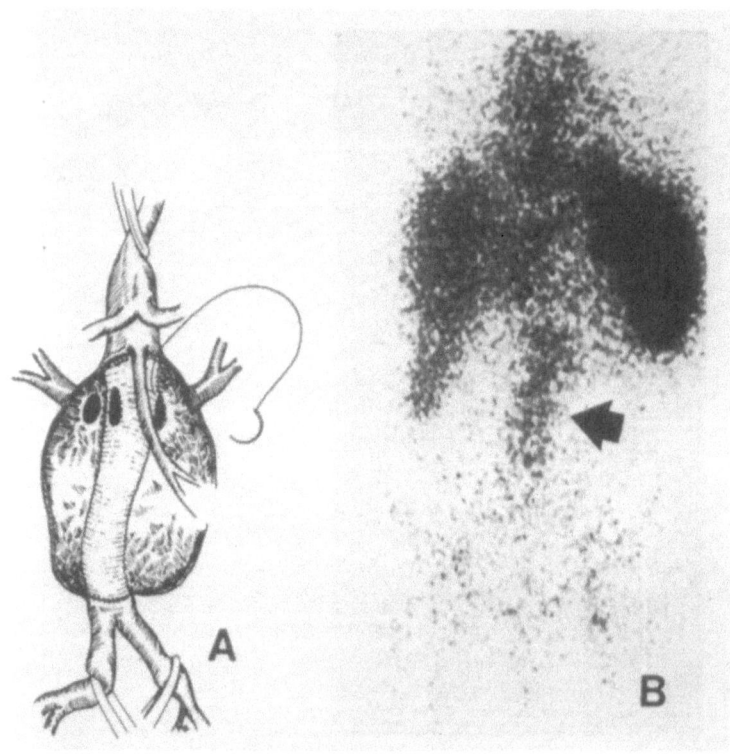

Fig 11
Surgical repair of aneurysm, anastomosis to adjoining arteries,
and Dacron graf+ (A). Scintigrams (8) of platelet thrombosis on
Dacron graft (black arrow) 24 hours after administration of III-
In-platelets. Note diffuse distribution of platelet deposition in
scintigram at 10 years post grafting; most of the vascular grafts
remain thrombogenic in the chronic phase. Robertson, J.S. (10)
Reproduced with permission from the publisher.

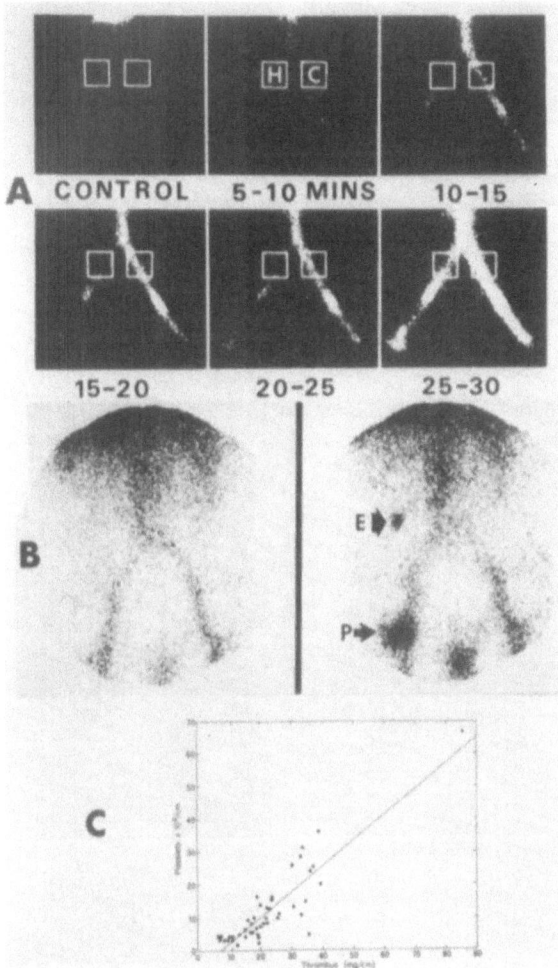

Fig. 12

Scintiphoto of platelet deposition at the site of puncture and
extravasation of blood at the site of catheter insertion.
A. Dynamics of platelet deposition on control (right), heparin-
coated polyethylene catheter (left) in dogs. Lipton M.J. (44).
Reproduced with permission from the publisher.
B. Scintiphotos were obtained in anterior view one hour pre and
post angiography in a patient. As the catheter is pulled out, the
adherent emboli (E) are left in circulation, the emboli could be
followed by imaging with a gamma camera. O'Connor M.K. (46).
Reproduced with permission from the publisher.
C. Correlation of linear platelet density and adherent thrombus
on polyethylene catheter inserted in carotid artery of goats.
Rodvien R. (45). Reproduced with permission from the publisher.

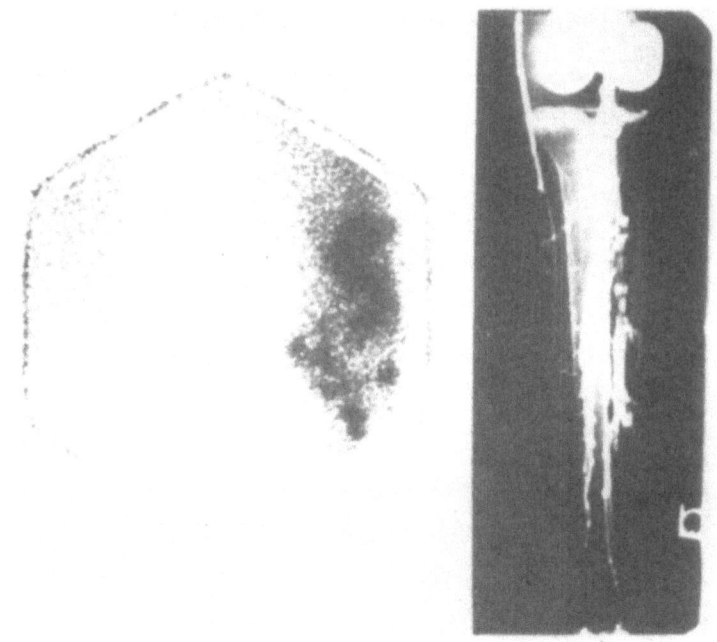

Fig 13

Scintiphoto (left) of platelet deposition (24 hour post injection) in both calves in a patient with deep vein thrombosis. The tortuous area of increased activity represents a large venous thrombus. The corresponding venogram (right) shows filling defects in the areas where higher platelet deposition was observed. Ezekowitz et al. (23). Reproduced with permission from the publisher.

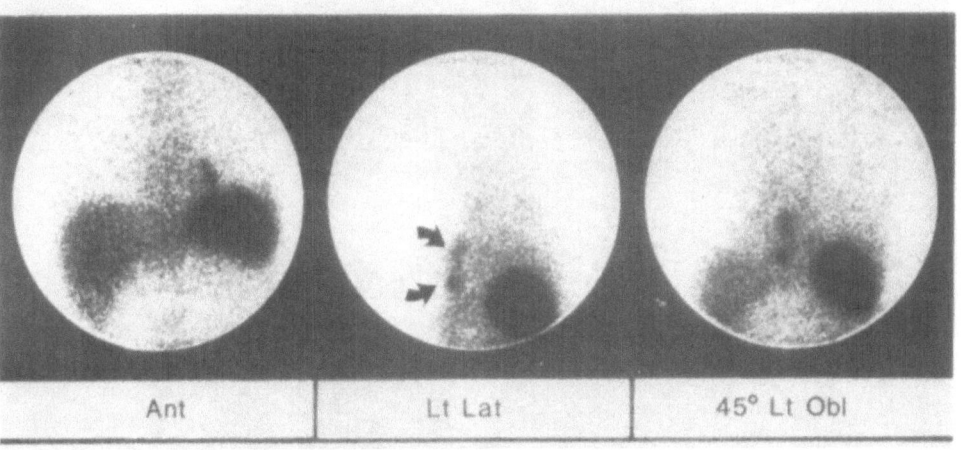

Fig 14

Scintiphoto of platelet deposition in left ventricular mural
thrombus in a patient with anterolateral transmural infarct, four
days after III-In-platelet injection. Note two focal spots of
platelet thrombus in the anterior (Ant), left lateral (Lt Lat),
and left anterior oblique view (Lt Obl). Proper positioning of
gamma camera could identify the two thrombi in the lateral views.

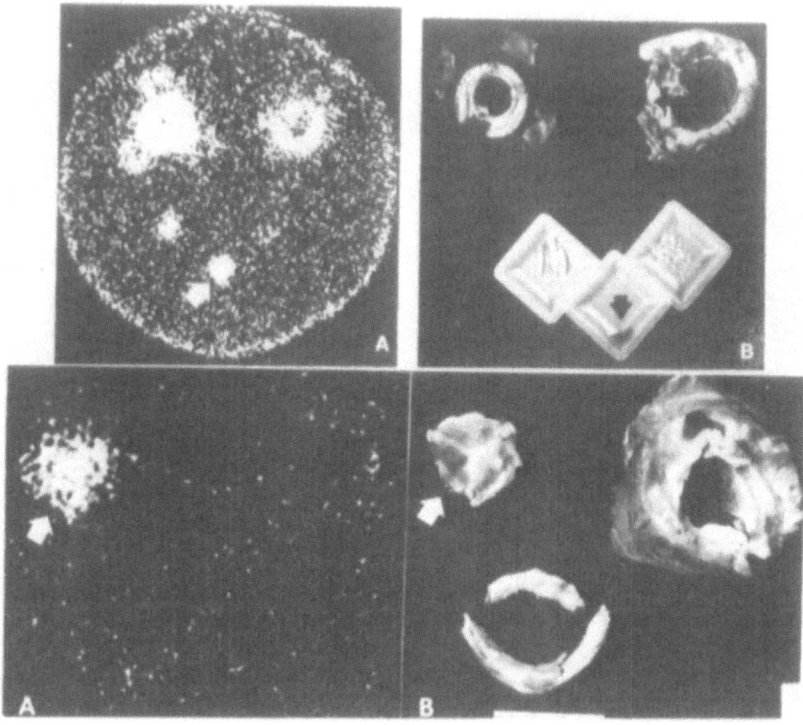

Fig 15b

(A) Scintiphoto (5,000 counts) of isolated components of tissue
valve prosthesis (Top) removed from a dog at 25 hours after
implantation and 24 hours after administration of labelled
platelets. White arrow indicates most intense radioactivity
[which comes from platelet thrombus (black arrow) on sewing
ring]. (B) Photograph of same objects; sewing ring with three
leaflets around it (upper left); perivalvular tissue (upper
right); stent supports, thrombus from sewing ring, and suture (in
trays below, left to eight). Thrombus from sewing ring amounted
to 31.44 mg (wet wt). Our recent studies suggest that detergent
treatment and diphosphonate immobilization reduce monocyte
infiltration and expedite endothelial cell coverage of tissue
valve and inhibit calcification. In the similar scintiphoto at 30
days. (Bottom) most of the platelet deposition occurs in the
leaflets, the sewing ring is covered with fibroblast and remains
nonthrombogenic. The dynamics of platelet deposition on
components of tissue valves in calves; unlike catheter in a small
vessel, the peak time is about 8 hours. Dewanjee M.K. et al.
(39). Reproduced with permission from the publisher.

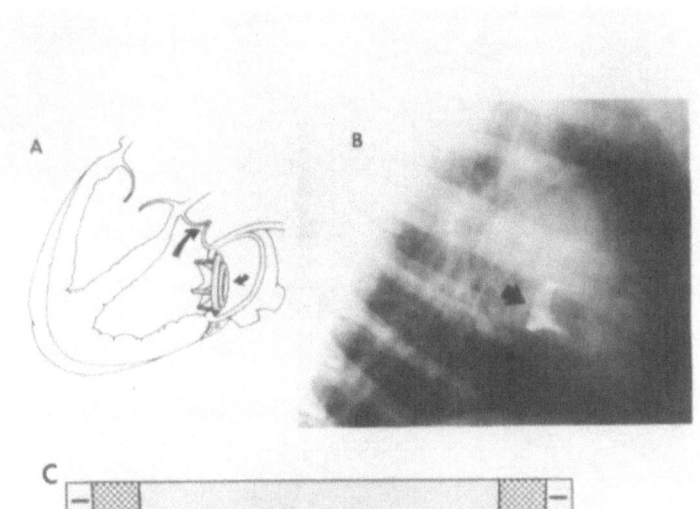

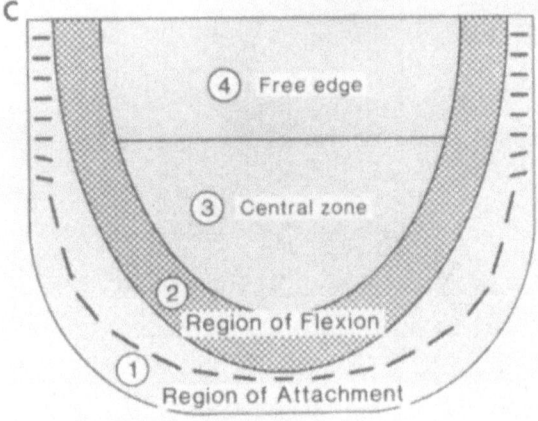

Fig 15a

A. Implantation of pericardial tissue valve in mitral annulus.
B. Radiograph of tissue valve in mitral annulus.
C. Four zones of each leaflet separated in such a way that regional platelet thrombosis and calcification could be quantified.

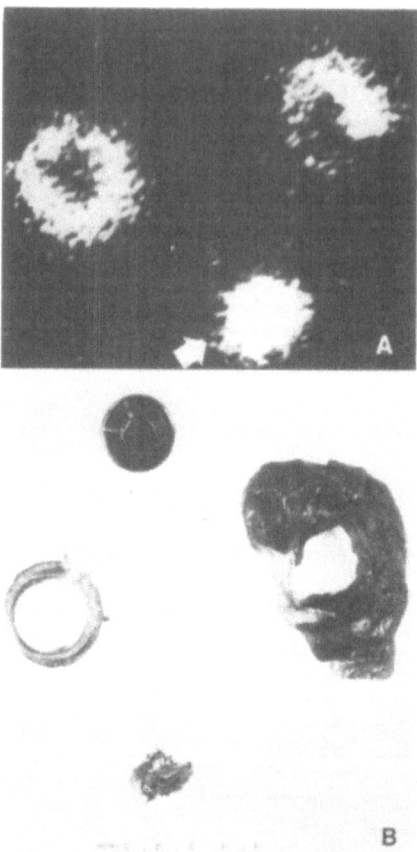

Fig. 16

Scintiphoto of platelet deposition on components of mechanical valve prosthesis 24 hours post injection of III-In-platelets and photograph in the same orientation. (A) Scintiphoto (25 hours after injection of III-In-platelets in a dog and 24 hours after implantation) of sewing ring (left), perivalvular tissue (right), and thrombus (arrow bottom). The disc and housing of the valve had few adherent platelets (top). (B) Thrombogenicity of tissue and mechanical valve is identical in the acute phase. Photograph of the same components in the same orientation. Dewanjee M.K.et al. (40). Reproduced with permission from the publisher.

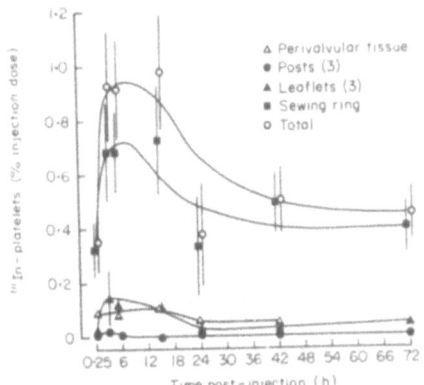

Fig 17

Quantification of platelet deposition on components of bovine pericardial tissue valve prosthesis implanted in calves. Note change in platelet deposition on all components with time as observed with other vascular prosthesis and conduits. Dewanjee M.K. et al. (41). Reproduced with permission from the publisher.

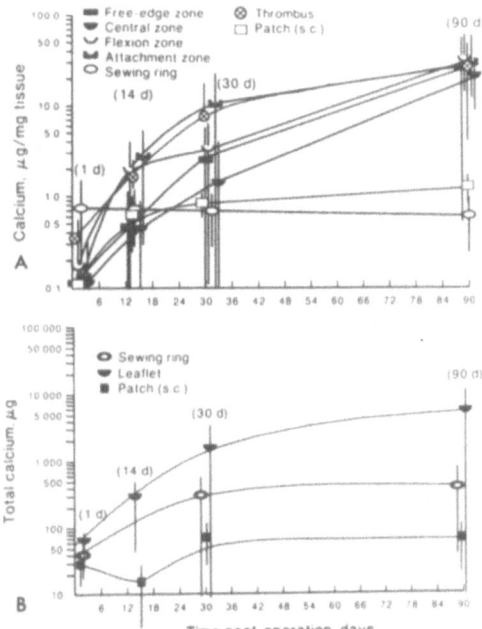

Fig 18b

Time course of exponential growth of regional calcification (A) and total calcium level (B) in components of tissue valve. The calcification of thrombus parallels that of collagen fibril in pericardial leaflet. Dewanjee M.K. (42) Reproduced with permission from the publisher.

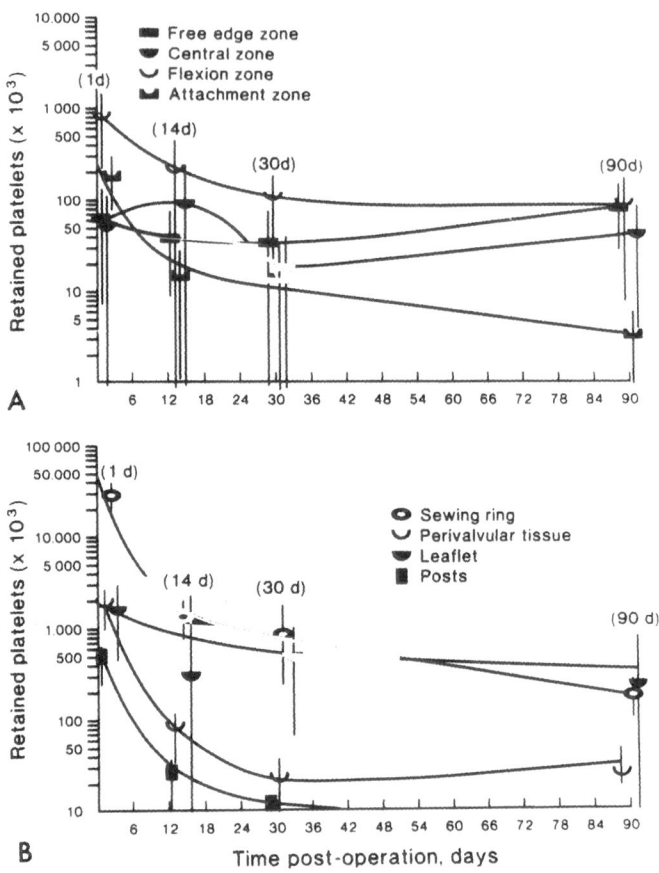

Fig 18a

Time course of 24-hour platelet deposition expressed as total number of platelets (mean -/+ standard deviation) on leaflet components at 1, 14, 30 and 90 days post implantation of 25 mm tissue valves in calves.

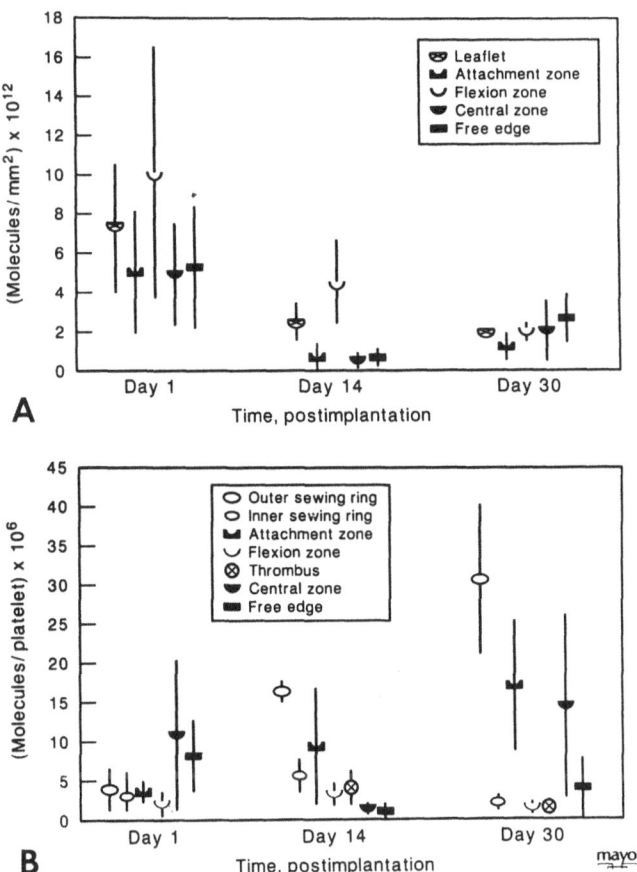

Fig 19a

Regional fibrin density on components of tissue valve at 1, 14 and 30 days post implantation.

Fig 19b

Regional distribution of fibrin monomer per platelet on components of prostheses. Although the fibrin density decreases, the fibrin/platelet tends to increase for outer sewing ring, attachment and central zone of tissue valve leaflet, Dewanjee et al. (48). Reproduced with permission from publisher.

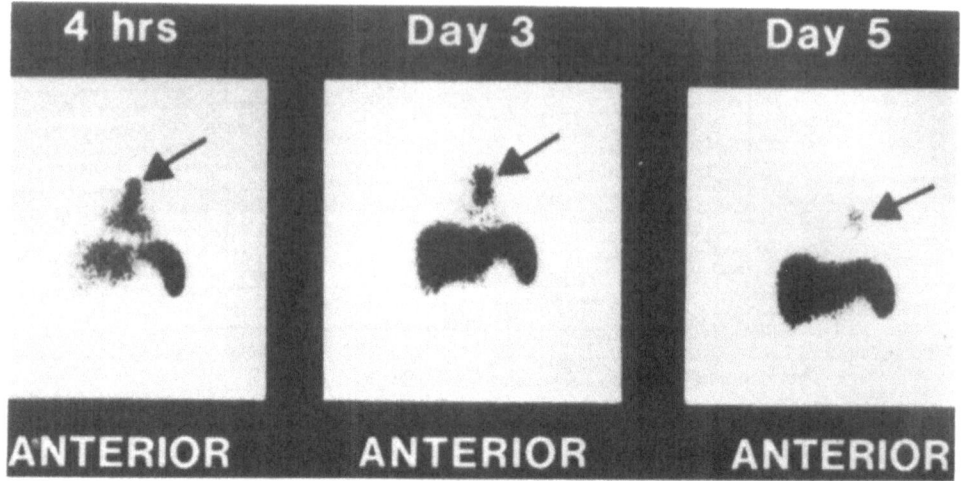

Fig 20

Scintiphoto of platelet accumulation in Hancock porcine valved-conduit at four hours to five days post injection; patient was treated with 75 mg of dipyridamole and 325 mg of aspirin (three times daily). Note uniform platelet deposition on conduit in the anterior view, optimum time of imaging is approximately 72 hours. Note lower platelet deposition possibly due to fibrinolysis and embolization at five days. Agarwal et al. (37). Reproduced with permission from the publisher.

DUAL ISOTOPE SUBTRACTION PLATELET SCINTIGRAPHY IN THE
DIAGNOSIS OF LEFT VENTRICULAR THROMBOSIS.

Freek W.A. Verheugt, M.D.
Albert J. Funke-Kupper, M.D.

INTRODUCTION

     Indium-111 platelet scintigraphy has proven to be a
highly specific technique for the detection of intracardiac
thrombosis.   Since platelets only incorporate in ongoing
thrombosis, platelet scintigraphy only identifies
hematologically active thrombi.   This unique aspect gives
this technique an outstanding feature in the study of
natural history of thrombi as well as pharmacological
intervention. A major drawback of platelet imaging is the
relatively long half life of circulating indium-111 labelled
platelets not incorporated in thrombi. They give rise to a
blood pool activity masquerading platelet sequestration in
intracardiac thrombi. Moreover, they might interfere in the
quantitation of platelet sequestration in the heart.
Therefore, attempts have been made to subtract the blood
pool activity of circulating non thrombus bound platelets
from sequestrated platelets.   Since technecium labelled
erythrocytes are the cells of choice for blood pool
labelling, techniques have been introduced for blood pool
subtraction in platelet scintigraphy in angiology (1,2) and
cardiology (3).   This so called dual isotope subtraction
technique in the diagnosis of left ventricular thrombosis
will be reviewed.

METHODS

     The technique of dual isotope subtraction for the
detection of cardiac thrombosis has been extensively
described elsewhere (3,4).   In brief, platelet labelling
according to Verheugt (3) is performed.   Immediately,
thereafter the labelled platelets are injected in the
patient. Forty - eight hours later an Indium image is made
of the cardiac area. During the imaging blood is drawn in a
syringe for Indium blood counts. With the patient and the
camera in the same position, Tc-99m is injected and the
camera is set to the Tc settings. Subsequently, a blood
pool image is made and simultaneously blood is drawn for
Technetium blood counts. Indium and Technetium blood counts
are measured with the syringe put on the camera, which is
set up to the Indium and Technetium settings respectively.

Ch. Kessler et al. (eds.), Clinical Application of Radiolabelled Platelets, 111–115.
© 1990 *Kluwer Academic Publishers.*

Subsequently, the Indium and Technetium images of the cardiac area are added and the areas of interest are drawn around the left ventricle, the left lung and the complete thorax. The Technetium image is subtracted (s) from the Indium image according to the following formula:

Indium image (s) = Indium image - K.Technetium image, in which K is the Indium/Technetium blood count ratio.

Subsequently, the areas of interest mentioned above are applied to the Indium (s) image. The Indium (s) is normalised for lung background and total thorax counts. Finally, the left ventricular count per pixel in the normalised subtracted (ns) image is expressed as follows:

$$\text{LV cpp (ns)} = \frac{\text{LV cpp(s)} - \text{lung cpp(s)}}{\text{thorax cpp(s)}}$$

RESULTS

The methodology described has been applied in two studies. Figs 1 and 2 represent quantitative data from both reports. Visually positive and negative images could easily be discriminated quantitatively. Also left ventricular platelet deposition in patients with transmural infarction was more pronounced than in those with subendocardial myocardial infarction. Systemic embolism seems to be correlated with a high left ventricular platelet sequestration.

However, in both studies quantitative platelet scintigraphy does not seem to be more sensitive than conventional platelet scintigraphy. The left ventricular counts per pixel in the normalised subtracted images are too low for clear-cut discrimination into quantitatively positive and negative images.

On the other hand, the dual isotope technique gives clear delineation of the right and left ventricle. Thrombi can be localised much easier and delineated from "hot" areas like the liver and the spleen.

DISCUSSION

For the diagnosis of intracardiac thrombosis Indium-111 platelet scintigraphy is the most specific technique. Its largest advantage over other techniques is its ability to estimate the hematological activity of thrombi. To quantify platelet sequestration blood pool subtraction must be

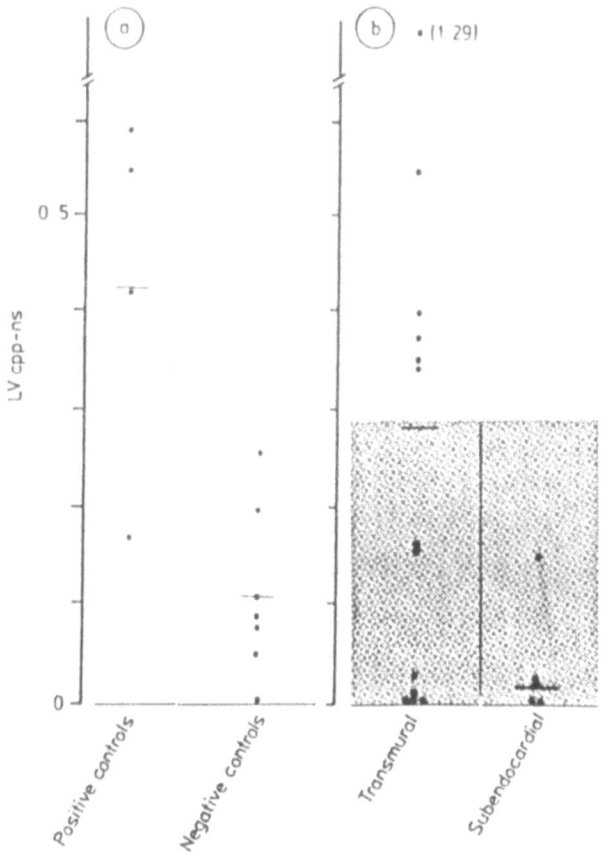

Fig. 1

Verheugt: DUAL ISOTOPE SUBTRACTION

Results of quantitative platelet scintigraphy in (a) patients with either positive (positive controls) or negative (negative controls) echocardiography for left ventricular thrombosis and in (b) patients with recent myocardial infarction. Shaded area represents mean ± SD of the negative controls. (reproduced by permission of the author [3]).

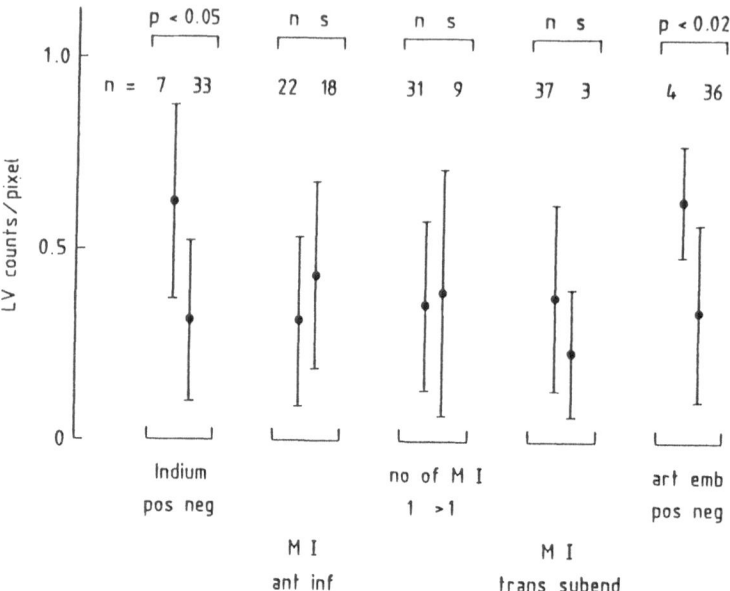

Fig. 2

Verheugt: DUAL ISOTOPE SUBTRACTION

Results of quantitative platelet scintigraphy in patients
with recent myocardial infarction in relation to results of
conventional platelet scintigraphy, infarct localisation,
number of infarcts and systemic embolisation. (reproduced
by permission of the author [4]).

performed. The use of a second isotope is necessary for that purpose, but carries two major disadvantages: differences in tissue attenuation of both isotopes and crossdown of the two isotopes. Crossdown has proven to be negligable (4). But the problem of differences in tissue attenuation cannot be solved and, therefore, blood pool subtracted platelet scintigraphy will always be semi-quantitative. Moreover, in the two clinical studies (3,4) using this technique it failed to be more sensitive than conventional platelet scintigraphy. Although pathological validation is lacking in both studies, it must be assumed, that very low counts in the left ventricle in the subtracted Indium images do not represent platelet deposition. In any case, these low counts cannot be the starting point for longitudinal quantitative studies on natural history or drug intervention.

In conclusion, dual isotope platelet scintigraphy is of limited value in the quantitation of left ventricle platelet deposition. Its only advantage over conventional platelet scintigraphy is its clear delineation of crucial landmarks in the Indium image of the cardiac area.

REFERENCES

1. Isaka Y, Kimura K, Yoneda S, Kusuncki M, Etani H, Uyama O, Tsuda Y, Abe H. Platelet accumulation in carotid atherosclerotic lesions : semiquantitative analysis with indium-111 platelets and technetium-99m human serum albumin. J.Nucl.Med.1984; 25:556-563
2. Kessler C H, Reutner R, Kinnig B, Pietzsch T. Dual isotope scintigraphy in stroke patients. Neuroradiology 1984; 26:113-7
3. Verheugt FWA, Lindenfeld JA, Kirch DL, Steele PP. Left ventricular platelet deposition after acute myocardial infarction. An attempt at quantification using blood pool subtracted indium-111 platelet scintigraphy. Br.Heart J. 1984; 52:490-6
4. Funke Kupper AJ, Verheugt FWA, Jaarsma W, Van der Wall EE, Van Eenige MJ, Den Hollander W, Roos JP. Detection of ventricular thrombosis in acute myocardial infarction : value of indium-111 platelet scintigraphy in relation to two-dimensional echocardiography and clinical course. Eur J.Nucl.Med.1986; 12:337-41.

FAILURE OF SULFINPYRAZONE TO PREVENT LEFT VENTRICULAR
THROMBOSIS IN PATIENTS WITH ACUTE MYOCARDIAL INFARCTION
TREATED WITH ORAL ANTICOAGULANTS: A RANDOMIZED TRAIL IN 100
PATIENTS

Funke-Kupper A.J., Verheugt F.W.A., den Hollander W.

Department of Cardiology and Department of Nuclear Medicine,
Free University Hospital, Amsterdam, The Netherlands

INTRODUCTION

Left ventricular thrombosis (LVT) has been known for a
long time as complication of acute myocardial infarction
(MI) (Garvin C.F., Hellerstein H.K.). Patients with LVT run
a risk for systemic embolism, which can contribute to
morbidity and mortality after MI (Visser C.A., 1985, Meltzer
R.S.). Previous studies have shown that LVT with subsequent
embolism can develop shortly after MI (Eigler N., Weinreicht
D). Administration of anti-thrombotic therapy to prevent
formation of a LVT should be started in the early phase of
MI. Despite early anti-throbotic therapy with oral
anticoagulants or heparin, LVT is still found in patients
with acute or recent MI (Weinreich D.J., Cokkinos D.V.,
Scholl J.< Friedman M.J., Gueret P., Ezekowitz M.D. 1984).
Two-dimensional echocardigraphy (2DE) and indium-III
platelet scintigraphy (IND) have proven to be valuable and
sensitive techniques in identifying LVT (Reeder GS, Stratton
J.R., Visser C.A., 1983, Ezekowitz M.D., 1981, 1982, 1983,
Asinger R.W., 1981 I, Verheugt F.W.A., Funke Kupper A.J.).
2DE provides anatomical information and detects the thrombus
mass. With IND hematological activity at the surface of the
thrombus is assessed.
The purpose of this study was to evaluate the value of
sulfinpyrazone (SFP), an antiplatelet drug, as prophylactic
therapy in patients with MI receiving early anticoagulation,
with respect to the incidence of LVT.

PATIENTS, STUDY DESIGN AND METHODS

One hundred consecutive patients, admitted to our
coronary care unit from July 1982 to November 1984 were
studied after informed consent. All patients, admitted to
the CCU within 24 hours after onset of symptoms of MI, were
eligible for the study. Patients on oral anticoagulants or
platelet active drugs were excluded as were patients with a
serum creatinine . 150 micro mol/L (normal value 70-120
micro mol/L).
A diagnosis of acute MI was made on the following
criteria: a typical history of anginal pain, characteristic

116

Ch. Kessler et al. (eds.), Clinical Application of Radiolabelled Platelets, 116–127.
© 1990 Kluwer Academic Publishers.

ECG changes and significant creatine kinase isoenzyme release. Electrocardiographic criteria included typical ST-segment and T wave changes and the development of new Q waves. A Q-wave MI as considered anterior if there were Q waves in leads I, AVL and/or V1 to V6 and was considered inferior or posterior if there were new Q waves in leads II, III, AVF and/or the RS-ratio in V1 was .1. A MI was called a non-Q wave infraction if only T wave changes were present.

All patients received coumadin as oral anticoagulant directly after admission and during hospital stay. Heparin 5000 U B.I.D. subcutaneously was given till mobilization (3 to 4 days). The beginning coumadin dose was 6 mg on the first day and 4 mtg on the second and third day. Thereafter the dose was determined depending on the thrombo test results. Thrombo test was kept between 120-180 second (normal value under 40 seconds) and was checked daily during the first week and every second day thereafter during hospital stay. Patients were randomized double blind to SFP 200 mg 4 times a day or placebo 4 times a day. The first dose was given within 24 hours after onset of symptoms.

Clinical data including: age, sex, history of previous MI site and type of MI (anterior versus inferior, Q wave versus non-Q wave), laboratory data, systemic embolism, time between first symptoms and echocardiographic and scintigraphic imaging, were recorded of all patients. Laboratory data included hemoglobin hematocrit blood platelets count, enzyme peak values (creatinine kinase, creatinine kinase isoenzyme, lactate dehydrogenase) and serial thrombo test. Because SFP can give significant rise to serum creatinine, special attention was paid to serial serum creatinine levels during the study. 2DE and IND were performed 10 to 14 days after entering the study. Unblinding of the study medication was carried out after completion of the results in all patients.

ECHOCARDIOGRAPHIC TECHNIQUE

Two-dimensional echocardiography was performed with a commercially available mechanical 90 degrees wide angle sector scanner (ATL mark 300 with a 2.5 mHz transducer) and a phased array 90 degrees wide angle sector scanner (HP 7720A with a 3.5 mHz transducer). Images were obtained with patients in the left lateral supine position from multiple parasternal long- and short axis views and apical two and four chamber views. Images were stored on videotape and interpreted by two independent investigators. In case of equivocal images the interpretation of a third investigator was decisive. To avoid a false positive diagnosis of LVT, previous established guide lines were used (Asinger RW 1981 II). Left ventricular function was judged in two ways using echocardiography: Firstly the overall impression in good, moderate or poor left ventricular function. Secondly the left ventricular wall was divided into 13 segments (Gibson RS). A total score was made depending on the degree of asynergy of each segment: normal 0, hypokinesia +1, akinesia +2, dyskinesia +3, hyperkinesis -1.

INDIUM-III-PLATELET SCINTIGRAPHY

The method used to label platelets with indium-III-oxine was described previously (Ezekowitz MD 1981, Stratton JR 1981, Funke Kupper A.J., Verheugt F.W.A., Thakur M.L.). Between 48 to 72 hours after injection of the labelled platelets imaging was performed with a Picker Dyna 4 gamma camera with a 3000 holes medium energy collimator in a 30 degrees right anterior oblique and a 45 degrees left anterior oblique position. The gamma camera was set up to use a 20% window for both 173 Kev and 247 Kev peak activity of indium-III. The IND was judged positive if a clear "hotspot" was visible with the left ventricular region. All images were interpreted by two investigators. Discrepancies were resolved by consensus (interobserver analysis agreement was 90%) To correct the blood pool activity of still circulating labelled platelets a dual isotope-subtraction method with IND and technetium-99m blood pool scan was used (Funke Kupper AJ). After the IND in the 45 degrees left anterior position the patients and the gamma camera remained in the same position. After labelling of the red cells in vivo by intravenous injection of 10 mg stanous pyrophosphate, 2.5 to 15 mCi technetium-99m pertechnetate was injected. The gamma camera was adjusted to a 20% window of the 140 Key peak activity of technetium-99m and image time was 5 minutes. During both the IND and technetium-99m blood pool scan 19 ml venous blood was drawn and collected in a 20 ml syringe containing 1 ml citrate acid dextrose solution. Both blood samples were placed subsequently on the collimator in the same way, and activity was measured during 5 minutes with the gamma camera in the previous peak settings. After correction for differences in image time (15 versus 5 minutes), decay of activity and background activity, the indium-III/technetium-99m blood count ratio (=k) was measured.

After addition of the indium-III and the technetium-99m image on a video screen, regions of interest were made of the left ventricle, lung (=background) and thorax (see Fig 1). Subsequently a subtraction image was obtained by subtracting the technetium-99m image from the indium-III image using the indium-III/technetium-99m ratio (=k): subtraction image = indium-III image - k x technetium-99 image (see figure). The previous regions of interest were applied to this subtraction image and the counts per pixel were determined in region of the left ventricle (LVcpp-s), lung (lung cpp-s) and thorax (thorax cpp-s). Left ventricular platelet deposition in the left ventricle was expressed as left ventricular counts per pixel (LVcpp-s) after correction of the counts per pixel in the lung (lung cpp-s) and thorax (thorax cpp-s): LVcpp-ns = LVcpp-s -lung cpp-s/thorax cpp-s).

Statistics

Student's test and used for the analysis of paired or unpaired data and X-square test for frequency distribution analysis. Analysis of the results in the evaluable patients was according the intention to treat principle.

RESULTS

In 90 out of total number of 100 patients who entered the study, data could be analyzed. Three patients died before the echocardiography and indium imaging could be performed, 2 patients refused participation after previous informed consent and in 5 patients indium-III-platelet labelling or scintigraphy could not be performed, because of technical problems. Both the two 2DE and IND were performed 12 about 2 days (mean about SD, range 8-17 days) after onset of symptoms. Efficiency of labelling was 60 about 24% (mean about SD), which resulted in a dose of platelet bound indium-III-oxine of 213 about 84 micro Ci (mean about SD). Time between injection of the labelled platelets and imaging was 61 about 13 hours (mean about SD, range 40-76 hours).

Of the 90 evaluable patients, 45 received SFP and 45 placebo. No differences in relevant baseline characteristics were noted between SFP group (N=45). Both the SFP and placebo group were comparable with respect kto site and type of MI enzyme peak values, level of oral anticoagulation as assessed with the thrombo test and other collected clinical data. Twenty-four patients had previous MI, 19 in the SFP group and 5 in the placebo group. Left ventricular wall motion score as well as platelet labelling efficiency were similar in both groups.

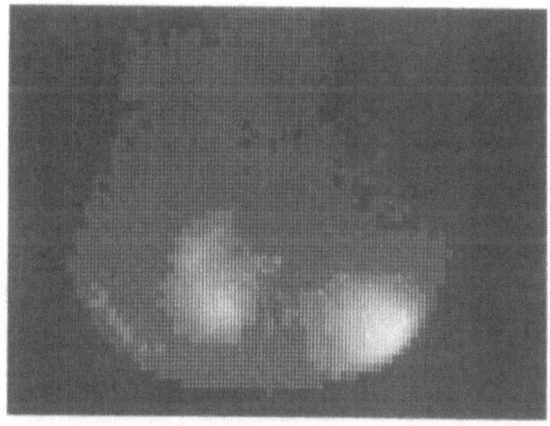

Fig 1a.
Indium-III-platelet scintigram of a patient with a large anterior infarction and "active" left ventricular thrombus.
a) Indium scan in the 45 degrees LAO position 60 hours after injection of the labelled platelet showing a hot spot.

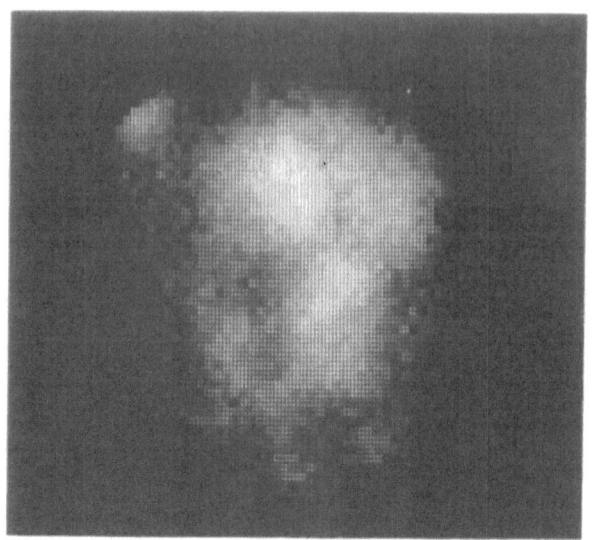

Fig 1b
Technetium-99m blood pool scan in the same 45 degrees LAO
position.

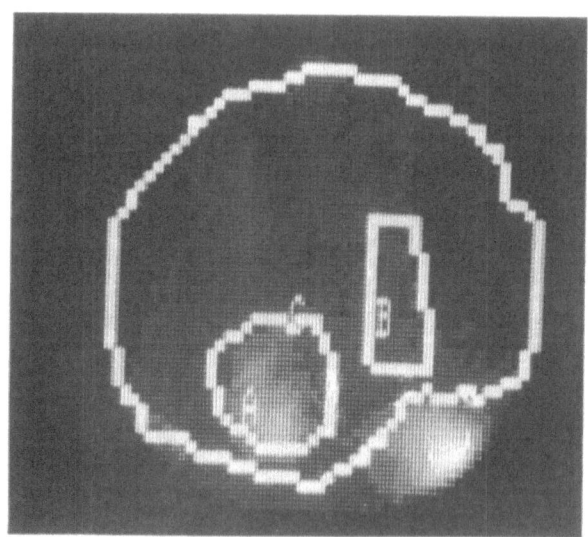

Fig.1c
Subtraction image with regions of interest of left ventricle
(A), lung (B) and thorax. In the left ventricular region the
hot spot is visible.

Effect of sulfinpyrazone on the incidence of
thrombosis. There was no difference in the incidence of LVT
between

patients receiving SFP and placebo. In 18 patients LVT was detected on 2DE and/or IND. In table 1 a comparison of 2DE and IND results and trial medication is given.

Among all patients 16 patients had a positive 2DE and all LVT were situated in the left ventricular apex. Seven patients showed a positive IND. Five patients had both positive 2DE and Ind. Eleven patients had a negative IND and positive 2DE and two patients had only positive IND. An uniform distribution of the use of SFP or placebo was noted in these findings.

SIDE EFFECTS OF SULFINPYRAZONE

A total of seven patients developed serum creatinine levels above 150 micromol/L and all these patients received SFP (p<0.02 versus placebo). A serious rise in serum creatinine level (>250 micromol/L) was only observed in 3 patients and in these patients SFP was discontinued prematurely.
Creatinine levels returned to the pre-=study level after discontinuation of SFP within three weeks in all cases.

TABLE 1.
Comparison of the two-dimensional echocardiography and Indium-III platelet scintigraphy results

---

A.   PATIENTS RECEIVING PLACEBO (n=45)

	positive indium scan	negative indium scan
positive echocardiogram	3	5
negative echocardiogram	1	36

==

PATIENTS RECEIVING SULFINPYRAZONE (N=45)

	positive indium scan	negative indium scan
positive echocardiogram	2	6
negative echocardiogram	1	36

QUANTITATIVE IND-III-PLATELET IMAGING

In figure 1 an example of positive IND is shown: a) indium scan in 45 degrees LAO position, 60 hours after injection of the labelled platelets, b) subsequent technetium-99m blood pool scan, c) subtraction image with regions of interest of left ventricle, lung (background) and thorax. Platelet deposition in the left ventricle is expressed as left ventricular counts per pixel as described in methods. There was no difference in left ventricular counts per pixel between patients using SFP or placebo (0.32 -/+ .22 vs 0.26 -/+ .22), patients with positive or negative IND (0.36 -/+ .24 vs 0.29 -/+ .21) and positive or negative 2DE (0.23 -/+ .22 vs 0.31 -/+ .21).

CLINICAL CORRELATIONS

Clinical characteristics of patients with and without LVT are given in table 2. LVT is almost exclusively observed in anterior MI with left ventricular apical akinesia or dyskinesia and poor left ventricular function. In the 24 patients with previous MI 3 had a positive IND (2 SFP, 1 placebo) and 4 had a positive 2DE (2 SFP, 2 placebo). In 18 of the 39 patients with and in one of the 51 patients without left ventricular apical akinesia or dyskinesia LVT was detected.

There were no differences in left ventricular counts per pixel and left ventricular wall motion score between patients with LVT receiving SFP or placebo. No clinical embolic events were noted during hospital admission in any patient.

DISCUSSION

Formation of LVT in the setting of acute MI is an early phenomenon (Asinger R.W. 1981 I, Spirito P., Sharma B). Most thrombi in acute MI are visualized by 2DE in the first week. So anti-thrombotic therapy to prevent LVT should be started early after onset of symptoms. In this study we assessed the effect of SFP, which has an almost immediate antithrombotic effect, with respect to the incidence of LVT in patients with an acute MI treated with early anticoagulation.

SFP did not reduce the incidence of LVT compared to placebo. There was also no difference in hematological activity of the thrombi, as assessed with IND, in patients receiving SFP or placebo. This last observation is in contrast with previous findings (Stratton J.R., 1984, Ritchie J.L.). Stratton et al. (1984) showed inhibition of platelet deposition during short term therapy with SFP 200 mg q.i.d. in 5 out 7 patients with chronic thrombi in remote MI. A presumable explanation of this contrasting finding is that the hematological activity between freshly formed (2 weeks) thrombi and chronic thrombi may differ.

Another interesting finding in our study is the

difference in the 2DE and IND results. Only five of sixteen patients with positive 2DE have a positive IND. Thus in 70% of the patients on oral anticoagulants with a "fresh" LVT, independent of the use of SFP there is no detectable platelet sequestration 12 days after MI. This discrepancy between 2DE and IND is in contradiction with other studies (Stratton J.R., 1981, Ezekowitz M.D., 1982, 1983, Verheugt F.W.A.). A very important difference between those studies and our study is the use of oral anticoagulants. In the Clinical characteristics of patients with or without left ventricular thrombosis as assessed by two-dimensional echocardiography and/or indium-III platelet scintigraphy.

	thrombus n=18	no thrombus n=72	p value
anterior MI (n=55)	94%	53%	0.03
inferior MI (n=35)	6%	47%	0.03
transmural MI (n=74)	100%	81%	ns
max LDH	663 -/+ 328	631 -/+ 352	ns
max CPK	1128 -/+ 932	1204 -/+ 896	ns
max CKMB	138 -/+ 119	143 -/+ 108	ns
LV function (echo)			
good (n=19)	0%	27%	
moderate (n=25)	6%	34%	
poor (n=46)	94%	39%	<0.0001
LV wall motion score	13 -/+ 3	3 -/+ 5	<0.001
LV apical dyskinesia	61%	11%	<0.0001
Cor-thorax ratio > 0.5	50%	22%	ns

CKMB = creatine kinase insoenzyme
CPK = creatine phosphokinase
LDH = lactate dehydrogenase
LV   = left ventricle
MI = myocardial infarction

study of Ezekowitz (1982) most patients and in the study of Verheugt all patients received heparin, but did not receive oral anticoagulants, which might explain this contrasting finding. Only in the study of Stratton (1984) IND and 2DE were compared in a serial study with respect to the hematological activity, size and resolution of chronic LVT. In this study in 3 of the 4 patients the platelet scan changed from positive to negative after using warfarin for several weeks. But as mentioned before the thrombi were much older (range 4 to 60 months) compared with our study and all patients had a positive IND before the drug intervention. Numerous studies have been published concerning 2DE and oral anticoagulation therapy in the prevention and treatment of LVT and subsequent embolization (Visser C.A., 1983, 1984, 1985, Weinreich D.J., Cokkinos D.V., Friedman M.J., Funke Kupper A.J., Stratton J.R., 1984, Keating E.C., Nordrehaug J.E., Kothari A.J., Davis M.J.E.). Unfortunately most studies deal with small numbers of patients, are retrospective, no randomized or anticoagulation was started after assessment of the diagnosis of LVT. Although there seems a beneficial trend in patients with an acute MI treated with oral anticoagulation with respect to the incidence and resolution of LVT, a definite answer cannot be given. A large prospective randomized trial in patients with MI who are at risk for LVT is warranted.

The performance of simultaneous IND and technetium-99m blood pool scintigraphy as a dual isotope subtraction method was helpful in identifying the left ventricular region. Distinction between sometimes confusing activity of spleen or liver and a "hotspot" indicating a LVT was much easier. No difference was observed between the left ventricular counts per pixel in the group receiving SFP or placebo. There was also no difference in counts per pixel between other subgroups as could be defined by site or type of MI. Diagnostic accuracy of platelet scintigraphy was not improved by the subtraction method.

In concordance with previous studies, this study indicates that patients with an acute anterior MI and severe apical-wall motion abnormalities and poor left ventricular function run a risk for developing LVT (Weinreich D.J., Keating E.C., Johanessen K.A., Visser C.A., 1984, Nordrehaug J.E.). We found detectable LVT in 46% of our patients with such an MI. All thrombi visualized by 2DE were situated in the left ventricular apical region. So stasis of blood in the apical region together with injured endocardium caused by a large transmural anterior MI are the most important pathological features for the formation of LVT suggested before (Garvin C.F., Asinger R.W., 1981).

This study represents to the best of our knowledge the first large randomized controlled trial of antiplatelet therapy in the prevention of LVT in acute MI. It is shown that despite early oral anticoagulant therapy LVT can develop in patients with acute MI and that SFP does not reduce the incidence of LVT. Furthermore, SFP has no effect on hematological activity of fresh ventricular thrombi. Further studies on the prevention of LVT should be focussed on patients with large acute anterior transmural MI with severe apical wall motion disturbances.

REFERENCES

1. Asinger R.W., Mikell F.L., Elsperger J., Hodges M. (1981) Incidence of left-ventricular thrombosis after acute myocardial infraction. Serial evaluation by two-dimensional echocardiography. N. Engl. J. Med. 305: 297-302 (I).

2. Asinger R.W., Mikell F.L., Sharma B., Hodges M. (1981) Observation on detecting left ventricular thrombus with two dimensional echocardiography: emphasis on avoidance of false positive diagnoses. Am. J. Cardiol. 47: 145-56 (II).

3. Cokkinos D.V., Ioannou N., Dellos C., Salpeas D., (1984) Failure of anticopagulant therapy to prevent left ventricular thrombus formation in acute myocardial infarction. Eur. Hear J. (Abstr. suppl. 1) 5: 203.

4. Davis M.J.E., Ireland M.A. (1986) Effect of early anticoagulation on the frequency of left ventricular thrombi after anterior wall acute myocardial infarction. Am. J. Cardiol. 57: 1244-47.

5. Eigler N., Maurer G., Shah P.K. (1984) Effect of early systemic thrombolytic therapy of left ventricular mural thrombus formation in acute anterior myocardial infarction. Am. J. Cardiol. 54: 261-63.

6. Ezekowitz M.D., Leonard J.C., Smith E.O., Allen E.W., Taylor F.B. (1981) Identification of left ventricular thrombi in man using Indium-III labelled autologous platelets. A preliminary report. Circulation 63 : 803-10.

7. Ezekowitz M.D., Wilson D.A., Smith E.O. et al. (1982) Comparison of Indium-III platelet scintigraphy and two-dimensional echocardiography in the diagnosis of left ventricular thrombi. N. Engl. J. Med. 306: 1509-13.

8. Ezekowitz M.D., Burrow R.D., Heath P.W., Streitz T., Smith E.O. Parker D.E. (1983) Diagnostic accuracy of Indium-III platelet scintigraphy in identifying left ventricular thrombi. Am. J. Cardiol. 51: 1712-16.

9. Ezekowitz M.D., Kellerman F.C.C.P., Smith E.O., Streitz T.M. (1984) Detection of active left ventricular thrombosis during acute myocardial infarction using Indium-III platelet scintigraphy. Chest 1984: 86.

10. Friedman M.J., Carlson K., Marcus P.I., Woolfenden J.M. (1982) Clinical correlations in patients with acute myocardial infarction and left ventricular thrombus detected by two-dimensional echocardiography. Am. J. Med. 72: 894-98.

11. Funke Kupper A.J., Verheugt F.W.A., Jaarsma W., van der Wall E.E., van Eenige M.J., Den Hollander W., Roos J.P. (1986) Detection of ventricular thrombosis in acute myocardial infarction; value of Indium-III platelet scintigraphy in relation to two-dimensional echocardiography and clinical course. Eur. J. Nucl. Med. 12: 337-341.

12. Garvin C.F. (1941) Mural thrombi in the heart. Am.

Heart J. 21: 713-20.
13. Gibson R.S., Bishop H.L., Stamm R.B., Crampton R.S., Beller G.A., Martin R.P. (1982) Value of early two-dimensional echocardiography in patients with acute myocardial infarction. Am. J. Cardiol. 49: 1110-19.
14. Gueret P., Ferrier A., Farcot J.D. et al. (1984) Influence of heparin on left ventricular thrombi formation during the first episode of acute transmural myocardial infarction. A prospective randomized study. JACC (abstr) 3: 600.
15. Hellerstein H.K., Martin J.W. (1947) Incidence of thromboembolic lesions accompanying myocardial infarction. Am. Heart J. 33: 443-51.
16. Johannessen K.A., Nordrehaug J.E., Lippe v.d. G. (1984) Left ventricular thrombosis and cerebrovascular accident in acute myocardial infarction. Br. Heart J. 51: 533-6.
17. Keating E.C., Gross S.A., Schlamowitz R.A. (1983) Mural thrombi in myocardial infarctions. Prospective evaluation by two-dimensional echocardiography. Am. J. Med 74: 969-95.
18. Kothari A.J. Paczkowski K., Baker K. et al. (1984) Ventricular thrombi in acute myocardial infarction: incidence complications and effects of anticoagulation. JACC (abstr) 3: 601.
19. Meltzer R.S., Visser C.A., Kan G., Roelandt J. (1984) Two-dimensional echocardiography appearance of left ventricular thrombi with systemic emboli after myocardial infarction. Am. J. Cardio. 53: 1511-13.
20. Nordrehaug J.E., Johannessen K.A., Von der Lippe G. (1985) Usefulness of high-dose anticoagulation in preventing left ventricular thrombus in acute myocardial infarction. Am. J. Cardiol. 55: 1491-93.
21. Reeder G.S., Tajik A.J., Seward J.B. (1981) Left ventricular mural thrombus. Two dimensional echocardiographic diagnosis. Mayo Clin. Proc. 56: 82-86.
22. Ritchie J.L., Stratton J.R., Thiele B. et al. (1981) Indium-III platelet imaging for detection of platelet deposition in abdominal aneurysms and prosthetic arterial grafts. Am. J. Cardiol. 47: 882-89.
23. Scholl J.M., Castillo-Fenoy A., Morice J.C. et al. (1984) Does heparin prevent left ventricular thrombus formation in acute myocardial infarction? Eur. Heart J. (abstr. suppl.) 5: 53.
24. Sharma B., Carvalho A., Wyeth R., Franciosa J.A. (1985) Left ventricular thrombi diagnosed by echocardiography in patients with acute myocardial infarction treated with intracoronary streptokinase followed by intravenous heparin. Am. J. Cardiol. 56: 422-25.
25. Spirito P., Bellotti P., Chiarella F., Domenicucci S., Sementa A., Vecchio C. (1985) Prognostic significance and natural history of left ventricular thrombi in patients with acute anterior myocardial infarction: a

two-dimensional echocardiographic study. Circulation 72: 774-80.

26. Stratton J.R., Ritchie J.L., Hamilton G.,W., Hammermeister K.E., Harker L.A. (1981) Left ventricular thrombi: in vivo detection by Indium-III platelet imaging and two-dimensional echocardiography. Am. J. Cardiol. 47: 874-81.

27. Stratton J.R., Ritchie J.L. (1984) The effects of antithrombotic drugs in patients with left ventricular thrombi: assessment with Indium-III platelet imaging and two-dimensional echocardiography. Circulation 69: 561-68.

28. Thakur M.L., Welch M.J., Joist J.H., Coleman R.E. (1976) Indium-III labelled platelets: Studies on preparation and evaluation of vitro and in vitro functions. Thrombosis Research 9: 345-57.

29. Verheugt F.W., Lindenfeld J., Kirch D.L., Steele P.P. (1984) Left ventricular platelet deposition after acute myocardial infarction: an attempt at quantification using blood pool subtracted Indium-III platelet scintigraphy. Br. Heart J. 52: 490-6.

30. Visser C.A., Kan G., David G.K., Lie K.I., Durrer D. (1983) Two-dimensional echocardiography in the diagnosis of left ventricular thrombus. A prospective study of 67 patients with anatomic validation. Chest 83: 228-32.

31. Visser C.A., Kan G., Meltzer R. (1984) Long-term follow-up of left ventricular thrombus after acute myocardial infarction. A two-dimensional echocardiographic study in 96 patients. Chest 86: 532-36.

32. Visser C.A., Kan G., Melzer R.S., Dunning A.J., Roelandt J. (1985) Embolic potential of left ventricular thrombus after myocardial infarction: a two-dimensional echocardiographic study of 119 patients. JACC 5: 1276-80.

33. Weinreich D.J., Burke J.F., Pauletto F.J. (1984) Left ventricular mural thrombi complicating acute myocardial infarction, long-term follow-up with serial echocardiography. Annals of intern Med. 100: 789-94.

CARDIAC INDIUM-III PLATELET SCINTIGRAPHY IN STROKE PATIENTS

Rosch M., Bihl H., Reuther R.

Departments of Neurology and Nuclear Medicine, University of Heidelberg.

Henningsen H.

Department of Neurology, Mannheim-Hospital.

Kessler Ch.

Department of Neurology, Medical University of Lubeck.

INTRODUCTION

The incidence of cardiac embolic events in stroke patients has often been underestimated. Recent research has shown that it ranges from 15% to 35% (1, 11, 14, 17). In most cases, the diagnosis of cardiac embolism can be established by using clinical criteria along - for example, the presence of atrial fibrillation, valvular disease, cardiomyopathy or rheumatic heart disease (3, 6, 8). A direct positive detection of intracardiac thrombi is, however, not to be expected often, even when using two-dimensional echocardiography (2, 7, 10, 13). The diagnostic techniques mentioned above including chest-ray, ECG and echocardiography provide the means of splitting the patient population into groups with a high risk of cardiac embolism, with a low risk of cardiac embolism and with heart diseases without an enhanced risk or cardiac embolism.

Heart diseases with a high risk or cardiac embolism include absolute arrhythmia, mitral valve diseases, anterior wall infarction and lateral wall infarction, aneurysms, endocarditis with vegetations on the valves, cardiomyopathy and myxoma.

Heart diseases with a lower risk or cardiac embolism comprise aortic valve diseases, coronary heart disease, mitral valve prolapse and mitral annulus calcification (4, 12, 15, see table 1).

Recent research was therefore aimed to establish a technique that would allow identification of the source of embolism directly. The scintigraphy with indium-III oxine labelled platelets has proven to be a useful in vivo method for thrombus detection. Clinical studies demonstrated the

128

Ch. Kessler et al. (eds.), Clinical Application of Radiolabelled Platelets, 128–136.
© 1990 Kluwer Academic Publishers.

high sensitivity of 65% and specifity of 99% for platelet scintigraphy in the evaluation of cardiac thrombi in patients with heart disease (5, 9, 16, 18).

In this study, the considerable diagnostic efficiency of indium-III platelet scintigraphy for the detection of intracardiac thrombi in stroke patients with a clinical risk of cerebral embolism was proved in 39 patients.

Table 1

CARDIAC DISEASES WITH A LOW RISK OF CARDIAC EMBOLISM	CARDIAC DISEASES WITH A HIGH RISK OF CARDIAC EMBOLISM
1. AORTIC VALVE DISEASE	1. ATRIAL FIBRILLATION
2. CORONARY HEART DISEASE	2. MITRAL VALVE DISEASE
3. MITRAL VALVE PROLAPSE	3. MYOCARDIAL INFARCTION OF THE ANTERIOR OR LATERAL WALL
4. MITRAL ANNULUS CALCIFICATION	4. ANEURYSMA
	5. ENDOCARDITIS WITH VEGETATIONS
(EASTON JD ET AL. 1980, NISHIDE M ET AL. 1983, ROBBINS JA ET AL. 1983)	6. CARDIOMYOPATHY
	7. MYXOMA

PATIENTS

The patient population, 31 male and 8 female, was constituted by 19 patients with transient ischemic attacks and by 20 patients with completed stroke. The mean age was 57.2 about 11.0 years. The scintigrams were performed within 2 to 180 days after the stroke with a mean value of 23.2 days.

15 patients were suspected to have a high risk of cardiac embolism due to an underlying heart disease, 5 patients to have a lower risk of cardiac embolism and 19 patients were expected to have no enhanced risk of cardiac embolism.

PSC was performed when clinical symptomatology or computer tomography ruled out intracerebral hemorrhage and when angiographic findings did not reveal any evidence of arteriosclerosis or if a high risk of cardiac embolism was suspected due to an underlying heart disease.

METHODS

PLATELET LABELLING

The autologous platelets were labelled with indium-III oxine in ACD normal saline solution according to a modification of the method described by Thakdur et al.: 50 ml of venous blood was anticoagulated with an acid citrate dextrose (ACD-formula A) solution (1:7). A compact platelet pellet was obtained by two differential centrifugation steps (180 g for 15 min, 700 g for 7 min), washed once in an ACD-A normal saline buffer solution a pH 6.5 and incubated for 20 min at room temperature with 17.5 - 27.8 MBq (0.5 - 0.75 mCi) of a commercially available indium-III oxine solution. The labelled platelets were washed a second time with the buffer solution and injected intravenously after resuspension in patient plasma. The average labelling efficiency reached 64.4 -/+ 19.8%. The patients were injected with the mean activity of 15.7 -/+ 3.33 MBq (0.41-/+ 0.09 mCi).

IMAGE PROCESSING

Scintigraphic images were obtained with a conventional gamma camera using a medium-energy parallel-hole collimator. The images of the heart were obtained in the anterior-posterior and the 45° left anterior projection 1, 24, 48 and 72 h after injection of the autologous labelled platelets. The images were obtained for a total of 100,000 counts each.

HEART EXAMINATION

M-mode echocardiograms were performed in 37 patients and completed in 8 patients by two-dimensional echocardiography. Eight patients (21.7%) had technically poor echocardiograms that provided limited diagnostic information. Electrocardiography was performed in all 39 patients. The corresponding data were completed by continuous electrocardiographic monitoring in 11 patients.

RESULTS

PSC findings were positive in 15 patients and negative in 24. Platelet accumulations in the left atrium were diagnosed in 3 patients, in the left ventricle in 7 patients and in the region of the valves in 8 patients. In 3 patients, the PSC findings provided evidence of 2 accumulations each.

Concerning the labelling efficiency, the recovery value and the injected activity, there were no significant differences between the two groups with positive and with negative PSC. The corresponding mean values with standard deviation in patients with positive PSC were 64.0 -/+ 15.0%,

56.3 -/+ 24.3% and 15.91 -/+ 2.96 MBq, in patients with negative PSC 64.7 -/+ 13.8%, 55.8 -/+ 16.3% and 13.43 -/+ 3.7 MBq (0.39 -/+ 0.1 mCi).

The accumulations could be identified best in the anterior-posterior projection in 4 patients and in the 45° left anterior position in 11 patients.

Positive diagnostic information was obtained on the third day after injection of the labelled platelets in 10 cases and after 4 days (k72h) in 5 cases.

Out of the 39 patients, 11 patients were submitted to PSC within one week after the last clinical neurological event. Positive scintigraphic findings could be observed in 3 cases. In the second week after the last neurological attack, 5 out of 10 patients had a positive PSC, in the third week 4 out of 9 and in the fourth week 1 out of 2. In seven patients, PSC was started more than 4 weeks after their last neurological attack. Within this group, positive findings were obtained in two cases. The largest interval for a positive scintigram was 60 days (see Fig. 1).

There were no differences due to the recurring or non-recurring character of the neurological event. Out of the group of 24 patients with negative PSC, 9 patients had no previous attack, 7 patients had a single attack and 8 patients had several attacks in their history. From the 15 patients with positive PSC, 6 patients had no previous neurological attack in their history, 5 patients had 1 and 4 patients had several attacks (see Fig. 2).

Based on the classification of table 1 15 patients were suspected to have a high risk of cardiac embolism (see Fig. 3 and 4). Ten out of them (66.7%) had a positive and 5 of them had a negative PSC. In the group of 5 patients with atrial fibrillation, there were 3 with a positive and 2 with a negative scintigram. The patient with mitral valve disease and atrial fibrillation showed a positive PSC. The patient with mitral valve insufficiency had a negative PSC. In both patients with endocarditis, the PSC was positive.

Out of the 3 patients with cardiomyopathy, 2 had a positive and 1 had a negative PSC. One patient with an aneurysm in the left ventricle had a positive PSC, whereas it was negative in a second one. The PSC of the patient with an akinetic apex was positive.

The group with lower risks of cardiac embolism due to the underlying heart disease comprised 5 patients. For one of them, we obtained a positive PSC, while PSC findings were negative in 4 cases. Out of the two patients with coronary heart disease one had a positive PSC. The two patients with aortic valve disease and the patient with an enlargement of the left atrium had a negative PSC. Based on cardiological examination, 19 patients were expected to have no enhanced risk of cardiac embolism. 4 of them had a positive and 15 (79%) had a negative scintigram (see Fig. 5).

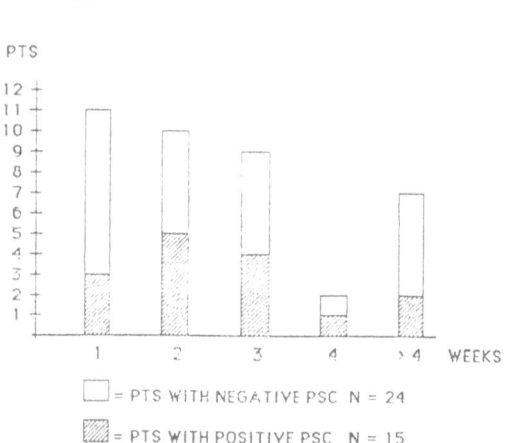

□ = PTS WITH NEGATIVE PSC N = 24

▨ = PTS WITH POSITIVE PSC N = 15

Fig.1   Interval between last neurological attack and
         beginning of PSC

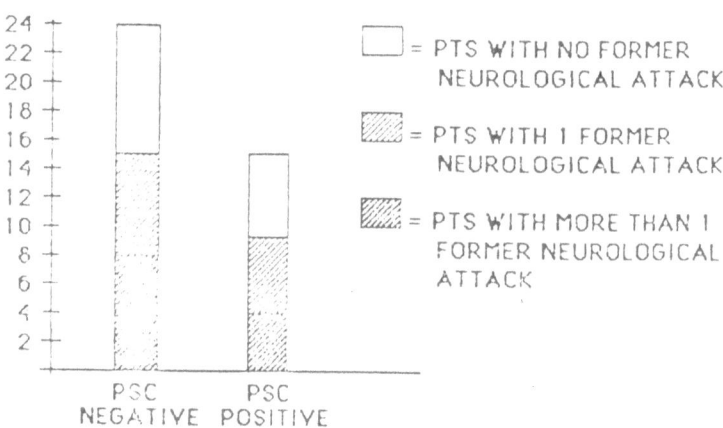

□ = PTS WITH NO FORMER
     NEUROLOGICAL ATTACK

▨ = PTS WITH 1 FORMER
     NEUROLOGICAL ATTACK

▨ = PTS WITH MORE THAN 1
     FORMER NEUROLOGICAL
     ATTACK

Fig.2   Incidence of neurological attacks in the history of
         39 Patients

CARDIAC EMBOLISM	TOTAL NO	PSC POSITIVE	PSC NEGATIVE
HIGH RISK	15	10	5
LOW RISK	5	1	4
NEGATIVE	19	4	15
	39	15	24

Fig.3 Platelet scintigraphy [PSC] with 111-Indium oxine in 39 stroke Patients

HEART DISEASE	TOTAL	PSC POS	PSC NEG
ATRIAL FIBRILLATION	5	3	2
MITRAL VALVE DISEASE WITH ATRIAL FIBRILLATION	1	1	-
MITRAL VALVE INSUFFICIENCY	1	-	1
ENDOCARDITIS	2	2	-
CARDIOMYOPATHY	3	2	1
ANEURYSMA	2	1	1
MYOCARDIAL INFARCTION	1	1	-
	15	10	5

Fig.4 PSC findings in Patients with a high risk of cardiac embolism

PSC FINDINGS IN PATIENTS WITH A LOW RISK
OF CARDIAC EMBOLISM OR WITH A NEGATIVE
HEART INVESTIGATION

HEART DISEASE	TOTAL	PSC POS	PSC NEG
AORTIC VALVE DISEASE	2	-	2
CORONARY HEART DISEASE	2	1	1
LEFT ATRIAL ENLARGEMENT	1	-	1
	5	1	4
NEGATIVE	19	4	15
	24	5	19

Fig 5

Echocardiography showed a thrombus in 5 cases. 4 of these thrombi could also be identified by PSC, i.e. in the two patients with florid endocarditis, in the patient with an aneurysm and in the patient with an akinetic apex after myocardial infarction. The existence of a suspected thrombotic accumulation on the aortic valve in one patient suffering from aortic valve disease could not be confirmed by PSC.

Two patients underwent cardiac surgery, one 6 days and the other 8 days after PSC. The PSC findings were positive in both patients. One had and accumulation in the region of the valves and the other in the left ventricle. In the patient with florid endocarditis, the aortic valve was replaced prothetically after a third-degree atrioventricular block.

Cardiac surgery revealed a perforation of the sinus valsalvae and two minor aneurysms at the basis of the coronary valves with fresh vegetations.

The second patient had a resection of an aneurysm with a reddish, soft thrombotic tumour without any organization. This patient had a myocardial infarction three years before, and 2 months before PSC investigation, he had suffered a completed stroke.

DISCUSSION

Scintigraphic imaging with indium-III oxine labelled autologous platelets has proved to be a valuable technique for detecting intracardiac thrombi in stroke patients. PSC findings were positive in 15 out of 39 patients (38.5%). Positive scintigrams correlate with the occurrence of heart diseases with a high risk of cardiac embolism. In 10 out of 15 (66.7%) patients with a high risk of cardiac embolism, the PSC was positive. In 19 out 24 patients (79.2%) with low risk or with no enhanced risk of cardiac embolism due to the underlying heart disease, the PSC was negative.

What seems to be remarkable is the fact that the PSC was positive in 4 out of 19 cases, where echocardiographic and electrocardiographic findings were negative. It should, however, be borne in mind that these patients were examined at a time, when two dimensional echocardiography and continuous electrocardiographic monitoring were not yet a routine practice.

With this restriction, we can say that the scintigraphic detection of intracardiac thrombi was successful in two patients, where cardiological investigation, including two-dimensional echocardiography, had not revealed any pathological findings. Taking into account the high specify of 99%, it must be concluded that an active thrombotic process was developing in these two patients, which would not have been detected by other diagnostic techniques.

To evaluate the clinical importance of a positive PSC finding, further studies are necessary. In our patients, there were no differences due to the recurring or non-recurring character of the neurological event.

REFERENCES

1. Caplan L.R., Hier D.B., D'Cruz J.D. (1983) Cerebral embolism in the Michael Reese Stroke Registry. Stroke 14 : 530-536.
2. Donaldson R.M., Emanuel R.W., Earl C.J. (1981) The role of two-dimensional echocardiography in the detection of potentially embolic intracardiac masses in patients with cerebral ischemia. J. Neurol. Neurosurg. and Psych. 44 : 803-809.
3. Dorndorf W. Schlagafalle-Klinik und Therapie, pp. 271-273, 2nd edition, Thieme, Stuttgart, New York.
4. Easton J.D., Sherman D. (1980) Management of cerebral embolism of cardiac origin. Stroke 11 : 433-440.
5. Ezekowitz M.D., Burrow R.D., Heath P.W., Streitz T., Smith O.E. (1983) Diagnostic accuracy of Indium-III platelet scintigraphy in identifying left ventricular thrombi. Am. J. Cardiol. 51 : 1712-1716.
7. Gagliardi R., Benvenuti L., Rosini F., Ammanati F. Barletta G.A., Fantini F. (1985) Frequency of echocardiographic abnormalities in patients with ischemia of the carotid territory - a preliminary report. Stroke 16 : 118-120.
8. Gautier J.C., Morelot D. (1977) Cardiac embolism and arterial hypertension as risk factors of cerebral

infarction; in Zulch K.J., Haufmann W., Hossmann K.A., Hossmann V. (eds.): Brain and Heart Infarct - Springer Berlin, Heidelberg New York, pp. 201-205.

9. Kessler Ch., Henningsen H., Reuther R., Kimmig B., Rosch M (1987) Identification of Intracardiac thrombi in stroke patients with indium-III platelet scintigraphy. Stroke 18: 63-67.

10. Lovett J.L., Sandok B.A., Guliana E.R., Nasser F.N. (1981) Two-dimensional echocardiography in patients with focal cerebral ischaemia. Ann. Intern Med. 95: 1-4.

11. Mohr J.P., Caplan L.R., Melske J.W., Goldstein R.J., Duncan G.W., Kistler J.P., Pessin M.S., Bleid H.L. (1978) The Harvard Cooperative Stroke Registry: a prospective registry. Neurology 28: 754-763.

12. Nishide M., Irino T., Gotch M., Naka M., Tsuji K. (1983) Cardiac abnormalities in ischemic cerebrovascular disease studied by two-dimensional echocardiography. Stroke 14: 541-545.

13. Rem J.A., Hachinski V.C., Boughner D.R., Barnett H.J.M. (1985) Value of cardiac monitoring and echocardiography in TIA and Stroke patients. Stroke 16: 950-956.

14. Ringelstein E.B., Zenner H., Schneider R (1985) Der Beitrag der zerebralen Computertomographie zur Differentialtypologie und Differentialtherapy des ischamischen Groszhirninfarktes. Fortsch. Neurol. Psychiatr. 53: 325-336.

15. Robbins J.A., Sagar K.B., French M., Smith P.H.J. (1983) Influence of echocardiography on management of patients with systemic emboli. Stroke 14: 546-549.

16. Stratton J.R., Ritchie K.L., Hamilton G.W., Hammermeister K.E., Harker L.A. (1981) Left ventricular thrombi: in vivo detection by Indium-III platelet imaging and two-dimensional echocardiography. Am. J. Cardiol. 47: 874-880.

17. Wolf P.A., Dawber T.R., Thomas H.E., Kannes W.B. (1978) Epidemiologic assessment of chronic atrial fibrillation and risk of stroke: The Framingham-Study. Neurology 28: 973-977.

18. Yamada M., Hoki N., Ishikawa K., Yoshima H. (198) Detection of left atrial thrombi in man using indium-III-labelled autologous platelets. Br. Heart J. 51: 298-305.

MONITORING OF ANTITHROMBOTIC THERAPY WITH RADIOLABELLED PLATELETS

H. Sinzinger, P. Fitscha

Atherosclerosis Research Group (ASF) Vienna, Atherosclerosis and Thrombosis Research Group (ATK) of the Austrian Academy of Sciences, Vienna and 2nd Department of Internal Medicine, Policlinic Vienna, Austria.

INTRODUCTION

In the mid of the last century (1852) the head of the Department of Pathology at the Vienna University Medical School, Carl von Rokitansky (49) was the first to claim that material from the blood stream is incorporated ("incrustation theory") into the arterial wall. Bizzozero quite soon thereafter stressed the important role of platelets (3) in atherogenesis. The importance of parietal thrombus formation has been underlined again by J.B.Duguid (11) and got even more importance after the discovery of prostacyclin (prostaglandin (PG) 12) by Sir John Vane, Moncada and other (36). They claimed an important role in hemostasis via an action of platelet-cAMP (4) and a decreased in-vitro PG12-formation by the arterial wall in atherosclerosis (50).

Exactly at the same time, Mathew L. Thakur (73) reported on a new platelet label, III-Indium-oxine, allowing not only calculation of platelet survival, but also camera imaging of pathological platelet accumulation in parallel. Quite soon thereafter, this new technique was proven to be a very useful tool for the study of experimental lesions and the monitoring of drug effects in experimental animals (Table 1). Although the next step further has been done in methodology in the meanwhile by the use of various monoclonal antibodies, only a few groups proceeded to the routine application in humans (Table 2) in certain conditions, such as endarteriectomy, percutaneous transluminal angioplasty (PTCA) and after bypass grafting. Finally, the clinical use for the evaluation of drug efficacy and monitoring in humans has been only approached by a few groups so far (Table s 2, 3).

The approach we used was the identification of so-called active atherosclerotic lesions sites (51, 52) being characterized by an enhanced platelet trapping over certain vascular areas (53). Morphological control of a few of these areas revealed either parietal thrombosis (24, 41) or exulcerated atherosclerotic lesions (61), whereas advanced lesions were inactive in so far as the platelet uptake is

137

Ch. Kessler et al. (eds.), Clinical Application of Radiolabelled Platelets, 137–161.
© 1990 *Kluwer Academic Publishers.*

table 1:
Imaging of spontaneous and experimental atherosclerosis after
platelet labelling

species	vessel	cond.	tracer	author	year	ref.
dog	carotid	E	oxine	THAKUR	1976	(74)
human	carotid	S	oxine	DAVIS	1980	(6,8)
dog	coronary	E	oxine	BERGMANN	1982	(2)
rabbit	aorta	E	oxine	FINKELSTEIN	1982	(12)
human	carotid	S	oxine	GOLDMAN	1982	(18)
human	aneurysm	S	oxine	HEYNS	1982	(25)
human	carotid	S	oxine	KESSLER	1982	(28)
dog	endarteriect.	E	oxine	LUSBY	1983	(35)
human	carotid	S	oxine	POWERS	1982	(39)
macaques	carotid	E	oxine	POWERS	1982	(40)
human	carotid	S	oxine	ISAKA	1984	(27)
human	carotid	S	oxine	KIMURA	1984	(31)

E... experimental; S...spontaneous

table 2:
Monitoring of antiplatelet therapy in experimental animals.

species	vessel	tracer	drug	author	year	ref.
dog	aorto-cor. bypass	tropolone	ASA/DIP	FUSTER	1979	(17)
dog	coronary	oxine	strepto-kinase	BERGMANN	1982	(1)
baboon	PTFE	oxine	PGI2	CALLOW	1982	(5)
rabbit	carotid	oxine	dazoxiben ASA	RANDALL	1982	(46)
dog	PTFE	tropolone	ibuprofen	LOVAAS	1983	(34)
dog	aorto-cor. bypass	tropolone	ASA/DIP	DEWANJEE	1984	(9,10)
rabbit	aorta	oxine	13-azapro-stan. acid	LE BRETON	1984	(33)

vessel	lesion	tracer	drug	author	year	ref.
graft/ aneurysm	-	oxine	ASA,DIP, SP	HUANG	1981	(26)
aorto- femoral	Dacron	oxine	ASA/DIP	PUMPHREY	1982	(44)
shunt	-	oxine	SP	RITCHIE	1982	(48)
graft	Dacron	oxine	SP	STRATTON	1982	(65)
left vetricle	thrombus	oxine	SP	STRATTON	1982	(66)
graft	Dacron	oxine	ticlopidine	STRATTON	1984	(69)
femoral	lesion	oxine	PGI2	SINZINGER	1984	(57)
femoral	lesion	oxine	opt. PGI2- regimen	FITSCHA	1985	(15)
carotid	ascl	oxine	ASA	KESSLER	1985	(30)
femoral	lesion	oxine	iloprost	FITSCHA	1986	(16)
femoral	lesion	oxine	PGE1	SINZINGER	1987	(62)
femoral	lesion	oxine	ASA	SINZINGER	1987	(64)

ascl....atherosclerotic; SP....sulphinpyrazone;
DIP....dipyridamole

table 3:
Monitoring of antiplatelet agents in human.

concerned. Demonstrating that the platelet uptake remains rather constant for weeks, we tried to interfere with various antiplatelet agents and different methodology in order to achieve optimal follow-up data from patients suffering from latent or clinically manifest atherosclerosis.

MATERIAL AND METHODS

In patients suffering from clinically manifest atherosclerosis (peripheral vascular disease [PVD], cerebrovascular disease [CVD]) platelet half-life (T/2) calculation after labelling by means of III-In-oxine sulphate is a routine diagnostic procedure. Platelet preparation is done using the labelling kit (56, 58) developed by us (Fig 1). Briefly, blood is drawn from a non-occluded cubital vein using 2 Monovette-vials and acid citrate dextrose (ACD) as anticoagulant. After the addition of PG12 blood is allowed to sediment at room temperature. After preparation of a platelet rich plasma (PRP) and a pellet, the later is dissolved in 500-1000 μl tyrode-buffer (pH 6,2). Labelling is performed at 37°C for 5 minutes using 100 μCi (100 μl) of tracer (III-In-oxine sulphate). Immediately thereafter, the radiolabelled cells resuspended in autologous platelet poor plasma (PPP) are reinjected. Aliquots are removed for determination of labelling efficiency. Bloods is drawn into EDTA-coated vials for calculation of recovery (REC) and determination of platelet half life (T/2).

Gamma-camera imaging is routinely done using a 4-minutes exposure each. Repeated images daily have been done during therapy. For that purpose a portable infusion pump system is used allowing repeated imaging and free movement of the patients. For quantification, regions of interest (ROI) have been inserted and compared with areas of identical size over the contralateral side after background subtraction. The platelet uptake ratio (PUR) serves as measure for platelet trapping. MASK-programs described earlier have been used for improved imaging, being of help especially in the carotid artery region (60, 61).

Engymetric monitoring: In some patients to allow continuous monitoring of platelet trapping a portable detector system (NOVO, Danmark) is used (Fig 2)). The detectors are placed over the lesion sites (Fig 3) for the follow-up period to be programmed in advance. Thereafter, data analysis is performed (Fig 4) as described below.

General description: NOVO is an acquisition and analysis program (Fig 5) for a portable detector system. The backbone of analysis is the CURVE program allowing a curve manipulation program at low costs. Beside that, only the development of an acquisition program and storage in BGAMMA-like safe areas is necessary. For the final analysis the CURVE package includes a wide range of curve manipulation commands. Our package includes a PASCAL program

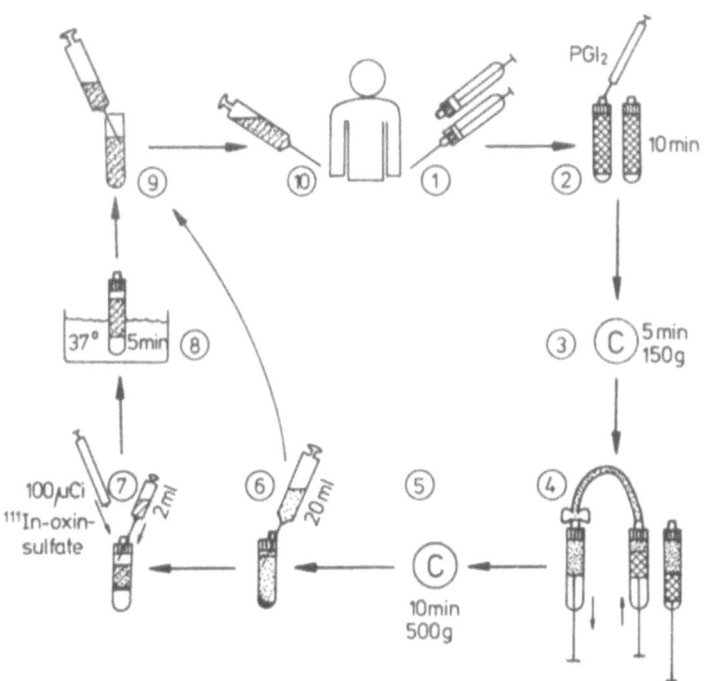

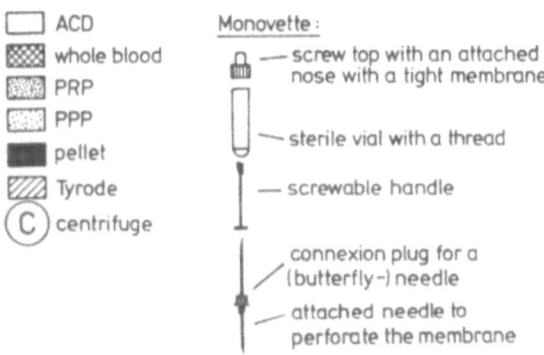

ACD
whole blood
PRP
PPP
pellet
Tyrode
(C) centrifuge

Monovette:

— screw top with an attached
  nose with a tight membrane

— sterile vial with a thread

— screwable handle

— connexion plug for a
  (butterfly-) needle

— attached needle to
  perforate the membrane

Fig 1:
Schematic presentation of the various steps of the labelling
method (56) developed and routinely used by us

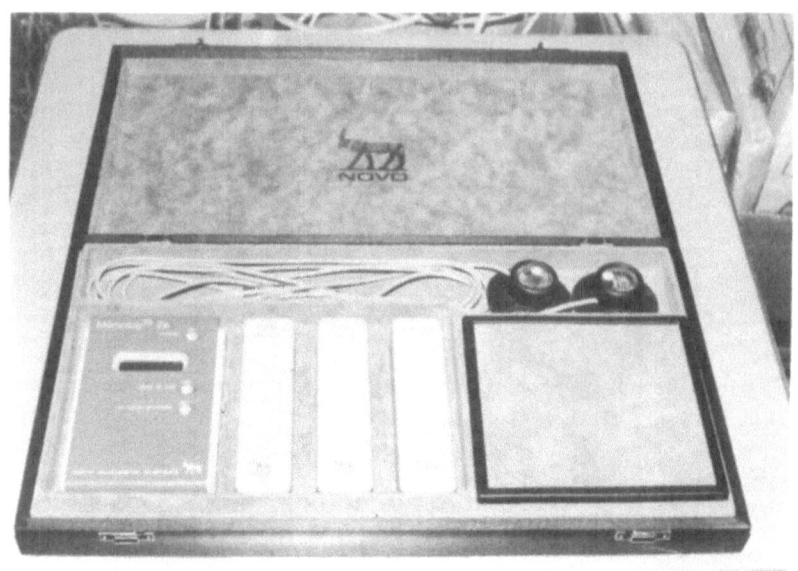

Fig 2:
Portable detector system (Novo-Memolog)

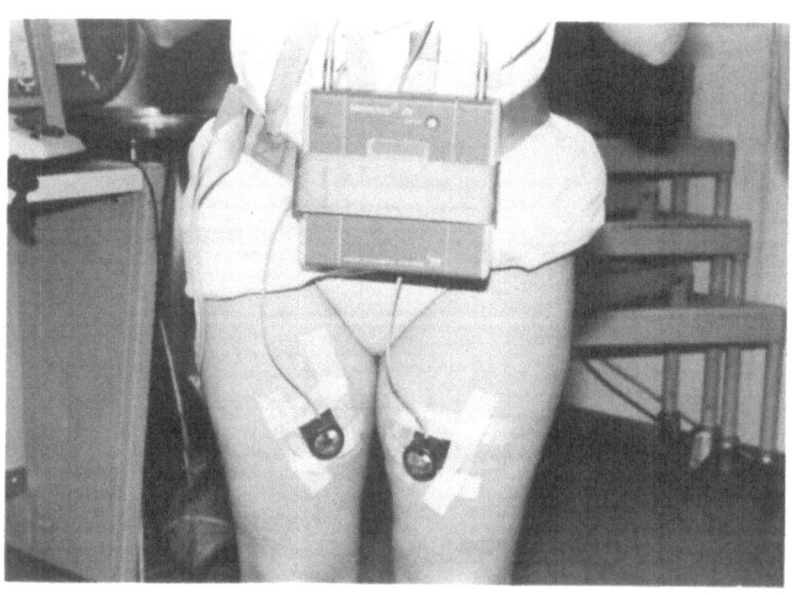

Fig 3:
Placement of detectors over femoral artery lesion site and
contralateral reference area

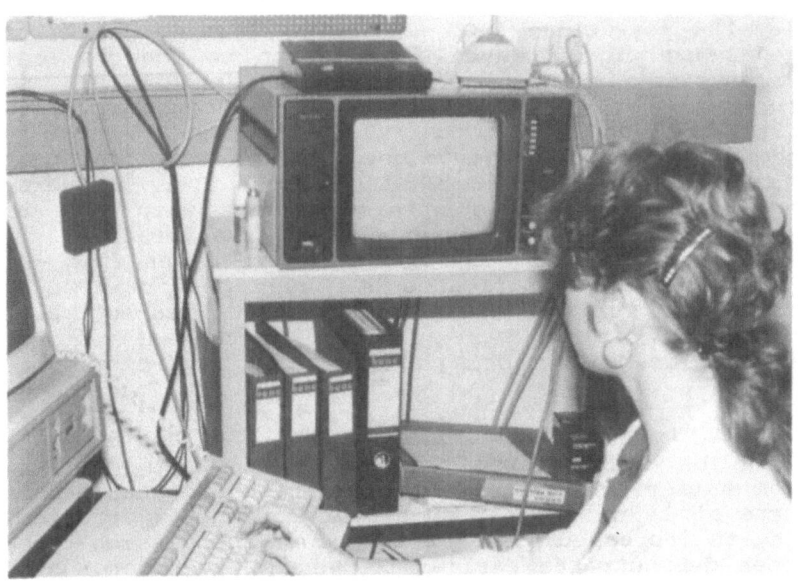

Fig 4:
Data analysis showing a 24-hours follow-up on the monitor

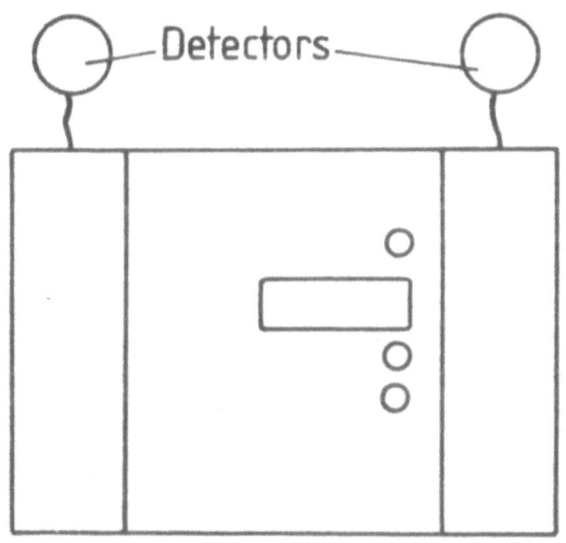

Fig. 5:
Scheme of hardware acquisition

to display the physical T/2 as a straight line (Fig 6). The
registered curve is displayed in relation to the physical
T/2. Our system is connected with the KERMIT to our
department computer (μ VAX II). So we are performing our
backup via KERMIT on TK 50 tapes (95 M Byte/tape). PASCAL is
the standard program language we use. The time critical part
of acquisition is written in MACRO, because it is not easy
to store an uninterruptable stream of data with 4800 Bd
under RT 11 over serial line on computer mass storage.
    Statistical analysis: All the data are given as x -/+
SD; calculation for significance has been performed using
Student's t-test for paired or unpaired data respectively.
The calculation of PUR was performed using analysis of
variance, Kapplan-Meier testing and WILCOXON rank-testing.

RESULTS

    It can be demonstrated that 5-10% of total patients
population suffering from clinical manifest atherosclerosis
demonstrate at least one hot spot over peripheral arteries,
reflecting an increased platelet trapping. Such lesion types
having been demonstrated earlier to persist even for months
have been used to assess the effect of various drugs and the
optimal therapeutic schedule.

1.   Optimal PGI2-infusion time as judged by influence on
      platelet deposition and platelet-T/2

a)   Patients and Methods
      18 patients suffering from PVD stage II according to
      Fontaine (26 males, 12 females) aged 47 - 71a) showing
      platelet deposition to active lesions with PUR-values
      higher than 1,30 received PGI2 i.v. at a rate of 5
      ng/kg/min. Infusion times lasted from 1 to 10 hours
      daily on 5 consecutive days (Table 4).

TABLE 4

PUR and T/2 during PGI2-infusion of different duration.

h	PUR before	PUR after	T/2 before	T/2 after	n
1	1,36 ± 0,09	1,26 ± 0,08*	72 ± 5	74 ± 5	6
2	1,37 ± 0,10	1,26 ± 0,07*	74 ± 4	75 ± 6	6
4	1,35 ± 0,09	1,20 ± 0,03*	73 ± 6	79 ± 4	6
6	1,40 ± 0,11	1,16 ± 0,05*	70 ± 6	82 ± 5*	4
8	1,38 ± 0,12	1,17 ± 0,08*	73 ± 7	81 ± 5*	10
10	1,37 ± 0,08	1,17 ± 0,04*	74 ± 5	82 ± 6*	6

x ± SD; * p < 0,01

b)   Results

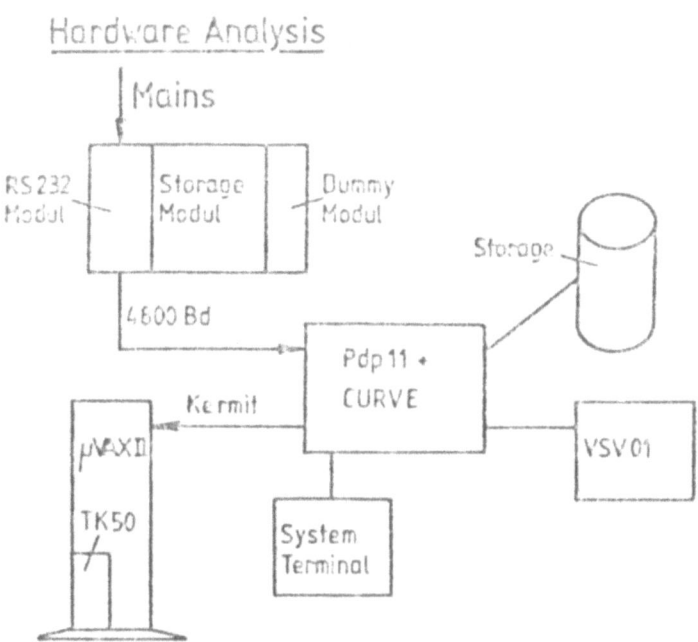

Fig. 6:
Hardware analysis

Details to software description

1. Acquisition:
The acquisition is done by an interrupt service MACRO-routine.
This stores all the data to a virtual device (VM: under RT 11).
After acquisition data are transferred into BGAMMA dynamic curves
format; the curves are stored an Mass-storage medium.

2. Transfer data from Mass-storage studies to the study currently
under evaluation.

3. Call the CURVE program (S. Forster).
With this part of the program the user is able to manipulate the
curve data. A help utility at curve level is to display the
physical T/2 in relation to biological T/2.

PG12 treatment resulted in a decrease of PUR (Table 4), the effect being not significant for infusion periods from 1 to 4 hours daily. However, infusion times of 6 to 10 hours provoked a significant decrease in platelet deposition to the active lesions as well as a significant prolongation of platelet T/2. The spleen-liver ratio was unchanged (Table 5).

TABLE 5

Spleen-liver-ratio during PGI2-infusion of different duration.

spleen-liver-ratio

h	before	after	n	o/o
1	1,03 ± 0,24	0,98 ± 0,24	6	4/2
2	1,08 ± 0,16	0,91 ± 0,35	6	4/2
4	1,09 ± 0,34	1,08 ± 0,25	6	5/1
6	0,97 ± 0,41	1,04 ± 0,42	4	3/1
8	1,11 ± 0,29	1,12 ± 0,26	10	7/3
10	1,15 ± 0,36	1,09 ± 0,33	6	4/2

x ± SD

2. Influence of different PG12-doses on platelet deposition and platelet T/2.

a. Patients and Methods
24 patients suffering from PVD stage II according to Fontaine since 2 - 11 years (19 males, 5 females; aged 52 -71a) showing active atherosclerotic lesions with a PUR higher than 1,30 were treated with 3 different doses of PG12. Group 1 (n = 7) received ng PG12/kg/min, group 2 (n = 8) 3 ng/kg/min and group 3 (n = 9) 5 ng/kg/min during 6 hours a day on 5 consecutive days.

b) Results
PG12 caused an immediate drop (Table 6) in the amount of platelets trapped over the active vascular lesions. However, the decrease and the time-course of the 3 different doses (1, 3 and 5 ng/kg/min) was similar. Moreover, a comparable prolongation in platelet T/2 (Table 6) could be detected. 1 month after therapy PUR-values were still diminished and T/2 prolonged exhibiting no differences between the doses examined. Again, no influence on the spleen-liver uptake has been seen (Table 7).

Table 6

Patients data, PUR and platelet half-life (before and after therapy).

PGI2 ng/kg/min	P U R before	after	T/2 before	after	n	♂/♀
5	1,36 ± 0,07	1,21 ± 0,06*	73 ± 6	82 ± 5*	9	7/2
3	1,38 ± 0,07	1,23 ± 0,06*	70 ± 5	81 ± 7*	8	6/2
1	1,35 ± 0,09	1,22 ± 0,07*	74 ± 7	83 ± 8*	7	6/1

x̄ ± SD; * p < 0,01

Table 7

Patients data and spleen-liver-ratio (before and after therapy)

PGI2 ng/kg/min h	spleen-liver-ratio before	after	n	♂/♀
5	0,89 ± 0,27	0,96 ± 0,32	9	7/2
3	0,96 ± 0,41	0,88 ± 0,25	8	6/2
1	0,92 ± 0,33	0,97 ± 0,40	7	6/1

x ± SD

3. Influence of PGE1 on platelet deposition and platelet T/2.

a) Patients and Methods
40 patients with PVD stage II according to Fontaine (27 males, 13 females; aged 46 - 75a) with PUR values as of more than 1, 30 were randomly allocated to receive either an i.v. infusion of PGE1 at a rate of 25 ng/kg/min or placebo during 6 hours on 5 consecutive days. After a 3 week interval the infusions were repeated. That second drug phase required the patients to receive either PGE1 or placebo (see Table 8).

Table 8

Table 8

PUR and platelet T/2 before and after PGE1- or placebo therapy, respectively.

therapy	P U R		T/2		n	♂/♀
	before	after	before	after		
placebo	1,34±0,04	1,35±0,04	75±7	74±6	8	6/2
PGE1	1,34±0,04	1,28±0,04*	76±7	81±5*	8	5/3
placebo after PGE1	1,27±0,03	1,27±0,04	79±6	80±7	6	4/2
PGE1 again	1,28±0,05	1,25±0,04	80±6	82±5	6	4/2
PGE1 after placebo	1,36±0,05	1,28±0,05*	73±8	79±5*	6	4/2
placebo again	1,34±0,06	1,35±0,07	76±5	74±7	6	4/2

$\bar{x} \pm SD$; * $p < 0,01$

Table 9

Spleen-liver ratio before and after PGE1- or placebo therapy, respectively.

therapy	spleen-liver-ratio		n	♂/♀
	before	after		
placebo	1,08 ± 0,31	1,02 ± 0,29	8	6/2
PGE1	1,00 ± 0,26	1,05 ± 0,33	8	5/3
placebo after PGE1	1,06 ± 0,19	1,04 ± 0,27	6	4/2
PGE1 again	1,05 ± 0,43	1,11 ± 0,41	6	4/2
PGE1 after placebo	1,09 ± 0,36	1,00 ± 0,33	6	4/2
placebo again	0,98 ± 0,39	0,99 ± 0,27	6	4/2

$x \pm SD$

b)   Results

All the patients had a PUR higher than 1, 30 prior therapy (Table 8); there was no significant difference between the groups. No change was observed during and after the placebo infusion. In contrast, a moderate, but significant reduction in platelet deposition was observed under PGE1-treatment. This effect persisted 3 weeks after having stopped the infusion. A repeated PGE1 induces a further drop in PUR and prolongation in T/2, however, not to a significant extent.

Platelet T/2 was shortened in all the groups prior to therapy reflecting a distributed hemostatic regulation in atherosclerosis; T/2 remained unchanged after placebo therapy. However, PGE1 provoked a significant prolongation in platelet T/2. Spleen-liver ratio remained unchanged under these therapeutic regimens too (Table 9).

Table 10

T/2 in PVD-patients before and after different dose of iloprost.

therapy	before	day 8	day 15
Placebo	72,8 ± 8,4	72,3 ± 9,0	72,5 ± 8,4
Iloprost			
1 ng/kg/min	69,4 ± 7,4	75,8 ± 6,7*)	76,1 ± 7,1*)
2 ng/kg/min	67,0 ± 9,4	72,3 ± 8,9*)	73,1 ± 9,4*)

$\bar{x}$ ± SD; *) p < 0,05

4. Influence of different iloprost doses on platelet deposition and platelet T/2

a) Patients and Methods
30 male patients with PVD stage II according to Fontaine (50 - 70a) with PUR values above 1,30 were randomly allocated to receive double-blind, placebo-controlled either an i.v. infusion of placebo or iloprost at two different doses (1 and 2 ng/kg/min) during 6 hours on 5 consecutive days. 10 Patients received the vehicle only.

b) Results
All patients had lesions with a PUR greater than 1,30 prior therapy. There was no significant difference in PUR pretreatment value between the 3 therapeutic groups. No change was observed during and after the placebo infusion. However, the infusion of iloprost provoked a significant decrease in platelet deposition to the active lesions (Table 11) with no significant difference between 1 and 2 ng/kg/min. The reduction in PUR values persisted up to 3 weeks after having stopped the infusions. Platelet T/2 was shortened in all the 3 groups of patients prior to therapy and did not change after treatment with placebo. However, a significant prolongation of platelet T/2 could be observed after the infusion with iloprost. It is noteworthy, that an increase in the dose of iloprost did not result in a further prolongation of platelet T/2 (table 10). 3 weeks after having stopped the infusion of iloprost platelet T/2 time still was prolonged to the same extent in both groups.

Table 11

PUR in PVD-patients during and after iloprost (1 or 2 ng) or placebo.

day	placebo	1 ng/kg/min	2 ng/kg/min
1	1,33 ± 0,03	1,33 ± 0,03	1,35 ± 0,03
2	1,33 ± 0,03	1,31 ± 0,04	1,32 ± 0,04
3	1,32 ± 0,03	1,27 ± 0,04	1,29 ± 0,04*
4	1,33 ± 0,03	1,24 ± 0,06*	1,26 ± 0,03*
5	1,33 ± 0,03	1,22 ± 0,05*	1,23 ± 0,02*
8	1,34 ± 0,03	1,21 ± 0,05*	1,23 ± 0,02*
15	1,32 ± 0,03	1,21 ± 0,05*	1,22 ± 0,02*
16	1,33 ± 0,03	1,21 ± 0,04*	1,22 ± 0,01*
17	1,33 ± 0,03	1,21 ± 0,05*	1,22 ± 0,03*
18	1,33 ± 0,03	1,22 ± 0,04*	1,22 ± 0,01*
19	1,33 ± 0,03	1,21 ± 0,05*	1,23 ± 0,02*
22	1,34 ± 0,03	1,21 ± 0,04*	1,23 ± 0,02*

$\bar{x}$ ± SD; * $p < 0,01$ (as compared to prevalue)

Table 12

PUR in PVD-patients during CG 4203-therapy and after 6 weeks (follow-up).

day	during therapy	after 6 weeks
1	1,34 ± 0,02	1,22 ± 0,05*
2	1,32 ± 0,05	1,24 ± 0,06*
3	1,25 ± 0,05*	1,22 ± 0,05*
4	1,23 ± 0,05*	1,22 ± 0,06*
5	1,21 ± 0,05*	1,21 ± 0,04*

$\bar{x}$ ± SD; * $p < 0,01$ (compared to prevalue)

Table 13

Effect of ASA, DIP and ASA plus DIP on platelet T/2 and spleen-liver ratio measured before and after 4 weeks treatment.

treatment	T/2		spleen-liver ratio		n
	before	after	before	after	
ASA	74 ± 6	75 ± 7	1,16 ± 0,27	1,11 ± 0,29	6
DIP	72 ± 7	70 ± 5	1,06 ± 0,35	1,10 ± 0,77	6
ASA/DIP	71 ± 6	75 ± 5	1,20 ± 0,39	1,17 ± 0,35	6

x ± SD; * $p < 0,01$

5. Influence of CG 4203 on platelet deposition and

platelet T/2.

a) Patients and Methods
15 male patients with PVD (risk factors: smoker 8,
hyperlipoproteinemia 7, hypertension 5) stage II
according to Fontaine (aged 49 - 68a) showing active
atherosclerotic lesions with PUR values higher 1,30
received CG 4203 i.v. at a rate of 25 ng/kg/min during
6 hours on 5 consecutive days.

b) Results
The infusion of CG 4203 provoked an immediate reduction
in platelet trapping to the active lesions. This
significant (p < 0,01) decrease in the PUR values could
still be demonstrated 3 weeks after having stopped the
infusions (Table 12). There was a significant (p <
0,001) prolongation in platelet T/2 after the CG 4203
infusions (67,1 -/+ 11 vs. 73,3 -/+ 10,3 hours)

6. Influence of 20mg aspirin in combination with
dipyridamole on platelet deposition and platelet T/2
(preliminary results).

a) Patients and Methods
18 patients with PVD stage II according to Fontaine
having an active atherosclerotic lesion characterised
by a PUR of greater than 1,20 were randomly divided
into 3 treatment groups receiving either 20mg aspirin
(ASA) daily, 75 mg DIP) 3 times daily or a combination
of 20 mg ASA daily together with 75 mg DIP 3 times
daily. Each treatment was administered for 5 weeks.

b) Results
All patients had lesions showing an initial PUR of >
1,20; there was no significant difference between the 3
treatment groups. No change was seen during the
observation period prior to therapy (Table 13). 4
weeks treatment with ASA alone and with DIP alone did
not cause any significant change in the PUR-values. In
contrast, treatment with a combination of ASA and DIP
resulted in a significant decrease in PUR (Table 14).
Platelet T/2 was shortened in all 3 groups of patients
before the therapy started and did not change
significantly after treatment with ASA or DIP alone.
However, a non-significant trend towards prolongation
of platelet T/2 was detected after the treatment with
the combination of ASA and DIP (Table 13).

Table 14

Effect of the drugs examined on PUR

treatment	P U R before	after	n
ASA	1,32 ± 0,05	1,28 ± 0,06	6
DIP	1,25 ± 0,06	1,28 ± 0,06	6
ASA/DIP	1,30 ± 0,05	1,21 ± 0,05*	6

$\bar{x} \pm SD$; * $p < 0,01$

Engymetric monitoring demonstrates steady state conditions after platelet injection (Fig 7) within a few minutes, thereafter, for 24 hours no alteration in spleen-liver ratio (Fig 8) is monitored. Reinjection of a new population of radiolabelled platelets causes an immediate increase over the investigated area (Fig 9). Computer manipulation allows to display activity curves over lesion and control as E-fit. This manipulation allows definite information about relative changes of lesional platelet uptake T/2-corrected.

DISCUSSION

Our findings indicate, that in human atherosclerosis the presence of areas with an increased platelet uptake is a not too rare feature (6, 32, 55). Morphological control revealed these lesions to be predominantly parietal thrombus of ulcerative lesions in nature. Interestingly enough, the follow-up of the spontaneous course of the lesion sites revealed that the vast majorities are unchanged through months (13). On the other hand, in contrast, some of the lesions have been shown to disappear within 4 weeks, whereas some others came up at other sites during the same time. The attempts to improve quality of images by subtraction after using a second radioisotope (42), especially 99mTC did not satisfy us at all. MASKing of interfering areas being close (61) improved the image quality somewhat. Comparing lesion sites with the contralateral area for reference may raise criticism. However, comparison performed using the heart, the lung or other vessel segments leads to even worse results. The most reliable test seems to be blood withdrawal for acute blood activity determination. The most promising experience we have so far with the preliminary use of 113In-

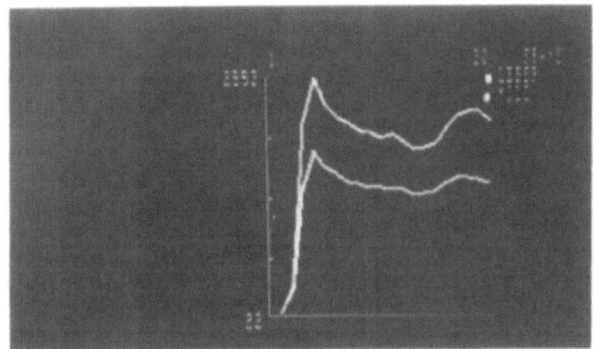

Fig 7:
Actual counts over liver and spleen during the initial phase
after reinjection of radiolabelled platelets.

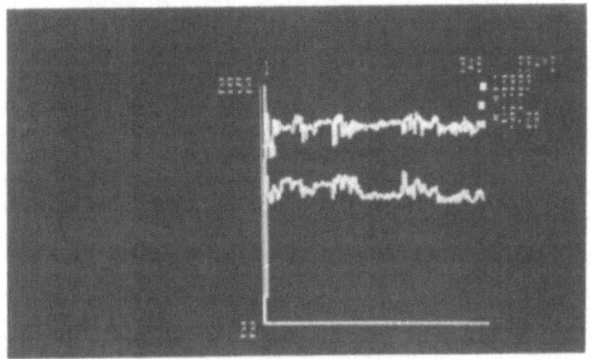

Fig 8:
24-hours follow-up of radioactive counts over spleen and
liver; no change is seen.

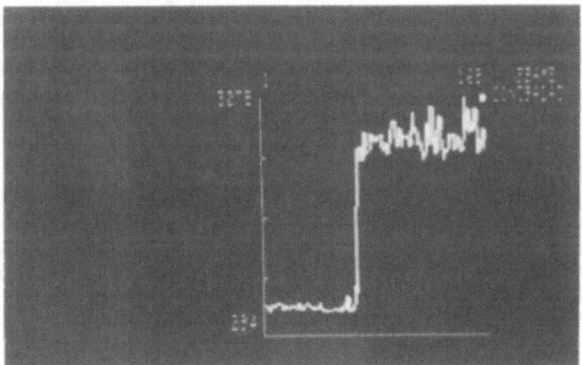

Fig 9:
Change of monitoring curve after repeated radiolabelling of
platelets.

labelled platelets. They seem not only to allow good quality subtraction, but may reflect much better the haemodynamic characteristics of platelets in circulation, thus allowing improved differentiation between still circulating and already resident platelets.

Treatment with a variety of antiplatelet agents, beside PGs, indicates, that these substances are capable of decreasing PUR and prolonging T/2, both being signs of improved haemostasis at a local and general level as well. Whereas certain PGs given i.v. have been shown to act within hours (70), some oral antiplatelet agents used need days or weeks to exhibit a clear effect (64). Surprisingly enough, no clear dose-response relation can be assessed (16, 70). Furthermore, the effect of a short-lasting single therapy, even with PG may be insufficient to retain the maximal effect (54). We were coming up rather quickly with the idea, that a clinically useful therapy (72) could be optimised by monitoring its effects on platelets. However, the mechanism of this action is by far unknown. The fact, that the beneficial effect persists over weeks points more to a vascular effect than to an action by platelets. At this time, as a matter of fact, the whole population of platelets is completely exchanged by a new family of cells delivered from the bone marrow. However, even at the vessel wall level, no morphological or biochemical sign for the mechanism of action has been discovered so far. Only a morphological experiment in rabbits after endothelial abrasion in abdominal aorta by Mustard's group revealed a decreased thrombogenicity (14) of subendothelium after various antiplatelet substances.

The phenomenon of platelet depositions on surfaces other than due to atherosclerosis and thrombi (24, 41) has been discussed in various directions: As a predictor of graft patency (22), after angioplasty (38), monitoring of antithrombotic therapy (37), evaluation of optimal therapeutic regimen (59, 60), thrombogenicity of grafts (19, 21, 43, 47, 54, 67, 68, 77) and bypass grafts (20, 45), detection of aneurysms (47, 71), clinical validation of carotid artery disease (18, 23, 29) and others. However, although the radiation dose (75) after platelet labelling using 100 μCi III-In is rather low, the routine use of radiolabelled platelets for single imaging and follow-up in patients is even nowadays limited world-wide to a few centers only. It may well be that preparation (63) and processing problems (56, 58) are responsible for the limited clinical application in cardiovascular medicine (76). However, we still need a wider clinical application and basic information to finally assess its indications and pitfalls as well.

REFERENCES

1. Bermann S.R., Mathias C.J., Sobel B.E., Welch M.J. (1982) Evaluation of thrombolytic therapy in coronary artery thrombosis; scintigraphic detection with the use of In-III-labelled platelets. In: Nuclear Medicine and Biology. C. Raynaud (ed.) Pergamon Press, Paris, pp 65-68.

2. Bergmann S.R., Lerch R.A., Mathias C.J., Sobel B.E., Welch M.J. (1983) Noninvasive detection of coronary thrombi with In-III-platelets; concise communication. J. Nucl. Med. 24; 130-134.

3. Bizzozero J. (1882) Uber einen neuen Formbestandteil des Blutes und dessen Rolle bei der Thrombose und der Blutgerinnung. Virchows Archiv Pathol. Anat. 90: 261.

4. Bunting S., Gryglewski R.J., Moncada S., Vane J.R. (1977) Arterial walls generate from prostaglandin endoperoxides a substance (prostaglandin x) which relaxes strips of mesenteric and coelliac arteries and inhibits platelet aggregation. Lancet i: 18.

5. Callow A.D., Connolly R., O'Donnell T.F., Gembarowicz R. (1982) Platelet arterial synthetic graft interaction and its modification. Arch. Surg. 117 : 1447-1452.

6. Davis H.H., Siegel B.A., Mathias C.A., Joist J.H., Sherman L.A., Welch M.J. (1978) Scintigraphic detection of atherosclerotic lesions and venous thrombosis in man by indium-III-labelled autologous platelets. Lancet 1: 1158.

7. Davis H.H., Siegel B.A., Sherman L.A., Heaton W.A., Naidich T.P., Joist J.H., Welch M.J. (1980) Scintigraphic detection of carotid atherosclerosis with indium-III-labelled autologous platelets. Circulation 61: 982-988.

8. Davis H.H., Siegel B.A., Welch M.J. (1980) Scintigraphic detection of an arterial thrombus with In-III-labelled autologus platelets. J. Nucl. Med. 21: 548-549.

9. Dewanjee M.K., Fuster V., Kay M.P., Josa M (1978) Imaging platelet deposition with III-In-labelled platelets in coronary artery bypass grafts in dogs. Mayo Clin. Proc. 53: 327-331.

10. Dewanjee M.K., Tago M., Josa M., Fuster V., Kaye M (1984) Quantification of platelet retention in aortocoronary femoral vein bypass graft in dogs treated with dipyridamole and aspirin. Circulation 69: 350-356.

11. Duguid J.B. (1946) Thrombosis as a factor in the pathogenesis of coronary atherosclerosis. Am. J. Pathol. Bacteriol. 58: 207-212.

12. Finkelstein S., Miller A., Callahan R.J., Fallon J.T., Godley F., Feldman B.L., Hinton R.C., Roberts A.B., Strauss H.W., Lees R.S. (1982) Imaging of acute arterial injury with In-III-labelled platelets: a comparison with scanning-electron micrographs. Radiology 145: 155-162.

13. Fitscha P., Kaliman J., Sinzinger H. (1984) Is gamma camera imaging of platelet deposition useful to assess the effectiveness of prostacyclin treatment? Biomed. Biochem. Acta 43: 403.

14. Fitscha P., Sinzinger H., O'Grady J. (1985) Does an antiplatelet therapy render active human atherosclerotic lesions less thrombogenic? Thromb. Haemost. 54: 85.

15. Fitscha P., Kaliman J., Sinzinger H. *1985) Gamma-camera imaging after autologus human platelet labelling with III-In-oxine-sulfate: a key for assessing the efficacy of prostacyclin treatment in active atherosclerosis: in: Prostaglandins and other eicosanoids in the cardiovascular system. K. Schor (ed), Karger-Verlag, Basel, p 352.

16. Fitscha P. (1986) Prostaglandine in Pathogenese und Therapie der peripheren arteriellen Verschluszkrankheit (PVK). in: Atherogenesis 7. O. Kraupp, H. Sinzinger, K. Widhalm (eds), Wilhelm Maudrich-"Verlag, Wien-Munchen-Bern.

17. Fuster V., Dewanjee M.K., Kaye M.P., Josa M., Metke M., Chesebro J.H. (1979) Noninvasive radioisotopic technique for detection of platelet deposition in coronary bypass grafts in dogs and its reduction with platelet inhibitors. Circulation 60: 1508.

18. Goldman M., Leung J.C.Y., Chandler S.T., Hawker R.J., McCollum C.N. (1982) Imaging carotid artery disease with III-in-labelled platelets: a combined clinical and theoretical study. In: Nuclear Medicine and Biology. C. Raynaud (ed.), Pergamon Press, Paris, pp 887-890.

19. Goldman N., Simpson D., Hawker R.J., Drolc Z., McCollum C.N. (1982) Indium-III labelled platelet accumulation on arterial grafts in man: a thrombosis model. In: Nuclear Medicine and Biology. C. Raynaud (ed.), Pergamon Press, Paris, pp 891-894.

20. Goldman M., Norcott H.C., Hawler R.J., Hail C., Drolc Z., McCollum C.H. (1982) Femoropopliteal bypass grafts - an isotope technique allowing in vivo comparison of thrombogenicity. Br. J. Surg. 69:380-382.

21. Goldman M., Norcott H.C., Hawker R.J., Drolc Z., McCollum C.H. (1982) Platelet accumulation on mature Dacron grafts in man. Brit. J. Surg. 69: 38-40.

22. Goldman M., Hall C., Rykes J. (1982) Does III-Indium-platelet deposition predict patency in prosthetic arterial grafts? Brit. J. Surg. 70: 653-658.

23. Goldman M., Leung J.O., Hawker R.J., Drolc Z., McCollum C.H. (1983) III-Indium platelet imaging, doppler spectral analysis and angiography compared in patients with transient cerebral ischemia. Stroke 14: 752.

24. Goodwin D.A., Bushberg J.T., Doherty P.W., Lipton M.J., Conley F.K., Diamanti C.I. Meares C.F. (1978) Indium-III-labelled autologous platelets for location of vascular thrombi in humans. J. Nucl. Med. 19:626-634.

25. Heyns Adup, Lotter M.G., Badenhorst P.N., Pieters H., Nel C.J.C., Minnaar P.C. (1982) Kinetics and fate of indium-III-labelled platelets in patients with aortic aneurysms. Arch. Surg. 117: 1170-1174.

26. Huang T.W., Harker L.A. (1981) In-III platelet imaging for detection of platelet deposition in abdominal aneurysms and prosthetic arterial grafts. Amer. J. Cardiol. 47: 882-889

27. Isaka Y., Kimaru K., Yoneda S., Kusunoki M., Etani H., Uyama O., Tsuda Y., Abe H. (1984) Platelet accumulation in carotid atherosclerotic lesions: semiquantitative analysis with Indium-III platelets and technetium-99m human serum albumin. J. Nucl. Med. 25: 556-563.

28. K e s s l e r   C . ,   T r a b a n t   R .   (1 9 8 2) Throbomozytenszintigraphie mit III-Indium. Arch. Psychiatr. Nervenkr. 231-449.

29. Kessler C., Reuther R., Berentelg J., Kimmig B. (1983) The clinical use of platelet scintigraphy with III-In-oxine. J. Neurol. 229:225.

30. Kessler C., Henningsen H., Reuther R., Antalics I., Kimmig B. (1985) Szintigraphie mit III-In-markierten Thrombozyten: Therapiekontrolle bei Acetylsalicylsaure (ASS)-behandelten Schlaganfallpatienten. Nuc. Compact 16: 30-31.

31. Kimura K., Isaka Y., Etani H., Kusunoki M., Yoneda S., Nagatsuka K., Yuama O., Abe H. (1982) In-III labelled autologous platelet scintigraphy for the detection of vascular thrombi in ischemic cerebrovascular disease. In: Nuclear Medicine and Biology, Raynaud D. (ed.), Pergamon Press, Paris, pp 1759-1761.

32. Lantieri R.L., Goodwin D.A., Guthaner D., Conley F., Goris M.L., Doherty P.W.: Static and dynamic studies of deep venous thrombosis and atherosclerosis in humans with indium-III-labelled platelets. Brit. J. Radiol. 53: 922-931.

33. LeBreton G.C., Lipowski J.P., Fernberg H., Venton D.L., Ho T., Wu K. (1984) Antagonism of thromboxane A2/prostaglandin H2 by 13-Azaprostanoic acid prevents platelet deposition to the deendothelialized rabbit aorta in vivo. J. Pharmacol. and Exp. Therap. 229: 80-84.

34. Lovaas M.E., Glovisczki P., Dwanjee M.K., Hollier L.H., Kaye M.P. (1983) Inferior vena cava replacement: the role of antiplatelet therapy. J. Surg. Res. 35: 234-242.

35. Lusby R.J., Florell L.D., Englestad B.L., Price D.C., Kipton M.J., Steney R.J., (1983) Vessel wall and In-III labelled platelets response to carotid endarterectomy. Argery 93: 424.

36. Moncada S., Gryglewski R.J., Bunting S., Vane J.R. (1976) An enzyme isolated from arteries transforms prostaglandin endoperoxides to an unstable substance that inhibits platelet aggregation. Nature 263: 663-665.

37. Moser K.M. (1985) Indium-III platelets in thromboembolism: can labelled platelets be used to evaluate antithrombotic therapy? In: Radiolabelled Cellular Blood Elements. Thakur M.L. (ed.), Plenum Publ. Corp., 155-176.

38. Pope C.F. Ezekowitz M.P., Smithe E.O. (1985) Detection of platelet deposition at the site of peripheral balloon angioplasty using III-Indium platelet scintigraphy. Amer. J. Cardiol. 55: 495-497.

39. Powers W.J., Siegel B.A., Davis H.H., Mathias C.J., Clark H.B., Welch M.J. (1982) Indium-III platelet scintigraphy in cerebrovascular disease. Neurology 32: 938-943.

40. Powers W.J., Mathias C.J., Welch M.J., Sherman L.A., Siegel B.A., Clarkson T.B. (1982) Scintigraphic detection of platelet deposition in atherosclerotic macaques: A new technique for investigation of antithrombotic drugs. Thromb. Res. 25: 137-143.

41. Powers W.J., Siegel B.A. (1983) Thrombus imaging with indium-III platelets. Sem. Thromb. Hemost. 9: 115-131.

42. Powers W.J., Hopkins K.T., Welch M.J. (1984) Validation of the dual radiotracer method for quantitative III-In platelet scintigraphy. Thromb. Res. 34: 135-145.

43. Price D.C., Lipton M.J., Lusby R.J., Engelstad B.L., Stoney R.J., Prager R.J., Hartmeyer J.A., Holly A.S. (1982) In vivo detection of thrombi with indium-III-labelled platelets. IEEE Trans. Nucl. Sci. 29: 1191-1197.

44. Pumphrey C.W., Dwanjee M.K., Chesebro J.H. Fuster V., Wahner H.W. (1982) A new method for quantifying human platelet-vascular graft interaction and the effect of platelet-inhibitor therapy. In: Nuclear Medicine and Biology. Raynaud C. (ed.), Pergamon Press, Paris, pp 895-897.

45. Pumphrey C.W., Chesebro J.H., Dewanjee M.K., Wahner H.W., Hollier L.H., Pairolero PC., Fuster V. (1983) In-vivo quantitation of platelet deposition on human peripheral arterial bypass grafts using Indium-III-labelled platelets. Amer. J. Cardiol. 51: 791-801.

46. Randall M.J., Wilding R.I. (1982) Acute arterial thrombosis in rabbits: reduced platelet accumulation after treatment with dazoxiben hydrochloride. Brit. J. Clin. Pharmacol. 15: 495

47. Ritchie J.L., Stratton J.R., Thiele B., Hamilton G.W., Warrick L.N. Huang T.W., Harker L.A. (1981) Indium-III platelet imaging for detection of platelet deposition in abdominal aneurysms and prosthetic arterial grafts. Amer. J. Cardiol. 47: 882-889.

48. Ritchie J.L., Lindner A., Hamilton G.W., Harker L.A. (1982) In-III oxine platelet imaging in hemodialysis patients: detection of platelet deposition at vascular access sites. Nephron 39: 334-339.

49. Rokitansky C. von (1852) Uber einige der wichtigsten Krankheiten der Arterien. K.K. Hof- und Staatsdruckerei Wien.

50. Sinziger H., Feigl. W., Silberbauer K. (1979) Prostcyclin generation in atherosclerotic arteries. Lancet II: 479.

51. Sinziger H., Silberbauer K., Fitscha P., Kaliman J. (1982) Wertigkeit des Nachweises atherosklerotischer Lasionen mit markierten autologen Thrombozyten. Acta med. Austr. 9: 181.

52. Sinzinger H., Fitscha P. (1983) Radioisotopic techniques for diagnosis of atherosclerosis. Giorn. Arterioscl. Suppl. 2: 31.

53. Sinziger H., Horsch A.K., Silberbauer K. (1983) The behaviour of various platelet function tests during long-term prostacyclin infusion in patients with peripheral vascular disease. Thromb. Haemst. 4: 885-887.

54. Sinziger H., O'Grady J., Cromwell M., Hofer R. (1983) Epoprostenol (prostacyclin) decreases platelet deposition on vascular prosthetic grafts. Lancet II: 1275-1276.

55. Sinziger H., Fitscha P. (1984) Scintigraphic detection of femoral artery atherosclerosis with III-indium-labelled autologous platelets. VASA 13: 350.

56. Sinziger H., Kobe H., Strobl-Jager E., Hofer R. (1984) A simple and safe technique for sterile autologous platelet labelling using "Monovette" vials. Eur. J. Nucl. Med. 9: 320.

57. Sinziger H., Fitscha P. (1984) Epoprostenol and platelet deposition in atherosclerosis. Lancet I: 905-906.

58. Sinzinger H., Strobl-Jager E., Pesl. H. (1984) Optimal labelling of human platelets. Film zur Markierungsmethodik (15 min.).

59. Sinzinger H., Fitsch P., Kaliman J. (1985) The optimal PG12 infusion as judged by autologous platelet-labelling in patients with active atherosclerosis. In: Prostaglandins and other eicosanoids in the cardiovascular system. K. Schror (ed.) Karger-Verlag, Basel. P 358.

60. Sinziger H., Fitsch P. (1986) The principles and application of treatment of atherosclerotic lesions with prostaglandins. In: Conf. Radionucl. Label. Cell. Blood Elements: Applications in Atherosclerosis and Thrombosis. A.duP. Heyns (ed.), South African Med. Res. Council. p 221.

61. Sinziger H., Fitscha P., Kaliman J. (1986) Imaging and monitoring of human atherosclerotic lesions with radiolabelled platelets. In: Conf. Radionucl. Label. Cell. Blood Elements: Applications in Atherosclerosis and Thrombosis. A. duP. Heyns (ed.), South African Med. Res. Council, p 153.

62. Sinziger H., Fitscha P. (1987) Influence of prostaglandin E1 on in-vivo accumulation of radiolabelled platelets and LDL on human arteries. VASA 17: 5-10.

63. Sinziger H., Fitscha P., Kaliman J (1987) Prostaglandin 12 during radiolabelling improves recovery, but does not change platelet half-life and platelet uptake over active human lesion sites. Prostaglandins (in press).

64. Sinziger H., O'Grady J., Fitscha P., Kaliman J. (1987) Diminished platelet residence time on active human atherosclerotic lesions in-vitro - evidence for an optimal dose of aspirin? J. Nucl. Med. (submitted).

65. Stratton J.R., Ritchie J.L., (1982) Sulfinpyrazone fails to inhibit platelet deposition on Dacron prosthetic grafts in man. Circulation 66: 55.

66. Stratton J.R., Ritchie J.L., Sisk E.J., McFadden K.W. (1982) McFadden KUW., Inhibition of indium-0III platelet deposition in left vetricular thrombi by platelet active drugs. Circulation 66: 342.

67. Stratton J.R., Thiele B.L., Ritchie J.L. (1982) Platelet deposition on dacron bifurcation grafts in man: quantitation with III-Indium platelet imaging. Circulation 66: 1287-1289.

68. Stratton J.R., Thiele B.L., Ritchie J.L. (1983) Natural history of platelet deposition on dacron aortic bifurcation grafts in the first year after implantation. Amer. J. Cardiol. 52: 371-374.

69. Stratton J.R., Ritchie J.L. (1984) Failure of ticlopidine to inhibit deposition of III-Indium-labelled platelets on dacron prosthetic surfaces in humans. Circulation 69: 677-683.

70. Strobl-Jager E., Fitscha P., Kaliman J., Sinzinger H. (1987) Monitoring of in-vivo platelet deposition in patients with peripheral vascular disease after different doses of prostaglandin I2 (PG12). In: Prostaglandins in Clinic and Research. H. Sinzinger, K. Schror (eds.F), Alan R. Liss Inc., Philadelphia-New York (in press).

71. Sutherland G.R., King M.E., Peerless S.J., Vezina W.C., Brown G.W., Chamberlain M.J. (1982) Platelet interaction within giant intracranial aneurysms. J. Neurosurg. 56: 53-61.

72. Szczeklik A., Nizankowski R., Skawinski S., Szczeklik J., Gluszko P., Gryglewski R.J. (1979) Successful therapy of advanced arteriosclerosis obliterans with prostacyclin. Lancet I: 1111.

73. Thakur M.L., Welch M.J., Joist J.H., Coleman R.E. (1976) Indium-III-labelled kplatelets: studies on preparation and evaluation of in vitro and in vivo functions. Thromb. Res. 9: 345.

74. Thakur M.L., Walsh L., Malech H.L., Gottschalk A. (1981) Indium-III-labelled human platelets: improved method, efficacy and evaluation. J. Nucl. Med. 22: 381.

75. Van Reenen C.R., Lotter M.G., Minnaar P.C.,, duHeyns
    A., Path F.F., Badenhorst P.N., Pieters H. (1980)
    Radiation dose from human platelets labelled with
    indium III. Brit. J. Radiol. 43: 790.
76. Vreeken J., Hardemans M.R., Vosmaer G.D.C., Royen van
    E.A., Schoot van der J.V., Duren D.R. (1982) Use of
    III-In-labelled platelets in cardiovascular disease.
    Nucl. Geneeskund. Bull. 4: 34-36.
77. Yui T., Uchida T., Matsuda S., Iwadya K., Umino M., Ono
    K., Muroi S., Owada K., Machii K., Kariyone S. (1982)
    Detection of platelet consumption in aortic grafts with
    III-In-labelled platelets. Eur. J. Nucl. Med. &: 77-79.

USE OF DUAL ISOTOPE PLATELET SCINTIGRAPHY FOR MONITORING
ANTIPLATELET THERAPY IN STROKE PATIENTS

Voosen P., Kessler Ch., Hipp M., and Petrovici J.N.

Department of Neurology, Cologne-Merheim Hospital, Cologne
F.R.G.

INTRODUCTION

The increase of therapeutic possibilities for the
management of patients with thromboembolic complications, as
e.eg. by fibrinolytic treatment or vascular surgery or the
use of new antiplatelet drugs, necessitate further
information as to the extent, age and activity of the
thromboembolic material causing clinical symptoms. Many
aspects concerning the clinical use of antiplatelet drugs in
stroke patients are as yet unsolved. It is for instance not
yet proven whether in vitro investigations can be compared
with the in vivo action of drugs (5). The ongoing discussion
on the amount of aspirin proper for an optimal prevention of
stroke highlights this problem (3, 22). Since the
introduction of the scintigraphic in vivo detection of
arterial thrombi with radiolabelled platelets platelet
scintigraphy (PSC) has been used as a diagnostic tool in
various thromboembolic diseases (15). It has a very high
specifity in diagnosing deep venous thrombosis (10) and has
been used in imaging pulmonary emboli (17) as well as
cardiac thrombi (8). PSC was further successful in imaging
atherosclerotic lesions in the peripheral arteries (1) as
well as in the coronary (7) and in the carotid arteries.
Davis et al. (6) were the first to demonstrate positive PSC-
findings at ulcerated carotid lesions. Since then several
investigations have been carried out concerning this
atherosclerotic aspect. The result of these studies shows
that pathological platelet accumulations can be visualized
predominantly in the area of the symptomatic carotid artery
and the double isotope technique, see 16). Using this
procedure, Isaka et al (13) were able to demonstrate that
aspirin treated patients, on average had a significantly
lower Pl-Exc than untreated patients. In a second study they
demonstrated that the Pl-Exc decreased in aspirin treated
patients if the PSC was performed twice. Because of the
radiation dose it is questionable whether recurrent scans
are not objectionable; this is why we sought for a new way
of measuring the drug effect in stroke patients.

TECHNICAL APPROACH

The platelets were labelled with Indium-III as

Ch. Kessler et al. (eds.), Clinical Application of Radiolabelled Platelets, 162–166.
© 1990 *Kluwer Academic Publishers.*

described elsewhere (14). 24 hours after injection of the radiolabelled platelets gamma-camera images of the neck vessels were performed in an anterior-posterior projection. Immediately after taking the platelet scan 5 mCi of Tc-99m labelled red cells were injected in an unchanged patients position, and a blood flow image could be scanned. 48 hours after injection of the radiolabelled platelets a second platelet image in an ap-projection was performed and once more 5mCi of Tc-99m-labelled erythrocytes were injected intravenously in an unchanged position. This procedure makes it possible to calculate the Pl-Exc at two different times and to observe drug induced changes of platelet incorporation by the thrombus.

DRUGS

We performed this dynamic platelet uptake study on 26 stroke patients. 21 were male, 5 female, all patients had symptomatic carotid lesions of varying degree. The 24 hour scan showed in all 26 patients a pathological Pl-Exc in the symptomatic carotid artery of more than 200 counts. In all patients the stroke was treated haemorrhologically by decreasing the haematocrit and by hydroxyethyl starch infusions. None of the patients had previously been treated with antiplatelet drugs. The patients were divided into three groups: Group 1 got no additional treatment up to the second scan (n = 8), group 2 was treated with 1000 mg/die aspirin orally starting immediately after the first 24 hour scan (n = 9), group 3 received infusions of 600 mg naftidrofuryl (NAF) immediately after the first scan and before the second scan (n = 9). All patients gave their informed consent for the participation of this study.

RESULTS

The results of our study are shown in fig. 1. The mean Pl-Exc 24 hours after the injection of the radiolabelled platelet was x = 260 cts. In the untreated patients (group 1) it was initially 262 cts. and increased during the next 24 hours (x = 380 cts.). This increase is statistically significant (t-test, p <0.005). The initial mean Pl-Exc in the ASS-treated patients (group 2) was x - 248 cts. and there was no statistically significant increase over the next 24 hours (x = 252 cts.; p = 0.9). In the NAF-treated patients the initial Pl-Exc was x = 270 cts. and the count after 48 hours was x = 304 cts., indicating a moderate blocking of the platelet uptake. This difference was also not statistically significant p = 0.17).

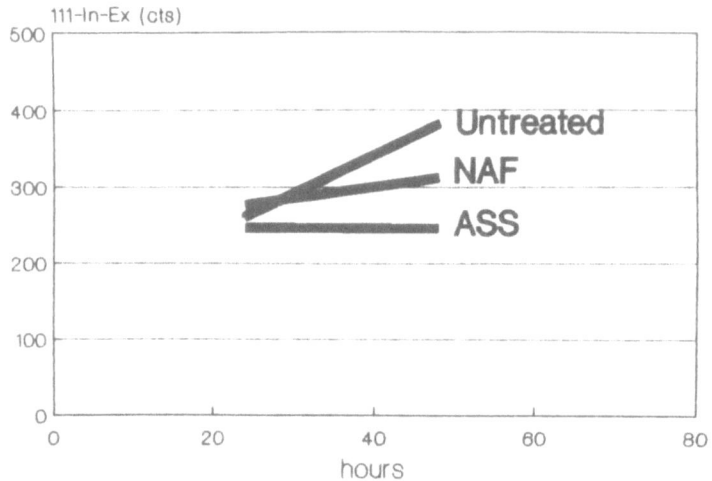

Fig 1.
III-In-EXC values in the symptomatic carotid bifurcations 24
and 46 h after injection of the radiolabelled platelets. In
the untreated patients a significant increase of the III-In-
Exc can be observed, both ASS and more moderate
Naftidrofuryl (NAF) enhance the increase of platelet bound
activity.

DISCUSSION

Aspirin enhances the collagen and ADP induced platelet
aggregation in vitro. Despite these laboratory findings, its
in vivo effect is discussed controversially. As aspirin
simultaneously inactivates the cyclooxygenase of platelets
as well as of the vessel wall, it has at the same time a
thrombogenic and antithrombotic effect. In spite of this
contradiction ASS has proven its positive effect on the
prevention of recurrent strokes in large clinical studies
(9). Up to now, PSC was used in only two studies to confirm
the ability of ASS for in vivo thrombus prevention. Stratton
et al. (21) showed that aspirin prevents pathological
platelet accumulations on Dacron grafts, and Isaka et al.
(13) reported a positive effect of 1000 mg/die aspirin on
thrombotic sites of the carotid arteries. We were able to
confirm these findings and to prove a decreased platelet
uptake in carotid atherosclerotic lesions of stroke
patients. For the present study we used the "high dose"-
aspirin dosage of 1000 mg/die because up to now it is the
most often used dosage and all large clinical studies were
performed with it. NAF is an antiserotogenetic drug which

acts as a vasodilatator. As a recent clinical trial showed, it has a positive clinical effect on acute cerebral hemispheric infarction (20). Recent investigations show that NAF has also an antithrombotic effect. Herrman et al. (11) demonstrated that NAF prevents the growing of thrombi in the area of the endothelial lesions, and Breddin (2) confirmed these findings in another animal model. In our study a decrease of platelet uptake in the atherosclerotic carotid lesions was evident which may explain the positive clinical effect of NAF, as published by Steiner et al. (20).

As our study shows, it is possible with Indium-III labelled platelets to monitor the antiplatelet effect of different drugs in vivo. The aim of further studies must be to compare the PSC-findings with the clinical effect and to select the drug and the dosage most useful for the treatment of stroke patients.

REFERENCES

1.   Bernard P., Bazan H., de Laforte C (1982) Labelled platelets in the detection of thrombotic process. Int. J. Rad. Appl. Instrum. 13; 165-171.
2.   Breddin
3.   Burch J.W., Baenzinger N.L., Stanford N., Majerus P.W. (1978) Selective cumulative inhibition of platelet thromboxane production by low dose aspirin in healthy subjects. Proc. Natl. Acad Sc.: 75: 5181-5184.
4.   Canadian Cooperative Study Group (1978) A randomized trial of aspirin and sulfinpyrazone in threatened stroke. New Engl. J. Med. 299: 53-59.
5.   deGaetano G., Gerletti C., Bertele V. (1982) Pharmacology of antiplatelet drugs and clinical trials on thrombosis prevention; A difficult link. Lancet 2: 974-977.
6.   Davis H.H., Siegel B.A., Mathias C.J., Joist J.H., Sherman L.A., Welch M.J. (1978) Scintigraphic detection of atherosclerotic lesions and venous thrombi in man by Indium-III-labelled autologous platelets. Lancet 2: 1183-1187.
7.   Dewanjee M.K., Fuster V., Kaye M.P., Josa M. (1978) Imaging platelet deposition with III-In-labelled platelets in coronary artery bypas grafts in dogs. Mayo Clin. Proc. 53: 327-331.
8.   Ezekowitz M.D., Smith E.O., Rankin R., Harrison L.H., Kraus H.P. (1982) Left arterial mass: Diagnostic value of transesophageal echocardiography and Indium-III platelet scintigraphy. Am. J. Cardiol. 51:1563-1564.
9.   Fields W.S., Lemak N.A., Frankowski R.F., Hardy R.J., Bigelow R.H. (1980) Controlled trial of aspirin in cerebral ischemia. Circulation 62 (Suppl. V) V90 - V96.
10. Goodwin D.A., Bushberg J.T., Doherty P.W., Lipton M.J., Conley F.K., Diamanti C.J., Meares C.F. (1978) Indium-III-labelled autologous platelets for location of vascular thrombi in humans. J. Nucl. Med. 19:626-634.

166

11. Herrmann K.S., Grosze-Heitmeyer A., Kreuzer H. (1986) Antithrombotic efficacy and its time course after application of Naftidrofuryl in vivo. Arch. Int. Pharmacodyn. Ther. 284: 145-150.

12. Isaka Y., Kinura K., Yoneda S., Kusunoki M., Etani H., Uyama O., Tsuda V., Abe H. (1984) Platelet accumulation in carotid atherosclerotic lesions; Semiquantitative analysis with indium-III platelets and technetium human serum albumin. J. Nucl. Med. 25: 556-563.

13. Isaka Y., Kimura K., Etani H., Uehara A., Uyama O., Toneda S., Kamada T., Kusunoki M. (1986) Effect of Aspirin and Ticlopidine on platelet deposition in carotid atherosclerotis: Assessment by Indium-III platelet scintigraphy. Stroke 17: 1215-1220.

14. Kessler Ch., Reutner R., Berentelg J., Kimmig B. (1983) The clinical use of platelet scintigraphy with II-In-oxine. J. Neurol. 229: 255-261.

15. Kessler Ch., Reutner R., Kimmig B., Pietzsch T. (1984) Dual isotope scintigraphy in stroke patients. Neuroradiology 26: 113-117.

16. Kessler Ch., Kniffort T., Reutner R., Kimmig B. zum Winkel L. (1984) Szintigraphie mit Indium-III-markierten Blut-plattchen. Dtsch. Med Wschr. 109: 1853-1859.

17. Moser K.M., Spragg K.G., Bender F., Konopka F., Hartman M.T. Fedullo P. (1980) Study of factors that may condition scintigraphic detection of venous thrombi and pulmonary emboli with indium-III-labelled platelets. J. Nucl. Med. 21: 1051-1058.

18. Powers W.J., Siegel B.A., Davis H.H., Mathias C.J., Clark H.B., Welch M.J. (1982) Indium-III platelet scintigraphy in cerebrovascular disease. Neurology 32: 938-943.

19. Powers W.J., Welch M.J., Mathias C.J. (1983) Improved scintigraphic detection of intravascular thrombi by a dual-radiotracer technique. In: Reivich M., Hurtig H.J. (Eds.) Cerebrovascular diseases. Raven Press, New York, pp. 337-346.

20. Steiner

21. Stratton J.R., Thiele B.L., Ritchie J.L. (1982) Platelet deposition on Dacron aortic bifurcation grafts in man; Quantitation with indium-III platelet imaging. Circulation 66: 1287-1292.

THE EVALUATION OF A NEW SPECIFIC THROMBOXANE A2 ANTAGONIST ON RADIOLABELLED PLATELET DISPOSITION IN PROSTHETIC GRAFTS

A.C. Meek, R.A. Harper, I.F. Lane, C.N. McCollum.

INTRODUCTION

Platelet inhibitory therapy has been found effective in the prevention of postoperative thrombosis following coronary artery bypass, and in the prevention of stroke in patients with cerebrovascular disease (1,2). It also reduces platelet adhesion and aggregation following arterial bypass using prosthetic material (3).
Unlikely autogenous vein, prosthetic bypass grafts do not develop a neointima with an anti-aggregatory endothelium and platelet deposition has been shown to continue up to 10 years following graft implantation. Existing platelet-inhibitory regimens use aspirin but patient compliance is limited by gastrointestinal side effects (6). We previously established a canine model in which PTFE grafts are implanted in the femoral artery and radiolabelled platelet uptake measured to calculate graft thrombogenicity (5). Using this model we tested a new specific thromboxane A2 inhibitor GR32191, (Glaxo Group Research), examining early post operative platelet accumulation, graft platelet uptake and pseudo-intimal thickening at 60 days.

MATERIALS AND METHODS.

Thirty greyhounds (wt 20 - 25 kgs) were randomised to receive GR32191, aspirin 150mg plus dipyridamole 50mg or placebo 12 hourly. Forty - eight hours following the commencement of therapy, a 6 cm length of thin walled 6mm diameter polytetrofluoroethylene (Gor - Tex) was used to replace an equivalent length of superficial femoral artery. On the 5th post operative day, the animals were injected with autologous radiolabelled platelets (7) and daily measurements of radioactivity over the graft using a highly collimated sodium iodide crystal and rate - meter were compared to the contralateral femoral artery. The daily increase in the ratio of radioactivity over the graft compared to the reference femoral artery was termed Thrombogenicity Index (TI). Graft patency was determined daily, and after 60 days radiolabelled platelets were again injected. Subsequently, the grafts were excised, sectioned at the mid point and 5mm from each anastomosis and under light microscopy the degree of intraluminal stenosis by

Ch. Kessler et al. (eds.), Clinical Application of Radiolabelled Platelets, 167–172.
© 1990 *Kluwer Academic Publishers.*

thrombus was measured by micron grid. This was expressed as the percentage of the total cross sectional area. Graft radioactivity was measured by well counter and expressed as the percentage of activity compared to 1ml of blood. Results for thrombogenicity, luminal stenosis and graft platelets uptake were compared statistically using the Mann-Witney U test for non parametric data.

RESULTS

All animals tolerated the medication and surgery, however three dogs, one from each group, developed early post operative wound infection and were excluded from subsequent analysis. Mean ($\pm$ S.E. mean) Thrombogenicity Index was reduced to 0.014 $\pm$ 0.012 by GR32191 and 0.088 $\pm$ 0.029 by ASA + DPM compared to 0.14 $\pm$ 0.07 significantly reduced to 16 $\pm$ 7.6% by GR32191 compared to both placebo at 57.7 $\pm$ 10.4 and ASA + DPM at 50.5 $\pm$ 13.5 (Fig. 2). Graft platelet uptake following a second infusion of 111-In platelets at 60 days was recorded as the percentage activity in the excised graft compared to 1ml of blood and was significantly reduced by the thromboxane A2 antagonist to 5.8 $\pm$ 2.4% compared to 21.1 $\pm$ 8.4% in the placebo group and 16.8 $\pm$ 5.5 with aspirin and dipyridamole.

DISCUSSION

In vivo assessment of platelet inhibitory therapy examines the natural incorporation of platelets into thrombus forming on the luminal surface of a prosthetic graft. This represents a far more physiological assessment compared to laboratory studies such as in vitro aggregation studies and artificial circuits requiring full anti-coagulation which may itself affect platelet function. This model allows platelet accumulation to be examined in the early post-operative period as well as measurements on the thrombus at 60 days. The Thromboxane antagonist significantly reduced luminal stenosis and graft platelet uptake compared to placebo and although both platelet inhibitory regimens appeared to lower Thrombogenicity Index compared to placebo this did not achieve statistical significance (0.1 $<p<0.05$). Thromboxane antagonists may have wide uses in the treatment of thrombotic and embolic events in patients if it can be shown to have few side effects.

In this canine model a thromboxane antagonist GR32191 was found to be at least as effective as the standard therapy of aspirin and dipyridamole in reducing thrombogenicity, graft platelet uptake and luminal stenosis

REFERENCES

1.   Canadian Co-operative Study Group. A randomised trial of aspirin and sulfinpyrazone in threatened stroke. New Eng.J.Med.1978;299:53-59

2. Chesebro JH, Clements IP, Fuster V, et al. A platelet-inhibitor drug trial in coronary artery bypass operations. New Eng.J.Med. 1983;307:73-78

3. Goldman M, Norcott HC, Hawker RJ, et al. Platelet accumulation on mature Dacron grafts in man. Br.J.Surg. 1982; 69:538-540

4. Goldman M, Norcott HC, Hawker RJ, et al.Femoro-popliteal Bypass Grafts - an Isotope Technique allowing in vivo comparison of thrombogenicity. Br.J.Surg. 1982: 69(7): 380-382

5. Lane IF, Irwin JTC, Jennings SA et al. The effect of the cyclo-oxygenase inhibitor Indobufen on platelet accumulation in prosthetic vascular grafts. Br.J.Surg.1986; 73: 563-565

6. Paris Study Group. Persantin and aspirin in coronary heart disease. Circ.1980: 449-461

7. Wilkinson AR, Hawker RJ, Hawker LM, 111-indium labelled canine platelets. Thromb Res 1978: 13; 175-182

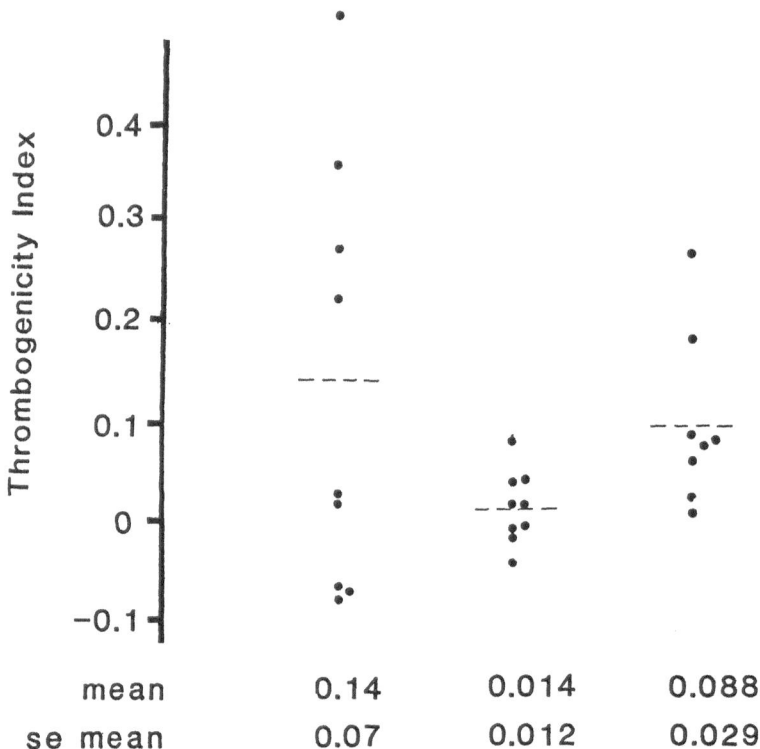

Fig 1   Early postoperative Thrombogenicity Index
         comparing GR 32191, ASA & DPM and placebo.

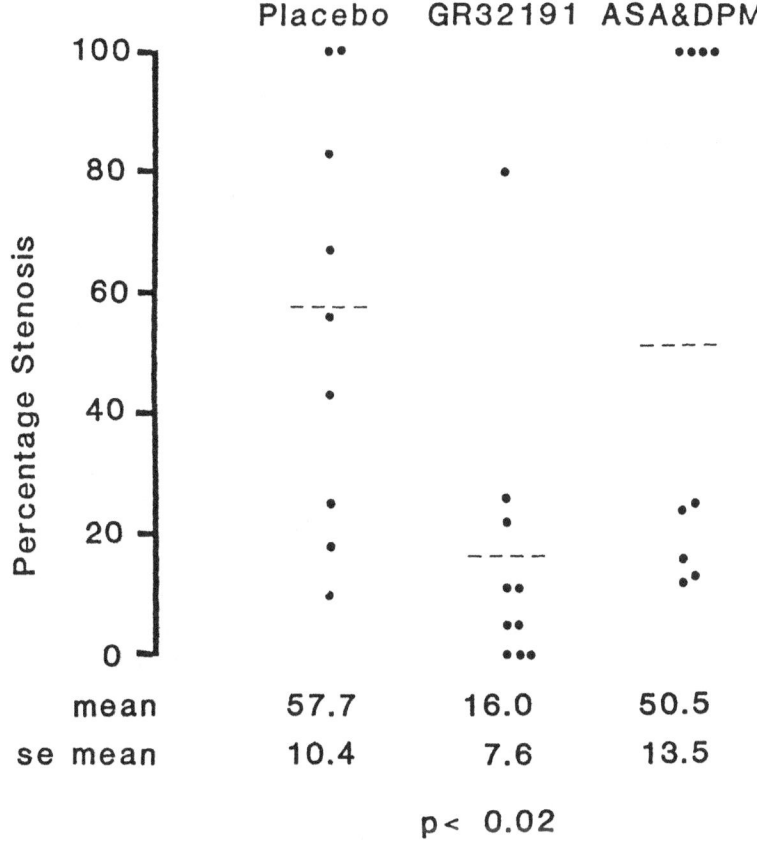

Fig 2   Percentage stenosis by intraluminal thrombus at
         60 days following implantation.

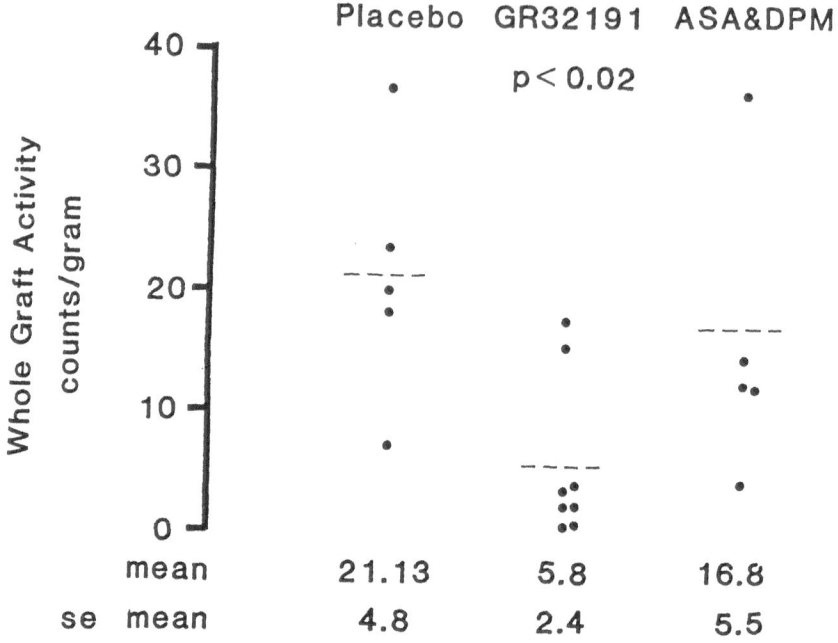

Fig 3   Graft platelet uptake measured by well counter
         after graft excision.

PLATELET SCINTIGRAPHY IN STROKE PATIENTS

Goldman M. Md FRCS.
Senior Lecturer in Surgery,
East Birmingham Hospital,
Bordesley Green East,
BIRMINGHAM, B9 5ST.
U.K.

INTRODUCTION

Stroke is the third commonest cause of death in Western Europe. The cost for those who survive with permanent neurological deficit is unmeasurable. Reducing risk factors such as diabetes, hypertension, obesity and stress may help to delay the onset of degenerative arterial disease, but are unlikely to help a patient whose carotid artery decay is manifest by transient loss of cerebral function (TIA) or vision (amaurosis fugax).

It has always been supposed that these temporary neurological deficits are a consequence of either cerebral hypo-perfusion due to carotid artery stenosis or emboli arising from disease at the carotid bifurcation. Eastcott (1954) advocated surgery for stenosis and Fisher's observations of platelet emboli occluding the retinal artery stimulated medical management. (2). Because either TIA or amaurosis fugax is frequently the harbinger of a completed stroke therapeutic intervention is justified. Unfortunately, it is not certain whether simple medication with an antiplatelet drug such as aspirin is more or less likely to prevent progression to a stroke than the more complex procedure of surgical endarterectomy to remove the diseased segment.

In practice the treatment offered to an individual patient is quite likely to be considerably influenced by empirical forces such as the particular prejudices of the physician in charge or the availability of local surgical expertise. Once it has been demonstrated that III-Indium labelled platelets could be used to identify thrombotically active carotid artery disease (3) the possibility existed, for the first time, that patients might be separated into treatment groups according to whether their symptoms were a consequence of stenosis or thrombo-embolism. Subsequently III-Indium platelet studies have been undertaken to establish:

1.   To what extent platelets accumulate on atherosclerotic carotid arterial lesions.

Ch. Kessler et al. (eds.), Clinical Application of Radiolabelled Platelets, 173–179.
© 1990 Kluwer Academic Publishers.

2.   Whether platelet scintigraphy offers a useful clinical investigation.

PLATELET DEPOSITION ON CAROTID ENDARTERECTOMY SPECIMENS

We studied eleven patients proceeding to carotid endarterectomy after injection of autologous labelled platelets (4). The surgical specimens were retrieved and radioactivity was calculated. It was notable that all the retrieved endarterectomy specimens showed measurable radioactivity. Platelet deposition was expressed as specimen activity, the ratio of emissions from the surgical specimen over those from 1 ml of blood taken simultaneously.

The most thrombogenic specimen was equivalent to 1,8 ml of blood (Fig. 1). Overall mean (-/+ s.e.m.) specimen activity was 0.65 -?+ 0.19 with the lowest activity being 0.10 found in a stenosis. Interestingly, four of the patients had ulcerated plaques and the activity in these at 1.12 -/+ 0.37 was considerably higher than that of 0.38 -/+ 0.10 which occurred in the 7 stenotic lesions.

In a similar study (5) four endarterectomy specimens were retrieved. Linear radioactivity profiles showed peaks coincident with thrombus located by serial histological sectioning. Both studies confirmed the platelet deposition was taking place. To determine whether this was sufficient to permit reliable interpretation by gamma camera we undertook a theoretical study (4).

THEORETICAL STUDY TO ASSESS GAMMA CAMERA SENSITIVITY

A phantom was constructed to represent a single carotid sheath in the neck (Fig. 2). The activities used were based upon blood samples and computer analysis of images from studies in 20 patients with peripheral arterial disease. To represent labelled platelet deposition III-In-oxine was added to the tapered tube based on endarterectomy specimen activities (maximum 851 Bq).

Images of the phantom were examined by two observers. Both observers regularly detected the addition of 3700 and 1850 Bq. They noted 925 Bq of activity on half the occasions that image was offered and failed consistently to detect a lesser amount of added activity. Given that the most active surgical specimen was equivalent to 851 Bq, it was perhaps predictable that clinical imaging studies would yield conflicting results.

THE USE OF GAMMA CAMERA IMAGING FOR DIAGNOSIS

Several clinical studies have assessed the potential of carotid artery imaging with III-In platelets. (3, 4, 5, 6, 7). In our study anterior neck images were obtained at 24 hour intervals up to a maximum of 5 days. Any increase in

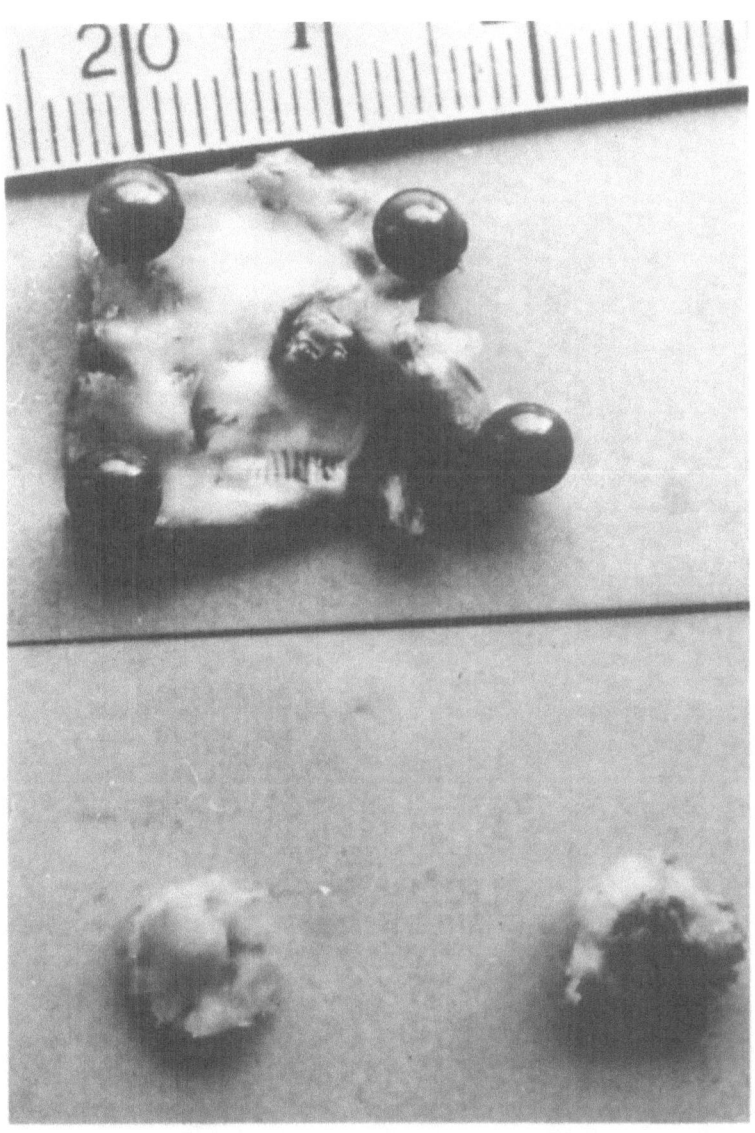

Fig 1.
The endarterectomy specimen had a total radioactivity count
of 17,323. The ulcerated plaque (bottom right) contributed
>95% of the total activity.

176

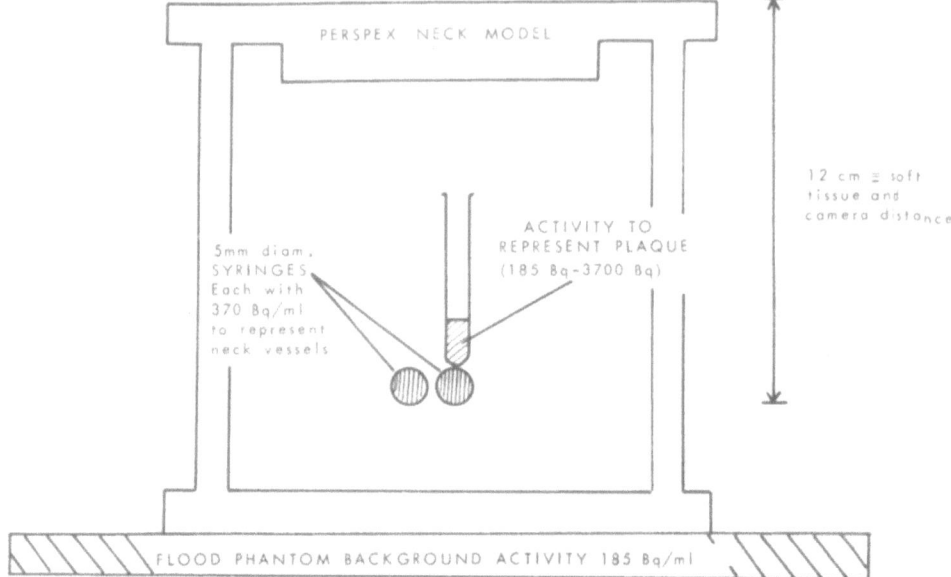

Fig 2.
In the phantom model various III-In activities could be introduced into the tapered tube to simulate platelet uptake.

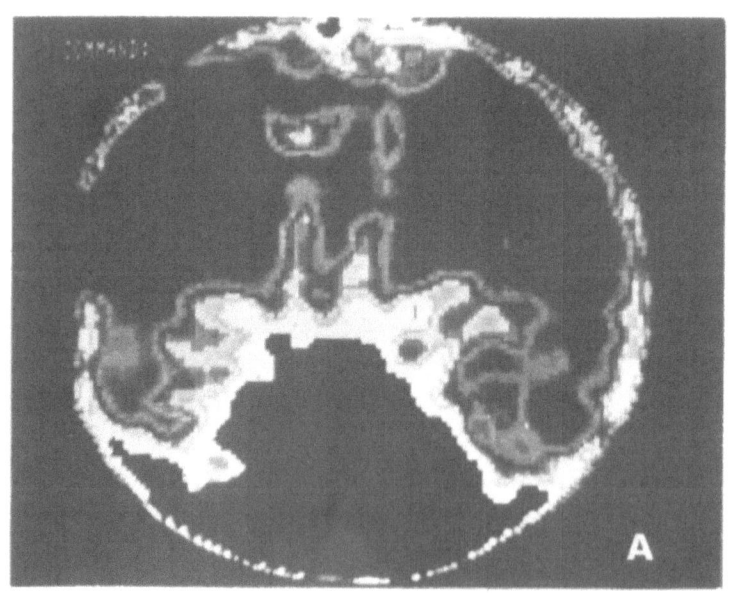

Fig 3
A clear "Hot Spot" is visible in the left carotid of a patient suffering right sided TIA

activity at either carotid bifurcation with respect to the surrounding tissue was considered to represent platelet accumulation and reported positive, giving rise to a possible maximum of 50 bifurcations. With these criteria two independent observers agreed in 38 of the 50 patients (22 positive, 16 negative). This was statistically significant (p<0.001 Chi squared).

Each individual observer identified a larger number of positive images thus reducing the sensitivity of the combined interpretation as noted by Davis et al (3) when comparing platelet images to angiographic abnomalities.

Different patient series have relied on interpretation by one, two or three observers sometimes independently and sometimes by consensus. In the Japanese study (6) semi-quantitative interpretation using Tc-99m for blood pool subtraction and region of interest analysis was considered more reproducible and sensitive than visual assessment. Amongst those studies relying on imaging alone, not only was the number of observers and the disciplines imposed on them variable, but also in some studies clinical information was withheld and in others made available. Thus the percentage of abnormal images detected visually has varied from as low as 23% by Powers et al (5) to as high as 60 (4) from essentially similar groups of patients using comparable techniques.

Several factors have been considered to influence the likelihood of demonstrating abnormal platelet accumulation (Fig. 3). All studies have shown a significant correlation with angiographic abnormalities and the collected results from four studies of 358 patients confirm the strength of this relationship (Table 1). More controversial has been the various results reported when considering the effect of the particular angiographic lesion on platelet accumulation.

Our study (4) showed lesions > 80% stenosis were less often imaged and accumulated less platelets when measured as endarterectomy specimens. Kessler et al (7) suggested that severe stenosis resulted in increased platelet uptake as did the group from St. Louis in their early study (3), but not subsequently in a larger series (5). We found symptomatic carotid arteries were more often positive on imaging, but others could not demonstrate this relationship. Similarly several studies have addressed the effect of anti-thrombotic medication. The results are conflicting and no firm conclusions can be made. Equally inconclusive reports concerning antiplatelet therapy have emerged from III-In platelet studies following carotid endarterectomy. McCollum's group showed a reduction in post-operative platelet uptake in patients receiving aspirin plus dypiridamole (personal communication). This did not occur in another virtually identical non-randomised series (8). Of note, the former study used an objective analysis whereas the latter relied on visual interpretation alone.

endarterectomy specimens. Kessler et al (7) suggested that severe stenosis resulted in increased platelet uptake as did the group from St. Louis in their early study (3), but not subsequently in a larger series (5). We found symptomatic carotid arteries were more often positive on imaging, but others could not demonstrate this relationship. Similarly several studies have addressed the effect of anti-thrombotic medication.

The results are conflicting and no firm conclusions can be made. Equally inconclusive reports concerning antiplatelet therapy have emerged from III-In platelet studies following carotid endarterectomy. McCollum's group showed a reduction in post-operative platelet uptake in patients receiving aspirin plus dypiridamole (personal communication). This
did not occur in another virtually identical non-randomised series (8). Of note, the former study used an objective analysis whereas the latter relied on visual interpretation alone.

CONCLUSION

The optimistic hope was that III-In platelet imaging would offer a reliable investigation to distinguish thrombotically active carotid artery lesions. In practice we now know that the levels of radioactivity deposited are at the limits of gamma camera resolution.

Image interpretation is difficult and controversy surrounds the possible effects of stenosis, ulceration, symptoms and medication. To date III-In platelet scintigraphy has not achieved the status of a useful clinical investigation.

TABLE 1

Combined platelet scintigraphy and angiography

n=358   refs. 4, 5, 6, 7.

Visual Interpretation

		Positive	Negative
Angiogram	Positive	85	82
	Negative	25	16

Sensitivity 51%

Specificity 87%

REFERENCES

1. Eastcott H.H.G., Pckering G.W., Rob C. (1954) Reconstruction of internal carotid artery in a patient with intermittent attacks of hemiplegia. Lancet 11: 994-998.
2. Fisher C.M. (1959) Observations of the fundus oculi in tranjsient monocular blindness. Neurology 9: 333-347.
3. Davis H.H., Heaton W.A., Siegal B.A., Mathias C.J., Joist J.H., Sherman L.A.,Welch M.J. (1978) Scintigraphic detection of atherosclerotic lesions and venous thrombi in man by Indium-III-labelled platelets. Lancet 1, 1185-1188.
4. Goldman M., Leung J.O., Auckland A., Hawker R.J., Drolc Z., McCollum C.N. (1983) III-Indium platelet imaging, Doppler spectral analysis and angiography compared in patients with transient cerebral ischaemia. Stroke 14: 752-756.
5. Powers W.J. Siegal B.A., Davis H.H., Mathias C.J., Clark H.B., Welch M.J. (1982) Indium-III platelet scintigraphy in cerebro vascular disease. Neurology 32: 938-943.
6. Isaka Y., Kimura K., Yoneda S., Kusunoki M., Etani H., Yuama O., Tauda Y., Abe H. *1984) Platelet accumulation in carotid atherosclerotic lesions: semi-quantitative analysis with Indium-III-platelets and Technetium-99m. Human serum albumin. J. Nuc. Med. 25: 556-563.
7. Kessler Ch., Reuther R., Berentelg J., Kimmig B. (1983) The clinical use of platelet scintigraphy with III-In-oxine. J. Neurol. 229: 255-261.
8. Lusby R.J., Ferrell L.D., Englestad B.L., Price D.C., Lipton M.J., Stoney R.J. (1983) Vessel wall and Indium-iii-labelled platelet response to carotid endarterectomy. Surgery 93: 424-432.

INDIUM-111-PLATELET SCINTIGRAPHY IN SYMPTOMATIC AND ASYMPTOMATIC CAROTID ARTERY DISEASE. PRELIMINARY FINDINGS OF A PROSPECTIVE STUDY

E.B. Ringelstein[1], A. Wicke[2], M.Holken[1], G. Fiedler[1], C. Weiller[1], U. Bull[2]

Department of Neurology[1] (Head: Professor Dr.K.Poeck)

Department of Nuclear Medicine[2] (Head: Professor Dr. U.Bull)

Klinikum RWTH,
Technical University
D-5100 Aachen, West Germany.

INTRODUCTION

The natural history of carotid artery occlusive disease (CAOD0 is still not known well enough so as to provide reliable information about the risk of stroke in the individual patient (15). Decision making in performing carotid endarterectomy is made particularly difficult in the case of moderate and low-grade carotid artery lesions, since one must weigh out the risk of this invasive procedure on the one hand and the spontaneous course of the lesion on the other hand (1,7,10,11).

It is generally accepted that an acute thrombotic process superimposed on a soft or ulcerated plaque at the origin of the internal carotid artery (ICA) is indicative of an impending arterial embolic stroke and/or acute thrombotic occlusion of the vessel with all its hazardous consequences (6,9,18). However, currently available imaging techniques (Doppler flow imaging of the carotid bifurcation, high resolution B-mode imaging, cerebral angiography) are not reliable enough in detecting this critical stage of the disease (2,3) This is understandable, since fresh thrombotic material, due to its low echogenicity (19), is hardly visible during B-mode imaging, yet can be identified and imaged with the help of platelet scintigraphy (4.5.13.17). This scanning procedure is not primarily a morphological technique but instead provides functional information about thrombotic activity at circumscribed sites.

It would seem logical to perform a prospective, open, non-randomized study in patients with asymptomatic and asymptomatic COAD for several reasons: (1) A comparison between symptomatic and asymptomatic patients would provide data for estimating the sensitivity of the scintigraphic technique and would also allow clinical validation. (2) In the asymptomatic cohort, platelet scintigraphy would deliver

180

Ch. Kessler et al. (eds.), Clinical Application of Radiolabelled Platelets, 180–194.
© 1990 Kluwer Academic Publishers.

information about the general frequency and extent of obviously active thrombotic processes at the affected carotid bifurcation. Additionally, the scintigraphic findings could be correlated to the severity of the disease as well as to ultrasound plaque morphology. This approach would also allow the prospective clinical validation of platelet scintigraphy if the scintigraphic findings turned out to be correlated to the clinical outcome of the patients during prospective follow-up studies.

With this in mind, the authors have started the present investigation. The preliminary findings in 36 patients are described here.

PATIENT SELECTION AND EXAMINATION TECHNIQUES

Cohort A: Twenty-one consecutive patients with known asymptomatic carotid artery occlusive disease were recruited for platelet scintigraphy. Individuals with severe concomitant internal diseases were excluded. All patients were asked to give common consent after they and their practitioners had been carefully informed about method, risks and potential clinical value of Indium-111 platelet scintigraphy. The patients also had to fulfill the following prerequisites: (1) They had to be completely asymptomatic with respect to carotid territory symptoms both transient or permanent. (2) They were not to have been treated with anti-platelet agents, particularly acetylsalicylic acid (ASA) for at least 10-days prior to scanning. (3) All of them had to have either unilateral or bilateral CAOD. Previous detection of the lesions was carried out with the aid of continuous-wave Doppler studies and/or high resolution (7.5 MHz) B-mode imaging of the carotid bifurcation.

Cohort B: A group of 15 consecutive symptomatic patients were also examined. All of them suffered from transient or permanent strokes within the carotid artery territory and, simultaneously, had been proven to have occlusive disease of the internal carotid artery on the corresponding side. The ischemic attacks had all occurred within the last 2 months prior to platelet scintigraphy, most of them within 10 days before scanning. Furthermore, these patients had not taken any antiplatelet agents during the last 10 days before scanning.

In fact, all patients underwent careful clinical examination and history taking, continuous-wave Doppler sonography of the extracranial brain supplying arteries, 7.5 MHz B-mode imaging of the carotid bifurcations on both sides and, finally, Indium-111 labelled platelet scintigraphy.

Platelet labelling was performed according to a slightly modified technique which had recently been described by Kessler et al (13). Details are listed in Table 1. In summary, the platelets, after being concentrated and washed,

Table 1: Platelet Labelling Procedure

45 ml venous blood in 0.8% Na-Citrate

First centrifugation (blood): 60 G, 20 min --> PRP

Second centrifugation (PRP): 160 G, 10 min --> pellet I

Pellet I resuspended in 10 ml washing solution.
(washing solution = 0.9% NaCl + 0.8% Na-Citrate, 9:1)

Third centrifugation (washing sol.): 160 G, 10 min --> pellet II

Pellet II resuspended in 2 ml washing solution.

Labelled with approximately 18 MBq (=approx.0.5 mCi) 111-In-Oxine

Incubation for 30 min and dilution with 4 ml PPP

Intravenous injection

PPP = platelet poor plasma
PRP = platelet rich plasma

were labelled with 111-Indium-oxine. The quantity of the tracer was calculated in such a way that, finally, a radiotracer dose of some 18 MBq (approximately 0..5 mCi) was injected intravenously into each patient.

The scanning procedure was performed with a computer-assisted, large field gamma camera with medium energy collimators. The 247 KeV peak with a window setting of 20 percent was used. Scans were obtained after 24 hours at 3 different projections (anterior and both lateral) during an acquisition time of 20 minutes each.

Findings during B-mode imaging were categorized according to the echogenicity of the plaques using the subgroups "hard", "soft", and "non-classifiable" lesions. During continuous-wave Doppler sonography, pathologic findings were classified as non-stenosing plaque (= < 50%, also considering the B-scan findings), medium-grade (= 50-70%) stenosis, high-grade (= 80-90%) stenosis, subtotal (= > 90%) stenosis and occlusion.

The routine quality check of the labelled platelets included two different procedures. (1) Measurement of the recovery in vitro, i.e. the number of platelets was counted immediately before intravenous injection and was compared with the platelet content of the platelet rich plasma (PRP). (2) Functional vitality check: ADP-induced platelet aggregation of the labelled platelets was performed with 0.5 molar ADP and was compared with the aggregation of non-labelled thrombocytes from the initial PRP. Details of this platelet aggregation measurement will be described elsewhere.

RESULTS

In 21 <u>asymptomatic</u> patients, a total of 37 ICA and/or ECA (=external carotid artery) lesions were found. The degrees of the 26 ICA lesions are listed in Table 2.

When correlating the degree of the asymptomatic internal carotid artery lesion to the findings during Indium-111 platelet scintigraphy, the ratio of positive findings increased with increasing severity of the stenosis, with the exception that complete ICA occlusions did not reveal any visible platelet accumulation whatsoever (Table 3). Four out of 11 ECA stenoses were also positive, however, three of then were associated with ICA or common carotid artery lesions. A total of 23% of the carotid bifurcations with asymptomatic occlusive disease were positive during Indium platelet scintigraphy, an illustrative example is shown in Figure 1.

Fifteen patients had 16 symptomatic carotid lesions. They had experienced amaurosis fugax (N=9), transient sensorimotor hemiparesis (TIA) (N=3), and completed strokes with hemiparesis and/or aphasia (N=4)

Scintigraphic scans were positive in 38% of the symptomatic carotid lesions (Fig. 2: Table 4). Within different subgroups of ICA lesions, the numbers of patients

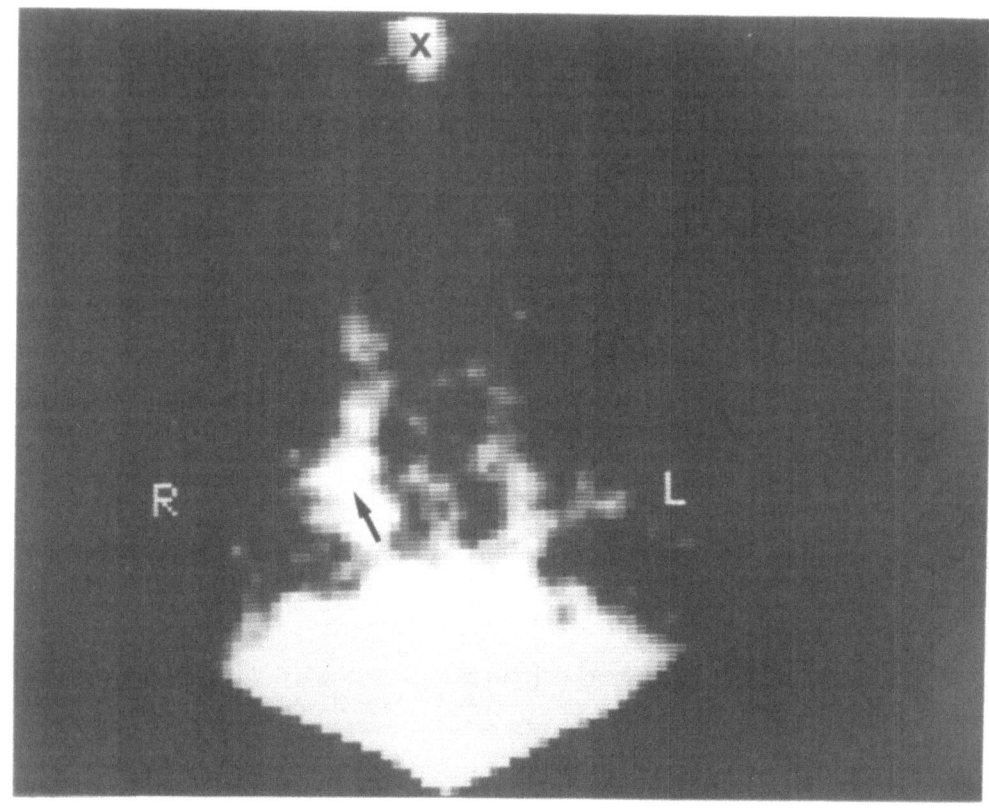

Fig 1: A.P.-view of the platelet-111 scintigram of a
patient with an asymptomatic carotid artery
disease on the right side. The arrow indicates
the hot spot. X corresponds to the nasopharyngeal
space.

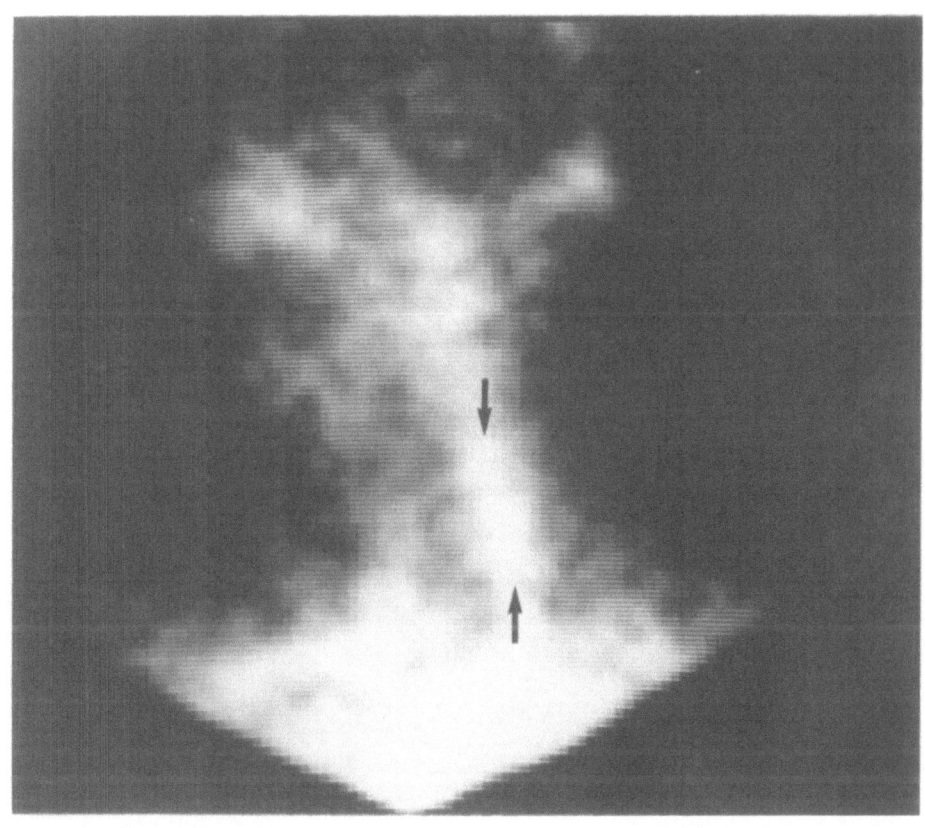

Fig 2: Lateral view of a positive platelet accumulation
in the left carotid arteries. The hot spot in
indicated by arrows.

Table 2: Number and Degrees of Asymptomatic Carotid Bifurcation
Lesions

---

37 ICA/ECA lesions
- 11 ECA lesions
- 26 ICA lesions

26 ICA lesions

-	non-stenosing	(< 50%)	1
-	medium degree	(50-70%)	10
-	high degree	(80-90%)	7
-	subtotal	(>90%)	4
-	occlusions	(100%)	4

26

ICA = internal carotid artery
ECA = external carotid artery

Table 3: In-111-Platelet Scintigraphy Findings in Asymptomatic
Internal Carotid Artery Lesions

Type of lesions	No.	positive	negative
non-stenosing ICA plaque	1	1	-
ICA medium degree stenosis	10	1**	9
ICA high grade stenosis	7	2	5
ICA subtotal stenosis	4	2*	2
ICA occlusion	4	-	4
	26	6 (23%)	20
ECA lesions	11	4 (3***)	7
"progressive" ICA lesions	3	1	2

*   One case associated with ECA stenosis

**   "progressive" lesion

***   Associated with CCA/ICA lesions (70% and subtotal ICA
       stenoses, CCA-Plaque)

Table 4: In-111-Platelet Scans in 16 <u>Symptomatic</u> Internal Carotid
          Artery Lesions

Type of lesions	No.	positive	negative
non-stenosing plaque	8	3	5
medium-grade stenosis (50-70%)	2	1	1
high-grade stenosis (80-90%)	2*	1	1
subtotal stenosis	2	-	2
occlusion	2	1	1
	16	6 (=38%)**	10

*   In one case with additional 90% ECA stenosis

**   One additional positive scan on the asymptomatic side
     with a 60% ICA stenosis

with positive scintigraphic findings were too small to draw any further conclusions.

When plaque morphology during B-mode scanning was correlated to the scintigraphic findings, a striking, though not significant, accumulation of positive scans within the subgroup of soft plaques was found in the asymptomatic group. There was only one positive scan among four hard and eight non-classifiable plaques. This trend, however, could not be confirmed among the symptomatic patients (Table 5).

Recovery in vitro revealed values of 40 - 50% in all cases. Functional vitality as demonstrated during ADP-induced platelet aggregation, was found to be intact in the vast majority of the cases. Data were not corrected in the case of a few patients where ADP-induced platelet aggregation was clearly disturbed.

DISCUSSION

The present report has a preliminary character, and, due to the limited number of cases, conclusions can only be drawn with caution. The ratio of positive findings was different in the subgroup of asymptomatic or symptomatic patients with a clearly higher number of positive scans in the latter group. However, due to the small numbers of patients, this difference was not statistically significant. From a clinical point of view, Indium-111 platelet scintigraphy does not allow one to differentiate sufficiently between symptomatic and asymptomatic carotid artery disease with respect to practical applicability. This means that the sensitivity of the method for the detection of actually active, i.e. symptomatic carotid artery lesions is not much higher than for the detection of any type of carotid lesion at all including the asymptomatic ones.

In comparison with currently available literature (4,5,13,14,16), the amount of positive platelet findings in the symptomatic group is relatively low. Other authors have found positive scans in 38 to 75% of the cases (Table 6) However, the lower amount of positive scans in this study might in part be attributed to selection artifacts. These are: (1) a relatively long period between the occurences of the last stroke symptoms and the performance of platelet scintigraphy. A comparably low incidence of positive platelet scans has also been found by Isaka et al. (12) in patients who also had relatively long intervals between the last ischemic attack or stroke and scanning (Table 6). (2) Nearly all patients had been pretreated with ASA and had experienced only a short interruption of ASA therapy of 10-day duration prior to platelet scintigraphy. It is known from the literature that ASA treatment has a long-lasting and irreversible effect on platelet function. It is unclear, however, whether this would only prevent "adult" labelled platelets to accumulate at the site of carotid artery thrombosis or also fresh vital platelets recruited

190

Table 5: Indium-111 Scintigraphy Findings Correlated with B-Scan
Plaque Morphology

	Plaque-morphology	No.	positive	negative	
	hard	1	-	1	
SY	mixed	7	2	5	N.S.* (P=1.0)
	soft	12	2	10	
	non-classifiable	2	1	1	
		22	5	17	
	hard	3	-	3	
	mixed	11	2	9	N.S.* (P=0.53)
AS	soft	15	7	8	
	non-classifiable	6	-	6	
		35	9	26	

SY = symptomatic ICA lesions

AS = asymptomatic ICA lesions

*   Fisher`s exact test

Table 6: Positive Platelet Scintigrams in Carotid Artery Disease

Authors	Type of lesion	positive platelet scans	
		N	%
Isaka et al 1984 (DIT)	34 carotid bifur-cations with angio-graphically proven occlusive disease	clearly positive N=13 probably positive N=22	38 65
Kessler et al 1984a (SIT)	20 symptomatic carotid bifur-cations	positive N=11	55
(DIT)	"	positive N=8	45
Kessler et al 1984b (DIT)	8 symptomatic carotid bifur-cations in amaurosis fugax	positive N=6	75
Davis et al 1980 (SIT)	33 symptomatic patients * 16 angiographically proven carotid lesions **	positive N = 16 positive N = 12	48 75
Powers et al 1982 (SIT)	21 symptomatic carotid lesions * 75 angiographically abnormal carotid arteries *	not specified positive N = 32	43

Table 6: (continued)

Authors	Type of lesion	positive platelet scans	
		N	%
Goldman et al 1983	25 (20```) symptomatic carotid bifurcations **/***/****	positive N = 16	64
(SIT)	14``` asymptomatic ICA lesions **/****	positive N = 17	50
Present study	26 asymptomatic ICA lesions	positive N = 6	23
(SIT)	16 symptomatic ICA lesions	positive N = 6	38

*	Large proportion of patients receiving aspirin and/or anticoagulant therapy
**	In the same patients
***	No. of abnormal findings during Doppler ultrasound and/or angiography
****	Two positive scans with no detectable arterial lesion

DIT = dual isotope technique, SIT = single isotope technique from the bone marrow (8).

Although our experience is still very limited, the findings suggest that the proportion of positive platelet scintigraphy findings increases with the severity of the arterial lesions. The highest ratio of positive scans was found among the subtotal ICA stenoses. By contrast. complete occlusions were found to be negative during PSC. This has already been described by other (13). Presumably, transportation of the labelled platelets to the site of actual thrombosis is no longer possible in these cases as the thrombotic process takes place at the downstream end of the thrombus, and/or the free edges of the thrombotic material have already been completely re-endothelialized.
A relationship between plaque morphology during B-mode imaging and pathologic platelet accumulation during platelet scintigraphy became suggestive during this study. Particularly, soft plaques in the asymptomatic group seem to react positively. The findings in the symptomatic patients are inconclusive, but a tendency is also visible in that hard and non-classifiable plaques are non-reactive with labelled platelets.

In conclusion, platelet scintigraphy seems to be a promising tool for the visualisation of otherwise non-detectable acute thrombosis superimposed on silent or symptomatic carotid artery plaques. It is not yet clear, however, whether these findings have a prognostic clinical meaning in that the positive scans are indicative of a higher stroke risk. This is to be demonstrated during the oncoming prospective clinical follow-up of the asymptomatic cohort.

REFERENCES

1. Barnett HJW, Plum F, Walton JN, Carotid endarterectomy. An expression of concern. Stroke 6: Editorial 941-943 (1984)
2. Boespflug OJM: Ultrasonography of supra-aortic trunks. Neuroradiology 27: 544-547 (1985)
3. Comerota AJ, Cranley JJ, Cook SE, Real-time B-mode carotid imaging in diagnosis of cerebrovascular disease. Surgery 89: 718-729 (1981)
4. Davis HH, Siegel BA, Sherman LA, Heaton WA, Naidich TP, Joist JH, Welch MJ: Scintigraphic detection of carotid atherosclerosis with Indium-111-labelled autologous platelets. Circulation 61: 982-988 (1980)
5. Goldman M, Leung JO, Aukland A, Hawker RJ, Drolc Z, McCollum CN: 111-Indium platelet imaging . Doppler spectral analysis and angiography compared in patients with transient cerebral ischemia. Stroke 14: 752-756 (1983)
6. Gunning AJ, Pickering GW, Robb-Smith AHT, Russel RR: Mural thrombosis of the internal carotid artery and

subsequent embolism. Q.J.Med.33: 155-195 (1964)

7. Guse F, Weiller C, Ringelstein EB, Zur Abhangigkeit des Hirninfarktrisikos vom Schweregrad Okkludierender Carotis Interna Lasionen. Nervenarzt 1987 in press

8. Harker LA, Fuster V: Pharmacology of platelet inhibitors. J.Amer.Coll Cardiol. 8: 21B-32B (1986)

9. Harrison MJ, Marshall J: The finding of thrombus at carotid endarterectomy and its relationship to the timing of surgery. Br.J.Surg. 64: 511-512 (1977)

10. Imparato AM, Riles TS, Mintzer R, Baumann G: The importance of hemorrhage in the relationship between gross morphologic characteristics and cerebral symptoms in 376 carotid artery plaques. Ann Surg.197: 195-203 (1983)

11. Imparator AM: Presidential address: The carotid bifurcation plaque - a model for the study of atherosclerosis. J.Vasc.Surg. 3: 249-255 (1986)

12. Isaka Y, Kimura K, Yoneda S, Kusunoki M, Etani H, Uyama O, Tsuda Y, Abe H: Platelet accumulation in carotid atherosclerotic lesions: Semiquantitative analysis with Indium-111 platelets and Technetium-99m human serum albumin. J.Nucl.Med.25: 556-563 (1984)

13. Kessler Ch, Reuhther R, Kimmig B, Pietzsch T: Dual isotope scintigraphy in stroke patients. Neuroradiology 26: 113-117 (1984a)

14. Kessler Ch, Reuther R, Rosch M: Dual isotope carotid scintigraphy in patients with amaurosis fugax attacks. Eur.Arch Psychiatr Neurol Sci 234: 106-111 (1984b)

15. Moore WS, Boren C, Malone JM, Roon AJ,Eisenberg R, Goldstone J, Mani R: Natural history of nonstenotic, asymptomatic ulcerative lesions of the carotid artery. Arch.Surg.113: 1352-1359 (1978)

16. Powers WJ, Siegel BA, Davis HH, Mathias CJ, Clark HB, Welch MJ: Indium-111 platelet scintigraphy in cerebrovascular disease. Neurology 32: 938-943 (1982)

17. Powers, WJ: In-111-platelet scintigraphy: Carotid atherosclerosis and stroke (Teaching Editorial) J.Nucl. Med.25: 626-629 (1984)

18. Ringelstein EB, Zeumer H, Angelou D: The pathogenesis of strokes from internal carotid artery occlusion. Diagnostic and therapeutical implications. Stroke 14: 867-875 (1983)

10. Wetzner SM, Kiser LC, Bezreh IS: Duplex ultrasound imaging: Vascular applications. Radiology 150: 507-514 (1984)

RADIOLABELLED PLATELET INTERACTIONS WITH DAMAGED ENDOTHELIUM
IN THE CAROTID ARTERY OF RABBITS

Meek A.C., Galvin D.A.J., Harper R.A., McCollum C.H.

Department of Surgery
Charing Cross and Westminster Medical School
Fulham Palace Road
London W6 BRF

INTRODUCTION

Animals have provided models in the field of research
into platelet kinetics and atherosclerosis with various
methods used to inflict endothelial damage on the arterial
wall. Isolation of the carotid artery with standardised
ischaemic time was advocated by Buchanan & Hirsch (3) and
balloon catheter damage has been used in the rabbit aorta
(5) and carotid artery (9). Constant infusion of
homocystine has been shown to cause endothelial damage (6)
as does dietary induced hyperchlorestolaemia (1). Carotid
interposition vein grafting produces a reliable model
producing intimal hyperplasia, but this resulted in a high
operative mortality (8).
    We have developed an inexpensive rabbit model to
evaluate platelet interaction with the damaged arterial wall
and have measured radiolabelled platelet deposition
following a standard intimal trauma. Effective methods of
labelling rabbit platelets with III-Indium oxine have been
described with minimal damage to the labelled cells (10, 11,
12). A proportion of the isotope is localised in the dense
bodies and to a lesser extent in the alpha granules of
platelets. This contrasts with human platelets which carry
the radionucleotide in the cytoplasm of the cell.
Theoretically this may result in the release of isotope
following platelet activation and aggregation, invalidating
results of platelet deposition (2), however sufficient
radioactivity remains in the aggregated platelet to allow in
vivo assessment of platelet deposition on the arterial wall
in the rabbit model, especially in short term experiments.
    It was the purpose of this study to develop and assess
a rabbit model of carotid intimal trauma using III-In
labelled platelets. The effect of low dose aspirin and
dipyridamole has been evaluated on these parameters.

195

Ch. Kessler et al. (eds.), Clinical Application of Radiolabelled Platelets, 195–203.
© 1990 *Kluwer Academic Publishers.*

MATERIALS AND METHODS

OPERATIVE PROCEDURE

Twenty young adult New Zealand white rabbits (2-2,5 kg) were randomised to receive either placebo or aspirin (ASA) 5mg/kg daily and dipyridamole (DPM) 5mg/kg twice daily. Drugs were administered by oro-gastric tube feeding, starting 48 hours prior to operation and continuing until the end of the study. Under general anaesthetic both carotid arteries were exposed over a distance of 2 cms. On one side, the carotid artery was crushed over a distance of 1cm for a 3 minute period using a serrated compression G clamp. The artery on the contralateral side was mobilised in a similar way, but left undamaged and used as a control. The wound was then closed and the animals allowed to recover from anaesthesia.

III-IN PLATELET LABELLING

Platelets were obtained from 30mls of blood from one donor rabbit which produced sufficient labelled cells for five study animals. This was anticoagulated with 4mls of 3.4% sodium acid citrate and centrifuged at 200G for 10 minutes to obtain platelet rich plasma (PRP). The PRP was then centrifuged again at 6400 to produce a platelet pellet and the resulting supernatant retained. The platelet pellet was resuspended in 5mls of calcium free Tyrode's solution with 70ng of PGE-1. This suspension was incubated with 250uCi of III-Indium oxine for 60 seconds and the radiolabelling reaction stopped by the addition of the plasma supernatant as remaining free nucleotide was bound to plasma proteins. Labelled platelets were then separated from the supernatant by centrifugation at 640G for 10 minutes and the platelets resuspended in 10mls of Tyrode's solution. Labelling efficiency was assessed by expressing the activity bound to labelled platelets as a percentage of the total activity in the platelets and supernatant. Cell function was confirmed by platelet aggregation studies. Each animal was then reinjected with III-In platelets containing approximately 50uCi activity, via the ear vein.

ASSESSMENT OF RADIOLABELLED PLATELET UPTAKE

Twenty four hours after reinjection of radiolabelled platelets, the animals were reanaesthetised and both carotid arteries excised. A 5ml blood sample was withdrawn for estimation of circulating blood activity and the animals were sacrificed. The excised carotid arterial lumen were cut to a length of 2cms with a 5mm section of normal artery proximal and distal to the traumatised segment. Reference undamaged arteries were removed, and prepared in an identical fashion. Radioactivity was estimated by well counter and the specimens weighed.

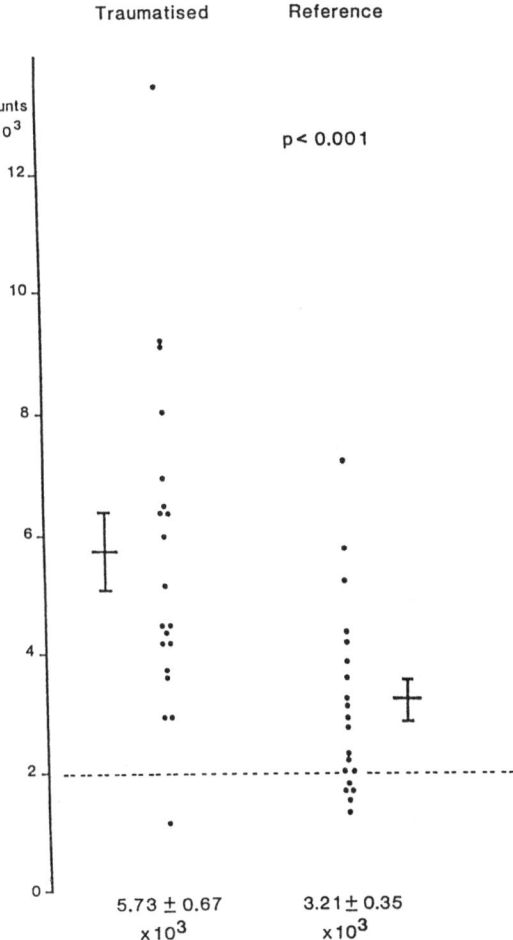

Fig 1   Specimen radioactivity comparing the traumatised
          carotid artery with the undamaged reference vessel

There were no differences due to the recurring or non-recurring character of the neurological event. Out of the group of 24 patients with negative PSC, 9 patients had no previous attack, 7 patients had a single attack and 8 patients had several attacks in their history. From the 15 patients with positive PSC, 6 patients had no previous neurological attack in their history, 5 patients had 1 and 4 patients had several attacks (see Fig. 2).

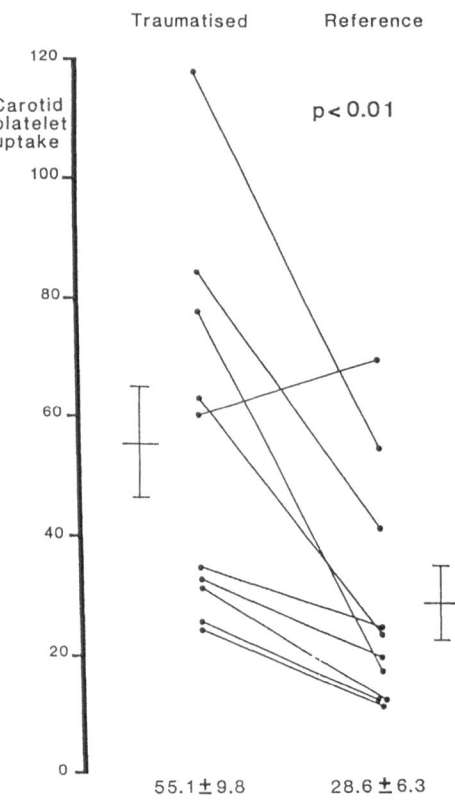

Figure 2

Fig 2   Carotid platelet uptake in animals receiving
          placebo

Carotid platelet uptake was estimated by expressing the counts from each specimen per gram as a percentage of the counts in 1ml of circulating blood at sacrifice.

Carotid uptake ratio was calculated by expressing the activity measured from the traumatised artery as a ratio of that obtained from the contralateral reference artery.

RESULTS

All the animals tolerated the surgery and on excision both the traumatised and reference arteries were patent.

SPECIMEN RADIOACTIVITY

Radioactivity counts from the reference artery of 3.2-/+ 0.3 x 10^3 were marginally higher than background at 2.0-/+ 0.07 x 10^3, but were much lower than that from the traumatised artery at 5.7 -/+ 0.7 x 10^3 (p<0.001) (Fig. 1). Counts expressed per gram of tissue were consistently higher in the traudmatised artery at 4.79 -/+ 0.39 x 10^5 compared to 3.11 -/+ 0.37 x 10^5 from the reference side (p<0.001).

CAROTID PLATELET UPTAKE

In the placebo group carotid platelet uptake showed consistently higher platelet accumulation on the traumatised artery of 55.1 -/+ 9.8 percent compared to 28.6 -/+ 6.3 percent from the reference side (p<0.01) (Fig. 2). This difference was seen to a lesser extent in the animals treated with aspirin and dipyridamole with platelet uptake of 43.7 -/+ 6.0 and 14.5 -/+ 5.3 percent respectively (p=0.05) (Fig. 3). There was no statistical difference in platelet uptake on the reference arteries in the treated and control groups at 34.5 -/+ 5.3 and 28.6 -/+ 6.3 respectively.

CAROTID UPTAKE RATIO

Carotid Uptake Ratio was significantly reduced in those animals treated with ASA+DPM at 1.35 -/+ 0.13 compared to 2.2 -/+ 0.29 in the placebo group (p<0.02) (Fig. 4).

DISCUSSION

A crush injury not only damages the intima, but will expose elements of the media to circulating blood allowing platelets to adhere to the collagen in this layer. Early platelet activity may also be expected in the arterial wall and tissue of the wound, but this should be stable by 24 hours. Intraluminal platelet uptake will continue until intimal regeneration occurs by approximately 2 weeks (6), but will be most intense in the days immediately following trauma. This is regarded as a dynamic process with

200

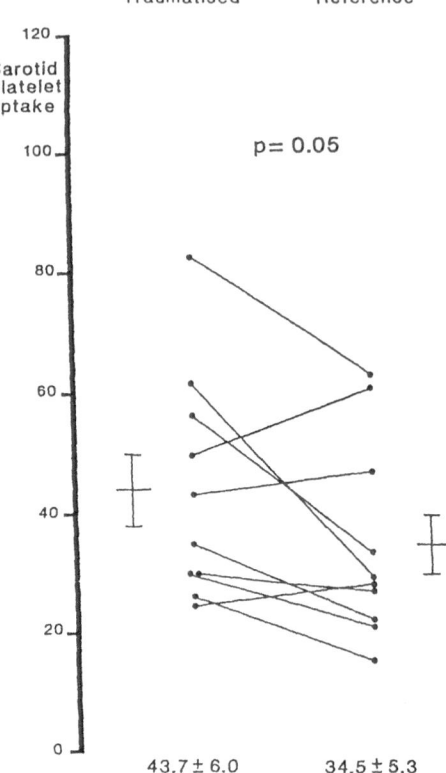

Figure 3

Fig 3   Carotid platelet uptake in animals receiving
           aspirin and dipyridamole

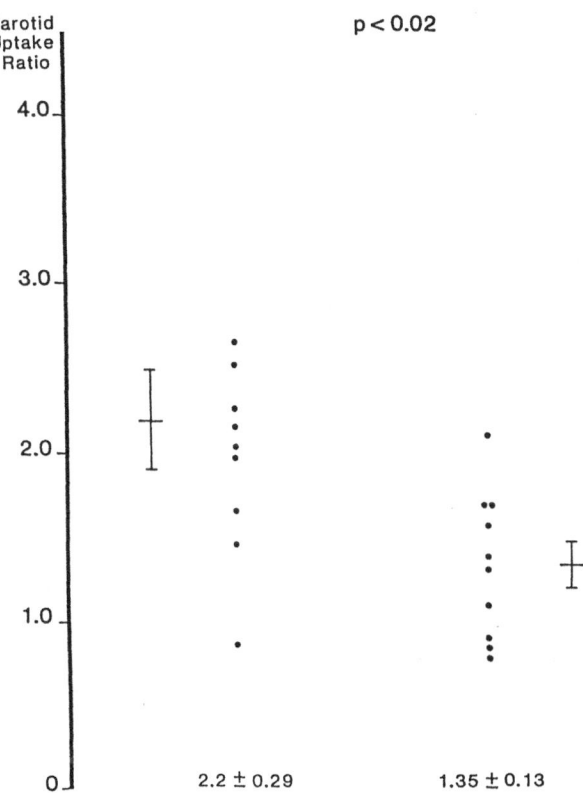

Figure 4

Fig 4   Comparison of Carotid Uptake Ratio in animals
          receiving placebo and platelet inhibitory therapy

continuing interaction between the circulating platelets, aggregated platelets and the connective tissue in the vessel wall. Using the contralateral artery as a reference allows for platelets adhering to the adventitia following mobilisation. As rabbit platelets carry a proportion of the isotope in the secretory granules some activity will be lost on aggregation. Part of this released radioactivity may be retained in the arterial wall as other alpha granule constituents have been identified within the vessel was following platelet deposition (4). Platelet uptake measured as Carotid Uptake Ratio is reduced in those animals receiving antiplatelet drugs. This suggests that the inhibition of thromboxane synthesis in platelets that results from acetylation of cyclooxygenase is more important than the influence of prostacyclin production in endothelium (7).

This model demonstrates a reproducible platelet response to carotid intimal trauma and may be useful in the assessment of platelets drugs. Oral aspirin at 5mg/kg reduced platelet accumulation in these areas of intimal damage.

REFERENCES

1. Armstrong M.L., Peterson R.E., Hoak J.C., Megan M.B., Cheng P.H., Clarke W.R.: Arterial platelet accumulation in experimental hyperchloesterolaemia. Atherosclerosis 1980; 36: 89-100.
2. Baker K.D., Eakins M.N., Pay G.F., White A.M.: Subcellular localization of III-In human and rabbit platelets. Blood 1982; 59 (2): 351-359.
3. Buchanan M.R., Hirsh J.: Effect of Aspirin in Salicylate on Platelet-Vessel Wall Interactions in Rabbits. Arteriosclerosis 1984; 4: 403-406.
4. Goldberg I.D., Stemerman M.B., Haudin R.I.: Vascular permeation of platelet factor 4 after endothelial injury. Science 1980; 209: 611-612.
5. Grove H.M., Kinlough-Rathbone R.L., Cazenaue J.P., Dejana E., Richardson M., Mustard J.F.: Effect of dipyridamole and prostacyclin on rabbit platelet adherence in vitro and in vivo. J. Lab. Clin. Med. 1982; 99: 548-558.
6. Harker L.A., Ross R., Slichter S.J., Scott C.R.: Homocystine-induced arteriosclerosis. The role of endothelial cell injury and platelet response in its genesis. J. Clin. Invest. 1976; 58: 731-741.
7. Kelton J.G., Hirsh H., Carter C.J., Buchanan M.R.: Thrombogenic effect of high-dose aspirin in rabbit. J. Clin. Invest. 1978; 62: 892-895.
8. Murday A.J., Gershlick A.H., Syndercombe-Court Y.D., Ledingham S.J., Betts N.J., Lewis C.T., Mills P.G.: Intimal hyperplasia in arterial autogenous vein grafts: a new animal model. Cardiovasc. Res. 1983; 17: 446-451.
9. Reidy M.A., Clowes A.W., Schwartz S.N.: Endothelial

regeneration : Inhibition of endothelial regrowth in arteries of rat and rabbit. Lab. Invest. 1983; 49: 569-575.

10. Schmidt K.G., Rasmussen J.W.: Labelling of human and rabbit platelets with III-Indium-oxine complex. Scand. J. Haematol. 1979; 97-106.

11. Schmidt K.G., Rasmussen J.W., Lorentzen M.: Function and morphology of III-In labelled platelets. Haemostasis 1982; 11: 193-203.

12. Wistow B.W., Grossmann Z.D., MdAfee J.G., Subramanian G., Henderson R.W., Roskopf M.L.: Labelling of platelets with oxine complexes of Tc-99m and In-111. Part. 1. in vitro studies and survival in the rabbit. Clin. Sci. 1978; 19: 483-487.

HEALING FOLLOWING CAROTID ENDARTERECTOMY MEASURED BY 111-IN PLATELET UPTAKE

AC. Meek, AD Chidlow, PM Jarvis, CN McCollum

INTRODUCTION

With recent improvements in prosthetic materials for arterial replacement or bypass and the widespread use of autologous vein,the indication for endarterectomy has progressively diminished. The carotid artery is the only vessel in which endarterectomy has been consistently retained as the operation of choices in the treatment of atherosclerotic disease.

Platelet deposition on the endarterectomised surface may cause thrombosis and the interaction between platelet derived growth factor and arterial smooth muscle cells has been suggested as a mechanism for the development of intimal hyperplasia and restenosis (1). This concept has defied further study as platelet accumulation has not previously been detectable in vivo. The development of 111-Indium platelet labelling techniques allows this problem to be investigated and has been shown to image prosthetic grafts in dogs (8) and in patients (5,6).

Carotid platelet uptake has been measured in patients to assess the thrombogenic characteristics of atherosclerotic lesions at the bifurcation (2,4) but we wondered whether this technique could also be used to evaluate platelet kinetics following operation.

In this study carotid platelet uptake following carotid endarterectomy was investigated in patients both immediately following surgery and at two months.

PATIENTS AND METHODS

Ten patients undergoing unilateral carotid endarterectomy were studied with 6 men and 4 women of a mean age 66.7 years (range 47-79 years). Standard endarterectomy was performed under general anaesthesia with heparin 5000 units administered prior to cross clamping the common carotid artery. A longitudinal arteriotomy was used in all cases and the arteriotomy was closed by direct suture with continuous 6/0 Prolene.

Autologous platelets from 26mls of blood were prepared on the second postoperative day by a method similar to that of Hawker et al (7) and labelled with approximately 200 Ci 111-Indium oxine. Carotid platelet uptake was measured by gamma camera two hours following reinjection and again at 24

204

Ch. Kessler et al. (eds.), Clinical Application of Radiolabelled Platelets, 204–209.
© 1990 *Kluwer Academic Publishers.*

and 48 hours. The labelling procedure was repeated 8 weeks later to assess platelet accumulation as intimal healing occurs. Using computer analysis of the gamma camera images, counts from the operated artery were compared as a ratio to those from the non operated side and expressed as the Carotid Uptake Ratio (CUR).

LABELLING EFFICIENCY

In the 10 early labelling procedures mean (+/-) efficiency was 93.6 +/- 0.8 percent with a mean injected activity of 258 +/- 16.4 μCi which was similar to efficiency of 94.5 +/- 0.5 percent and injected activity of 222.3 +/- 13.9 μCi at 2 months. In all cases labelled platelets showed a satisfactory response to ADP.

GAMMA CAMERA IMAGING

Three days after surgery the counts per gamma camera cell, calculated from an area of interest over the operated artery, were 46.3 +/- 4.3 per pixel. This was significantly higher than 38.6 +/- 3.9 on the non operated side (p<0.001) (Fig.1). By expressing the radioactivity from the operated artery as a reference ratio, the mean CUR was calculated at 1.22 +/- 0.04 in the early postoperative period.

At 2 months the counts per cell over the operated artery had fallen to 38,9 +/- 3,2 and were now equivalent to the reference counts of 39.1 +/- 3.1 (Fig.2). Mean CUR at 2 months was calculated at 1.01 +/-0.06. The comparison between CUR at 2 days and 2 months showed a significant decrease in carotid platelet uptake in the later examination (p<0.01) (Fig 3).

Radiolabelled platelet uptake was seen by an independent observer in 87 of the 10 early scans but was detected in only 2 patients at eight weeks. Both these latter patients had a persistently raised CUR indicating continued platelet accumulation.

DISCUSSION

These results demonstrate the accumulation of radiolabelled platelets at the site of carotid endarterectomy 72 hours after surgery. Early gamma camera pictures consistently showed higher levels of radioactivity on computer analysis when compared to the contralateral reference artery. Inaccuracies may occur as there may be thrombogenic atheromatous disease in the contralateral artery which has been used as our reference. It is likely however, that this platelet uptake on atheromatous plaque is relatively small especially as it is only in cases of atheromatous ulcer that gamma emissions are high for detection (4). The intensity of platelet uptake with such disease is recognisable on imaging.

The reduced thrombogenicity in 8 out of 10 cases at two

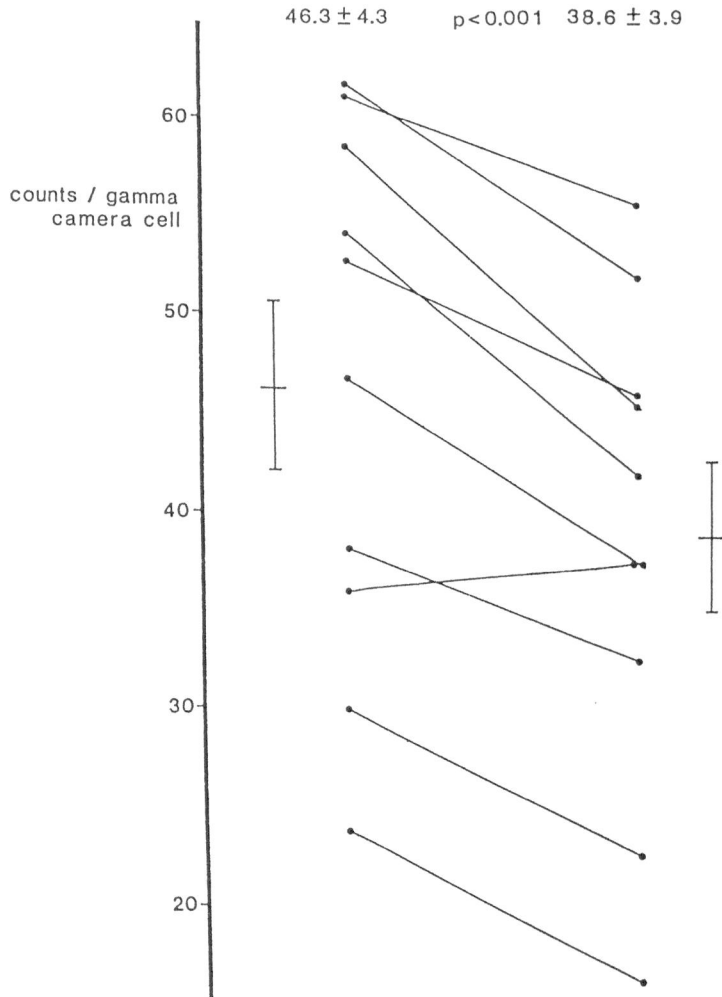

Fig.1   Comparison of counts per gamma camera cell from the operated and non-operated carotid artery 3 days after endarterectomy

ENDARTERECTOMY   REFERENCE

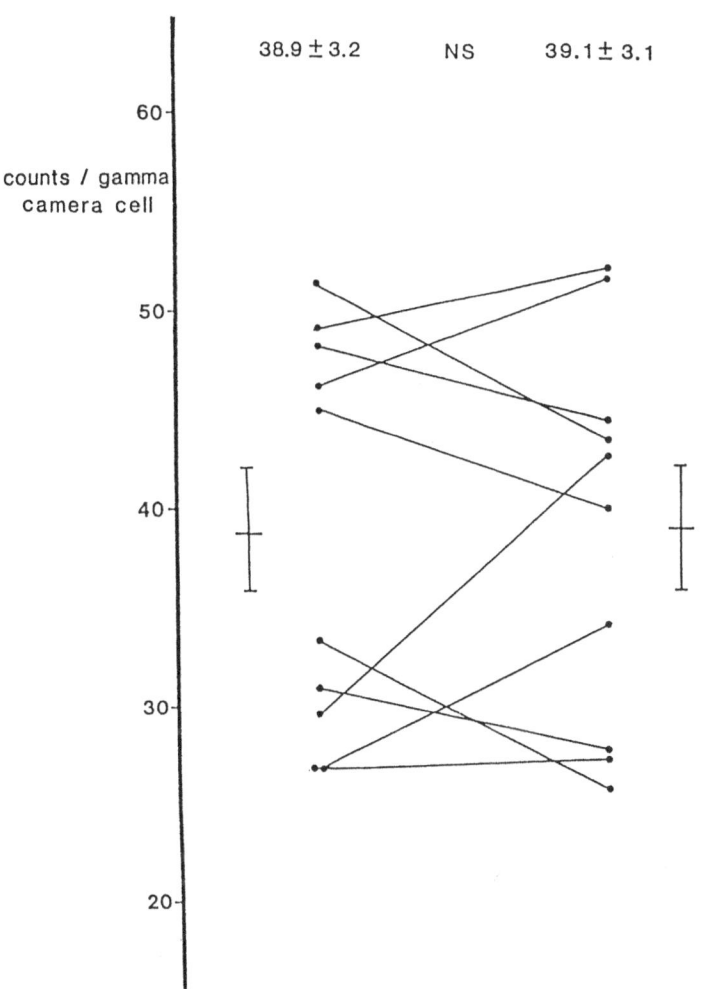

Fig.2   Counts per gamma camera cell from the operated and non-operated arteries 2 months following surgery

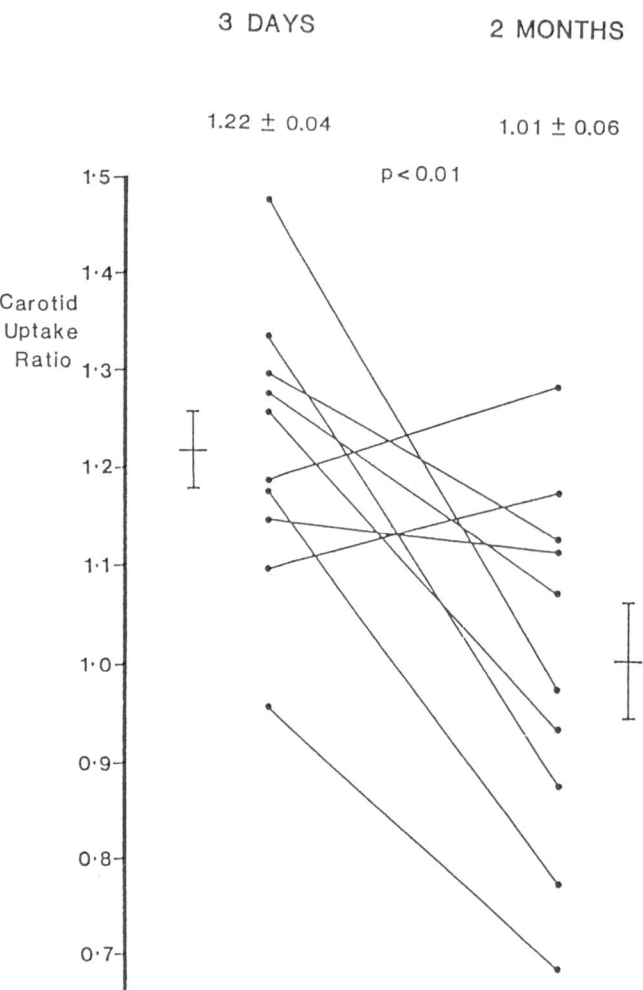

Fig.3   Carotid Uptake Ratio recorded 3 days and 2 months
         after surgery

months suggests that the endarterectomy has healed with neointimal covering the surface. This is consistent with the findings of French and Rewcastle (3) whose post-mortem study showed that the inflammatory reaction and mural thrombus associated with the trauma of endarterectomy had resolved by 30 days. Only 2 patients had consistently raised CUR at 2 months at 1.29 and 1.18. This may be caused by incomplete healing of the endarterectomy and resulting intraluminal thrombus could progress to stenosis or occlusion.

REFERENCES

1. Das MB, Hertzer NR, Ratcliff MD, O'Hara RJ, Beven EG: Recurrent Carotid Stenosis. Ann Surg. 1985; 202: 28-35

2. Davis HH, Siegel BA, Sherman LA, Heaton WA, Naidich TP, Joist JH, Welch MJ: Scintigraphic Detection of Carotid Atherosclerosis with Indium 111 labelled Autologous Platelets. Cir 1980; 61 (5): 982-988

3. French BN, Rewcastle NB: Sequential Morphological changes at the site of Carotid Endarterectomy. J. Neurosurg 1974: 41; 745-754

4. Goldman M, Leung JO, Auckland A, Hawker RJ, Drolc Z, McCollum CN: 111-Indium Platelet Imaging, Doppler Spectral Analysis and Angiography in Patients with Transient Cerebral Ischaemia. Stroke 1983; 14 (5) 752-756

5. Goldman M, Norcott HC, Hawker RJ, Drolc Z, McCollum CN: Platelet Accumulation on Mature Dacron Grafts in Man. Br.J.Surg.1982; 69 (Suppl): 538-540

6. Goldman M, Norcott HC, Hawker RJ, Hail C, Drolc Z, McCollum CN: Femoro-popliteal Bypass Grafts - an Isotope Technique allowing in vivo Comparison of Thrombogenicity. Br.J.Surg. 1982: 69 (7): 380-382

7. Hawker RJ, Hawker LM, Wilkinson AR: Indium (111-In)-labelled human platelets: Optimal method. Clin.Sci. 1980; 58: 243-248

8. Mergerman J, Christenson JT, Hanel KC, Strauss HW, Abbott WM: Imaging vascular grafts in vivo with Indium-111-labelled platelets, Ann.Surg. 1983: 198: 178-184.

Tc-99m-LABELED AUTOLOGOUS PLATELETS AS SCREENING IN PATIENTS WITH CEREBROVASCULAR DISEASE

M.Brenner *, R.Berberich **, A. Haass *, G. Huber ***,
H. Jäger

* Neurologie
** Nuklearmedizin
***Neuroradiologie
Universität des Saarlandes;6650 Homburg/Saar.

INTRODUCTION

In the recent years platelet scintigraphy with Indium-111 labeled autolologous platelets has been used in the detection of atherosclerotic lesions in extracranial feeding vessels (4-12,14,15). The aim of this study was to determine the reliability of the platelet scintigraphy with different gamma radiator, Tc-99 m-phytate, in the detection of atherosclerotic lesions, using a large collective of patients with cerebrovascular diseases as test group. Tc-99 m-phytate has the advantage of having a lower radiation load than indium-111 and is also not as expensive.

METHOD

45 ml of blood were withdrawn and the platelets labeled using the method described by Berberich et al. (1.3). The biological reaction of platelets labeled in this fashion was identical to that of 51 Cr labeled thrombocytes examined in healthy people. An occipital cerebral perfusion scan was followed by laterally right and left, occipital and frontal stationary images 10-30 min. p.i. and 2-3 hours p.i.
12 of the 149 examined patients, with a mean age of 49,9 ± 15,6 years and with no cerebral vascular process, served as control group. A second group consisted of 6 patients aged 44,7 ± 11,7 years, in whom a differential diagnosis could not be accurately performed. A third group comprised 131 patients with a mean age of 51,7 ± 11,8 years with a cerebrovascular disease. 39 patients had one or more transient ischemic attacks, 12 an infarction, preceded by one or more TIAs, 72 an infarction without TIAs, and 7 patients suffered from a cerebral vascular process without a laterally localized lesion. A further patient, aged 70, with a venous thrombosis in a sinus was also examined. Conventional angiography of the extra- and intracranial vessel was performed on 91 of the 149 patients.

Ch. Kessler et al. (eds.), Clinical Application of Radiolabelled Platelets, 210–213.

RESULTS AND DISCUSSION

An accumulation of platelets in the neck vessels was observed in 30 patients. In 18 cases this was on the clinically affected and in 5 patients on the unaffected side. In 1 of the 5 patients the angiogram revealed a plaque on the unaffected side. The remaining patients had clinical results which could not be brought into the relationship with the carotid feeding area. A 70 year old female patient with an angiographically evident left cavernous sinus thrombosis had a localized accumulation of thrombocytes in the region of the left orbit. This positive scintigraphic scan in a thrombosis of the sinus substantiates the findings of Kessler and colleagues (9). They detected the partial formation of a thrombosis in the superior sagittal sinus in a patient with a normal angiogram and computertomographic scan using indium-111 labeled autologus platelets. The thrombosis was postulated as the probable cause of transitory paralysis.

26 results were categorized as unclassified i.e. they were not normal observations yet irrelevant for this study. In 90 patients a localized extracranial accumulation of labeled platelets was not evident. In 2 patients an evaluation was not possible due to insufficiently labeled platelets.

40 of the 91 patients on whom angiography was performed had one or more atherosclerotic irregularities of the vessel walls and plaques. In 35 patients abnormalities, such as vascular occlusion, stenoses, aneurysms or tumour blush were evident without a plaque being discernible. In 29 of the 40 patients with angiographically discernible plaques the angiographical and neurological evidence was located on the same side. In these patients the neurological symptoms could thus have been embolically caused by an active plaque. Only 6 of the 29 patients with angiographically evident active plaques displayed a corresponding accumulation of labeled platelets. In 5 of them this accumulation was located on the clinically affected and in 1 on the unaffected side.

23 angiographically evident plaques with corresponding clinical symptoms were not accompanied by an abnormal scintigraphic scan. 36 patients and 7 controls had both a normal angiogram and scintigraphic scan. 6 patients without angiographically evident plaques had an abnormal scintigraphic scan, 4 of them on the clinically affected and 2 on the unaffected side. 15 patients on whom angiography was not performed had an abnormal scintigraphic scan, 8 of them on the clinically affected and 1 on the clinically unaffected side. 6 of them had no lateral clinical symptoms. Taking clinical and/or angiographical results into consideration, there was evidence of 20 correctly abnormal and 43 correctly normal as well as 5 falsely abnormal and 23 falsely normal scintigraphic scans. A partial explanation for the relatively high number (i.e.23) of normal

scintigraphic scans when there is angiographical evidence of a plaque lies in the fact that angiography enables the morphological detection of plaques, whilst scintigraphy is also dependent on the intensity of the platelet accumulation (2,15). The number of correctly normal scintigraphic scans could in fact be higher, as angiography was not performed on all patients. It is especially remarkable that, in a few patients, scintigraphy revealed plaques which were not evident on an angiogram. The influence of the acetylsalicylic acid and dextran administered to some patients can be considered minor, when taking the clinical findings and angiographical observations into account. This corresponds with observations made in other studies (5,7,13,14)

These results obtained show that scintigraphy using platelets labeled with Tc-99 m-phytate could be useful in the differential diagnosis of cerebrovascular diseases, especially as it is a less invasive type of examination than angiography.

It is however dissatisfying that both scintigraphic scans and angiography are apparently not sufficiently reliable in the determination of atherosclerotic lesions. To accurately determine the value and reliability of platelet labeling independently of the clinical findings and angiographical result the scintigraphic evidence must thus be compared with intra-operative morphological and histological results on a large collective. A corresponding statement is not possible due to the small number of patients in this study on whom vascular surgery was performed.

REFERENCES

1. Berberich R, Glöbel B: Markierung von Thrombozyten bei Verwendung kleiner Blutvolumina. 11. Jahrestagung d.G.f. Nuklearmedizin (1973). Hrsg.:Malamos B, Pabst HW; Hör G, Schattauer-Verslag, 1974:395-362
2. Erberich R,Wenig C, Schroth HJ, Huber G, Oberhausen E,Gutsfeld P:Der szintigraphische Nachweis von Angiopathien im Hals und Schädelbereich mit markierten hrombozyten. 18. Jahrestagung d.G.f. Nuklearmedizin. Schattauer- Verlag, 1980: 347-350
3. Berberich R, Schroth HJ, Oberhausen E: Scintigraphic detection of thrombosis and embolism with platelets labelled with technetium 99m-phytate. Brit J Radiol 1980; 53:925
4. Davis HH, Heaton WA, Siegel BA, Mathias CJ, Joist JH, Sherman LA, Welch MJ: Scintigraphic detection of atherosclerotic lesions and venous thrombi in man by indium-111-labeled autologus platelets. Lancet 1978; 1: 1185-1187
5. Davis HH, Siegel BA, Sherman LA, Heaton WA, Naidich

TP, Joist JH, Welch MJ: Scintigraphic detection of carotic atherosclerosis with indium-111-labeled autologus platelets. Circulation 1980; 61: 982-988

6. Ezekowitz MD, Smith EO, Burrow RD, Galloway DC: The detection of potential sources of embolic stroke by indium-111 platelet scintigraphy. Stroke 1982; 13: 114

7. Isaka Y, Kimura K, Yoneda S, Kusunoki M, Etani H, Uyama O, Tsuda Y, Abe H: Platelet accumulation in carotic atherosclerotic lesions: Semiquantitative analysis with indium-111 platelets and technetium-99m human serum albumin. J Nucl Med 1984; 25: 556-563

8. Jäger E, Kolbe H, Silberbauer K, Sinzinger H, Höfer R: Technik der radioaktiven Markierung autologer menschlicher Thrombozyten mit 111-indium-Oxin-sulfat und deren klinische Anwendung. Wien klin Wschr 1984; 96: 106-112

9. Kessler C, Kniffert T, Botsch H: Der Nutzen der Plättchenszintigraphie zur Aufklärung intrakranieller vaskulärer Prozesse. Akt Neurol 1980; 7: 27-29

10. Kessler C, Kniffert T, Reuther R, Kimmig B, zum Winkel K: Szintigraphie mit indium-111-markierten Blutplättchen. Dtsch med Wschr 1984; 109: 1853-1859

11. Kessler C, Reuther R, Berentelg J, Kimmig B: The clinical use of platelet scintigraphy with 11-in-oxine. J Neurol 1983; 229: 255-261

12. Kessler C, Trabant R: Thrombozytenszintigraphie mit 111- Indium.Arch psychiatr nervenkr 1982; 231: 449-457

13. Lusby RJ, Ferrell LD, Englestad BL, Price DC, Lipton MJ, Stoney RJ: Vessel wall and indium-111-labelled platelet response to carotic endarterectomy. Surgery 1983; 93: 424-432

14. Powers WJ, Siegel BA, Davis HH, Mathias CJ, Clark HB, Welch MJ: Indium-111-platelet scintigraphy in cerebrovascular disease. Neurology 1982; 32: 938-943

15. Sinzinger H, Silberbauer K, Fitscha P, Kaliman J: Wertigkeit des Nachweises atherosklerotischer Laesionen mit markierten autologen Thrombozyten. Acta medica Austriaca 1982; 9: 181-184

INDIUM-III LABELLED PLATELET IMAGING OF PROSTHETIC MATERIALS IN HUMANS

Stratton J.R., M.D.

Division of Cardiology
Seattle V.A. Medical Center
and
University of Washington

INTRODUCTION

Prosthetic materials are increasingly used in medicine. Currently, prosthetic materials are used in the construction of vascular catheters, arterial and venous substitutes, membrane oxygenators, dialysis machines, heart valves, ventricular assist devices and totally artificial hearts. The major complications of prosthetic materials are mechanical failure, infection, thrombotic occlusion due to thrombus formation on the prosthetic surface, and systemic embolization due to the breaking off of thrombotic deposits. Due to improved materials and fabrication techniques, mechanical failure is now extremely rare. The most common complications of prosthetic materials currently encountered are thromboemblic events. There is now abundant evidence that platelet mechanisms play a predominant role in the thrombotic and embolic events caused by intravascular prosthetic materials. All currently used prosthetic materials are thrombogenic when placed in humans.

To reduce the thromboembolic complications of prosthetic materials, research is focused on two broad strategies. The first strategy is the construction of improved, less thrombogenic materials, and the second is the development of improved, safe antithrombotic drug regimens. Testing of either new materials or new drugs prior to widespread clinical use is necessary. However, the assessment of the thrombogenicity of prosthetic materials in the past has been limited by the lack of suitable methods. In particular, in humans, commonly used measures of platelet function such as aggregation, adhesion, plasma levels of platelet specific proteins (platelet factor 4 or beta thromboglobulin), and the measurement of platelet survival have not accurately reflected platelet interaction with prosthetic surfaces. In addition, none of these tests anatomically localize the sites of abnormal platelet activation. Indium-III platelet imaging is a potentially useful new method of evaluating the thrombogenicity of new prostheses or the effects of new drugs, since it can semi

214

Ch. Kessler et al. (eds.), Clinical Application of Radiolabelled Platelets, 214–234.

quantitatively evaluate localized platelet uptake. Studies in animals have widely utilized indium-III platelet imaging to measure platelet uptake in vivo or in vitro following sacrifice. Animal studies have been recently reviewed (1). This chapter will be limited to a discussion of studies that have assessed platelet deposition on prosthetic materials in humans. First, the semi quantitative techniques that have been used to assess deposition will be reviewed, followed by a discussion of findings in acutely placed prosthetic grafts, chronically implanted prosthetic grafts, antithrombotic drug trials, and finally a review of trials that have compared different types of prosthetic materials.

SEMI-QUANTITATION OF PLATELET DEPOSITION

In man, no technique has been validated to absolutely quantitate indium-III labelled platelet uptake onto vascular grafts. However, numerous semi-quantitative methods have been developed. Virtually every investigative group that has studied platelet uptake onto grafts materials has used a different method of assessing the magnitude of platelet deposition. For example, Goldman, McCollum, and colleagues have used a "thrombogenicity index" in which nonimaging probe count data over a small portion of a grafts is compared to a reference non-graft region on a daily basis. The slope of the graft/reference counts over a 7 day period was calculated; the increase in the ratio per day was defined as the "thrombogenicity index" (2). Pumphrey and colleagues (3) used localized graft counts from several regions throughout the graft; they expressed graft platelet uptake as graft counts/100 pixels/injected dose, Kotze and colleagues used a background subtracted attenuation corrected measure of graft uptake in which radioactivity in the graft was expressed as a percentage of the injected dose (4). Sinziger and colleagues (5) used a platelet uptake ratio that compared radioactivity counts measured in a graft region of interest to counts over a contralateral region of interest at serial timepoints following platelet injection. Isaka and colleagues (6) used a dual tracer blood pool subtraction technique in which a platelet accumulation index (PAI) was calculated for each pixel in a graft region of interest. For quantitation of planar imaging results, we have used a graft/blood ratio (7). At each imaging time, aortofemoral graft and background count activities were derived from hand drawn regions of interest that encompassed the entire graft, as well as a separate adjacent background region. The graft/blood ratio was then derived by dividing the background corrected graft counts by the count activity in 0.1 ml of whole blood counted in a well counter (7). The same identical regions of interest for graft and background activities were applied to all planar images on a given patient. By dividing the graft counts by circulating whole blood activity, differences in injected dose, isotope decay, platelet survival and platelet recovery from study to study, as well as from one patient to the next, were normalized. Using planar imaging of vascular grafts, the test-retest reproducibility (r=9.88), the intra-observer reproducibility (r=0.97) and the inter-observer reproducibility (r=0.95) of this method were high (7).

For tomographic imaging of vascular grafts, we derived indium-III platelet activity in the graft from a computer generated circular region of interest that encompassed an area of 10.4 cm^2 (8). This region of interest was applied to each 6-18 mm thick transaxial slice throughout the graft. The proximal and distal ends of the graft were defined visually as well as by an increment in counts from the native vessel to the graft. Graft activity in all slices was summed to give the total graft activity. Graft activity was divided by whole blood counts at each imaging time to derive a tomographic graft/blood ratio. The intra-observer reproducibility of this technique was high (r=0.99)(8).

An example of the counts obtained using this tomographic technique of quantitation are shown in Fig 1. In this study, we compared 12 patients with chronically implanted Dacron aortic grafts who were receiving no antithrombotic medications to 9 normal subjects who did not have vascular grafts. The two groups received a similar amount of injected radioactivity, and both groups were imaged at 24 and 72 hours following labelled platelet injection. The normal subjects had a similar number of transaxial tomographic slices assessed for activity both above and below the aortic bifurcation, as did the graft patients. As can be seen, the counts within the "graft area" were significantly greater in the patients with prosthetic materials compared with the circulating aortofemoral blood pool activity in the normal subjects. Graft region counts increased by 34% between 24 and 72 hours in patients with prosthetic materials. In contrast, the normal subjects had a slight reduction in decay corrected aortofemoral blood pool counts between 24 and 72 hours as senescent platelets were removed from the circulation. In patients, the resulting graft/blood ratio increased from 6.2 at 24 hours to 11.4 at 72 hours, which was a significant increase (p<0.05). In contrast, normal subjects had no significant change in the tomographically determined ratio over time, as would be anticipated since the graft/blood ratio in normals is image determined vascular activity divided by well counted whole blood activity obtained from blood samples. This ratio is stable in regions without ongoing platelet deposition, such as the normal vasculature.

In humans, none of these semi-quantitative techniques have been adequately validated. Although Allen et al. (9) in animals noted an excellent correlation between platelet accumulation measured by a blood pool subtraction technique and well counting results following sacrifice of the animal, another study (10) suggested that a graft to reference region ratio was superior to a blood pol subtraction

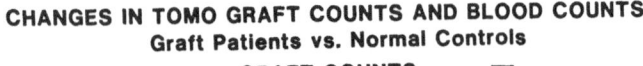

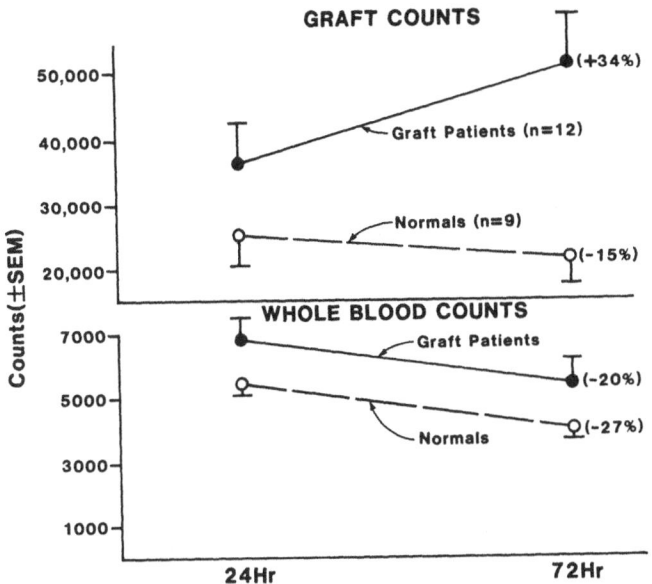

Fig 1

Tomographically determined graft counts from 12 Dacron aortic grafts are displayed in the upper panel. For comparison, results in 9 normal subjects without grafts are also displayed. Graft counts are decay corrected. In the normal subjects, the "graft" activity was obtained from an identical number of tomographic slices as in the patients with grafts. As shown, graft patients had significantly more activity in the graft region of interest at both 24 and 72 hours following labeled platelet injection. Moreover, activity in the graft region significantly increased over time in patients with prosthetic materials, while in normal subjects, activity in the aortofemoral area decreased over time as senescent platelets were removed from the circulation. The 34% increase in the graft region counts in patients with grafts between 24 and 72 hours occurred despite the fact that circulating whole blood counts decreased by 20% over the same time period.

technique in quantitating platelet uptake on grafts in dogs. Our findings suggested that the quantitation of platelet uptake on grafts was improved by tomographic imaging compared to standard planar imaging since tomographic imaging was able to detect a 36% reduction in the graft/blood ratio by drugs in twelve subjects, while a 50% reduction was necessary by planar imaging (8). This improvement was due to less measurement variability using the tomographic approach.

RECENTLY IMPLANTED GRAFTS

Multiple studies have demonstrated that virtually all recently implanted prosthetic arterial grafts have detectable indium-III labelled platelet uptake (2-5, 11-17). To determine whether platelet deposition decreased following graft implantation, we performed serial imaging on five patients at 1-2 weeks, 31 weeks, and 55 weeks following Dacron aortobifemoral graft placement (14). None of the patients received antithrombotic drugs. The mean graft/blood ratio progressively decreased from $4.4+4.1$ at 1-2 weeks to $3.0+1.8$ at 31 weeks (p<0.05). There was no further reduction at 55 weeks ($2.8+2.0$). The individual graft/blood ratios are shown in Fig 2. Although deposition decreased following implantation, it remained readily detectable in most patients studied at 1 year (14).

Additional evidence that deposition decreases over time was found in studies by Goldman and colleagues (12, 16). In one study, the mean thrombogenicity index decreased from 0.21 at 1 week following Dacron graft placement to 0.08 at 6-12 months (12). In a later study, patients with woven Dacron grafts had a reduction in the deposition index from 0.19 to 0.06 over 6-9 months following graft implantation (16).

Goldman, McCollum and colleagues made the important observation that platelet deposition at 1 week after implantation appeared to predict ultimate graft patency. Amount 21 femoro-popliteal grafts that occluded in the first year following implantation, the thrombogenicity index at 1 week was significantly greater than amount 36 grafts that remained patent ($0.19+0.02$ vs $0.07+0.01$, p<0.001). When grafts were split into those that had a thrombogenicity index below the median at 1 week following implantation vs those with a higher thrombogenicity index, there was a marked difference in the patency rate at 1 year by life table methods. Among patients with a low initial thrombogenicity index, the cumulative patency rate was 90% compared to a patency rate of only 39% in those with a higher initial thrombogenicity index (17).

In a cross-sectional study, Isaka and colleagues noted an inverse correlation between the age of the graft and their measure of platelet uptake (the platelet accumulation index) in patients with patent grafts (6). Thus four studies have reached a similar conclusion: platelet uptake onto

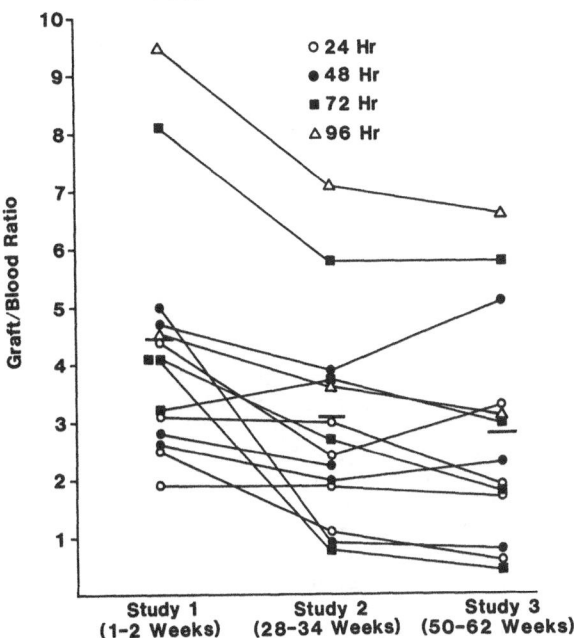

Fig 2

Individual graft/blood ratios obtained from planar images are displayed for patients studied serially in the first 1 year following graft implantation. The values obtained at 24, 48, 72 or 96 hours following labeled platelet injection at each of the three serial study times are connected by lines. Overall, the mean graft/blood ratio fell from 4.4±2.1 (±SD) at 1-2 weeks postoperatively to 3.0±1.8 at 31 weeks, and to 2.8±2.0 at 55 weeks.

prosthetic grafts significantly decreases over time following implantation in the absence of therapy in humans.

CHRONIC GRAFTS

Although platelet deposition decreases over time following implantation, the currently available data suggests that deposition onto the graft surface does continue, albeit at a lesser rate. Several studies have noted deposition on grafts that have been in place for periods of time between 1 month and 10 years (4, 6, 7, 12, 14, 16, 18) (Fig 3). For comparison to the deposition that occurs on a chronic graft, an example of the circulating platelet activity present in a normal subject without a graft is shown in Fig 4.

To semi-quantitatively assess platelet uptake onto chronic grafts, we studied 15 patients who had chronically implanted Dacron arterial grafts that had been in place between 9 months and 10 years. None of the patients were receiving antithrombotic drugs. For comparison, young healthy volunteers without grafts were also studied in order to gain an estimate of the circulating indium-III activity present in the native aortofemoral region (7). Images were both qualitatively analyzed by visual interpretation as well as semi-quantitatively analyzed using a planar derived graft/blood ratio. By blinded analysis, all 12 normal subjects had negative studies. In contrast 12 of the 15 patients with grafts had definitely positive studies and additional patient had a equivocal study; only two patients with grafts had visually negative studies. The graft/blood ratio showed an even greater separation between patients with chronically implanted grafts and the normal controls (Fig 5). In the case of the normal subjects, the graft/blood ratio was simply gamma camera derived aortofemoral blood pool activity divided by circulating whole blood activity. As expected, the ratio in normals was unchanged at the serial imaging times between 24 and 96 hours following platelet injection (2.0 -/+ 0.7, 1.8 -/+ 0.6, 1.7 -/+ 0.8, and 1.7 -/+ 0.9, respectively). In contrast, among the 15 patients with prosthetic grafts, there was a significant serial increase in the graft/blood ratio from 3.0 -/+ 1.6 at 24 hours to 7.8 -/+ 5.0 at 96 hours (all p<0.05 vs normals) (7).

Deposition was present in patients with grafts of all ages including one patient with a 10 year old graft. Most subjects had evidence of diffuse deposition. However, many also had relatively irregular foci of deposition, which occasionally changed over time (Fig 6). Overall, about two-thirds of patients had some irregularity of the deposition pattern detected visually. In several other patients with chronic grafts, we have detected increased deposition in areas of pseudoaneurysm formation (Fig 7).

Currently, we utilize tomographic imaging, since quantitative assessment may be improved (8). Examples of 6mm

DIFFUSE DEPOSITION—CHRONIC GRAFT

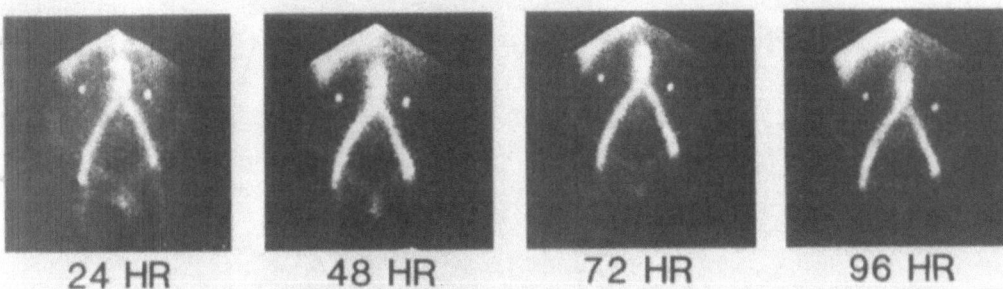

24 HR   48 HR   72 HR   96 HR

Fig 3

Diffuse platelet deposition was present throughout this 13 month old Dacron aortic bifurcation graft. The pattern was unchanged between the 24 and 96 hour imaging times. The two hot spots are anatomic markers located 8 cm to either side of the umbilicus; the markers are used to aid in reproducible patient positioning. (From Stratton JR, Thiele BL, Ritchie JL. Circulation 66:1287–1293, 1982. Used by permission of the American Heart Association.)

NORMAL ^{111}IN PLATELET ACTIVITY

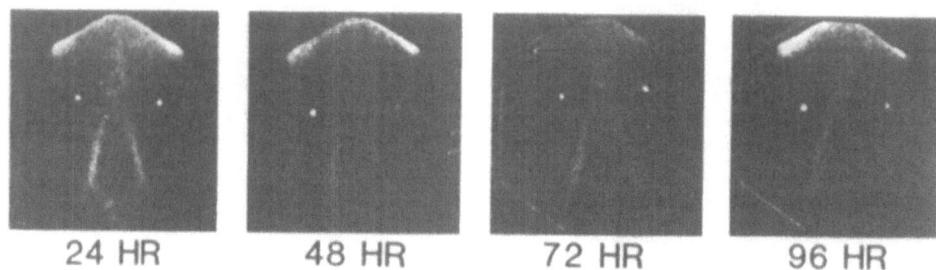

| 24 HR | 48 HR | 72 HR | 96 HR |

Fig 4

For comparison, anterior abdominal images of a young normal subject without a graft are shown. Large vessel blood pool activity is clearly seen on the 24 hour image. However, over the 96 hour imaging time, blood pool activity decreases as senescent platelets are removed from the circulation. The two hot spots are anatomic markers used for patient positioning. (From Stratton JR, Thiele BL, Ritchie JL. Circulation 66:1287–1293, 1982. Used by permission of the American Heart Association.)

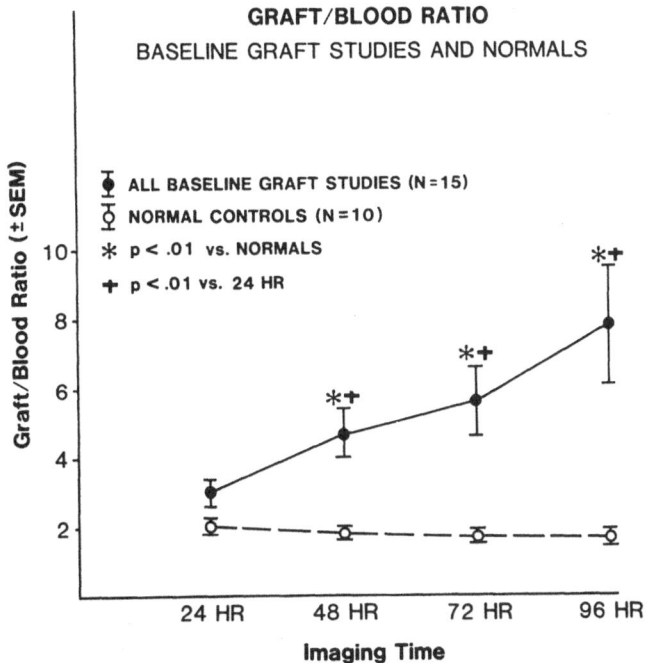

Fig 5

The mean graft/blood ratio of 15 patients with chronically implanted Dacron aortic bifurcation grafts was greater at all imaging times than a similarly obtained ratio in normal subjects without grafts. In patients with grafts, the ratio increased serially between 24 and 96 hours, while in normal subjects, the ratio was unchanged over time. These results suggest progressive indium-111 platelet uptake on prosthetic materials over the 96 hour imaging time, as demonstrated more convincingly by tomographic imaging techniques in Figure 1. (From Stratton JR, Thiele BL, Ritchie JL. Circulation 66:1287-1293, 1982. Used by permission of the American Heart Association.)

CHRONIC GRAFT - BASELINE
CHANGE IN PLATELET DEPOSITION OVER TIME

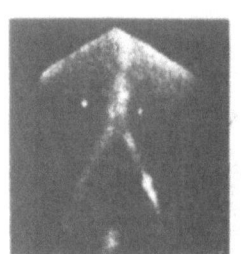 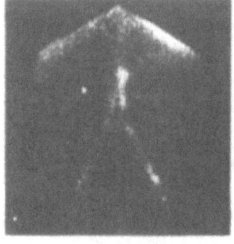 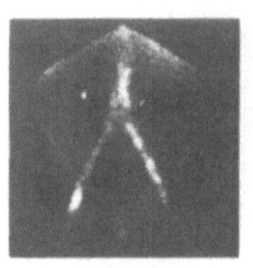 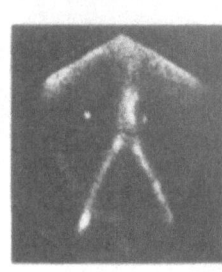

24 HR.   48 HR.   72 HR.   96 HR.

Fig 6

Although deposition was apparent diffusely throughout this graft, there was also irregular focal deposition. In addition, over time, new areas of increased uptake became apparent, particularly at the right distal anastomotic site. In approximately one-half of patients with chronically implanted grafts, new areas of uptake became apparent on later images. Much less commonly, areas of abnormal deposition occasionally decreased on serial imaging, suggesting disaggregation or downstream embolization of labeled platelets.

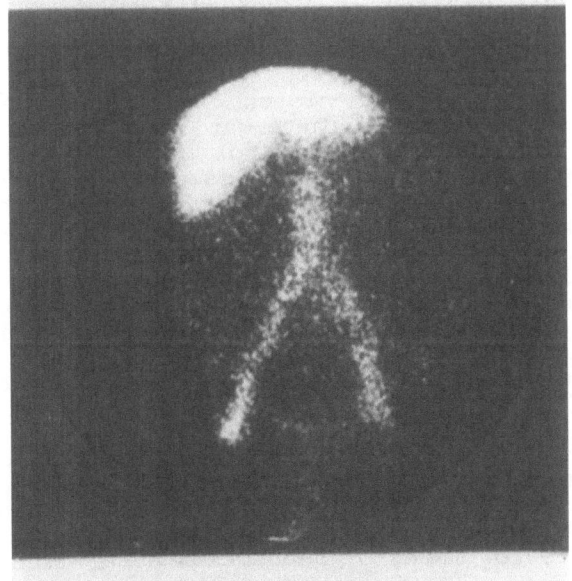

15 MOS. POST GRAFT

48 HR IMAGE

Fig 7

A pseudoaneurysm at the right distal anastomotic site was associated with particularly intense platelet uptake in this patient with a chronically implanted graft.

thick tomographic images of a chronic Dacron aortic graft are shown in Figure 8.

DRUG EFFECTS ON PLATELET DEPOSITION

The combination of aspirin plus dipyridamole has been most extensively studied in patients with either acute or chronic grafts. Pumphrey and colleagues (3) noted that aspirin (325 mg tid) plus dipyridamole (100 mg qid preoperatively and 75 mg tid postoperatively) decreased the counts/100 pixels/injected microcurie in all portions of Dacron aortofemoral grafts in eight drug treated patients compared to eight untreated control patients with recently implanted grafts. In contrast, the same drug regimen did not appear to have any benefit in five patients with polytetrafluoroethylene (PTFE) femoro-popliteal grafts.

Goldman and colleagues (19) randomized 47 patients with recently implanted Dacron, PTFE or vein grafts to either placebo or aspirin (300 mg tid) plus dipyridamole (75 mg tid), which was begun 48 hours prior to surgery and continued throughout the study. Among 12 patients with Dacron grafts, the drug regimen decreased the deposition index from 0.25 -/+ 0.09 to 0.16 -/+ 0.05 (p<0.05); similarly, among 15 patients with PTFE grafts, the deposition index was reduced from 0.16 -/+ 0.03 on placebo to 0.05 -/+ 0.01 on the combination of asprin plus dipyridamole (p<0.05). There was no reduction in deposition in patients with vein grafts; however, patients with vein grafts had very low rates of deposition even without therapy (0.03 -/+ 0.01). Therefore, in contrast to the study by Pumphrey et al, this study suggested that the combination of drugs also reduced deposition on recently implanted PTFE grafts as well as on Dacron grafts.

To determine whether inhibition of platelet deposition by aspirin plus dipyridamole was sustained on older grafts, we studied 18 patients who had Dacron aortic bifurcation grafts in place for 10-121 months (20). Patients were assessed before and during short-term (2-3 weeks) therapy with aspirin (325 mg tid) plus dipyridamole (75mg tid). By both planar and tomographic imaging, platelet accumulation was reduced. The mean drug induced decrease in the tomographic graft/blood ratio was 13+4%, and the decrease in the planar graft/blood ratio was 12+4%. The reduction in the graft/blood ratio in patients receiving aspirin plus dipyridamole was due entirely to a reduction in graft counts on therapy, since there was no significant difference in whole blood counts between the baseline and drug studies (Figure 10).

Prostacyclin (PGI$_2$) reduced platelet deposition on both recently implanted and chronically implanted grafts in humans as shown by Sinziger and colleagues (5). Although baseline pre-drug platelet deposition was significantly less in patients with older grafts compared with patients with younger grafts, prostacyclin significantly decreased

TOMOGRAPHIC IMAGING EXAMPLE
Dacron Aortic Graft

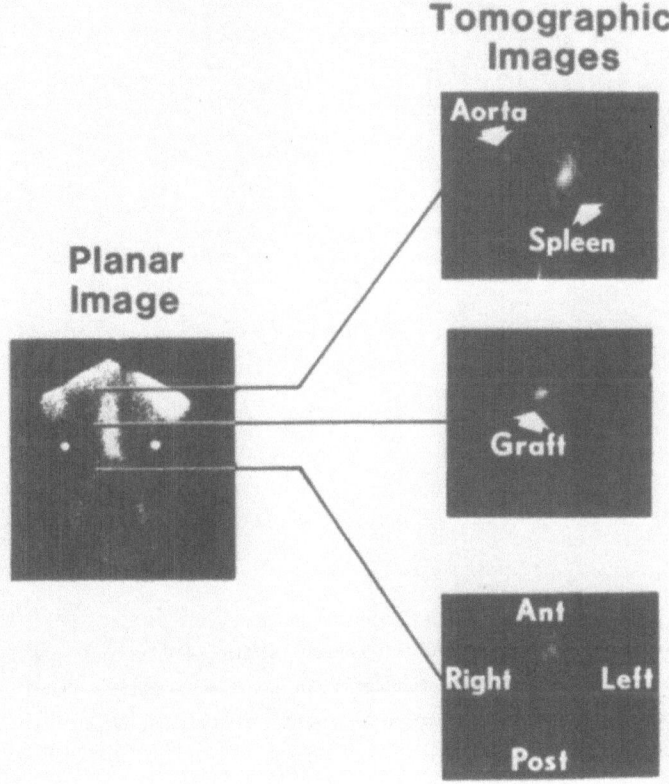

Fig 8

Planar and tomographic images obtained 72 hours following labeled platelet injection are displayed in this patient with a chronically implanted Dacron aortic graft. The approximate levels from which the 6mm thick tomographic slices were obtained are depicted on the planar image. The tomographic image recorded through the native aorta (top right panel) and below the graft (bottom right panel) revealed faint activity due to circulating labeled platelets in the native vessels. In contrast, a tomographic slice obtained through the mid portion of the graft (center right panel) showed intense platelet uptake compared with the native vessels. (From Stratton JR, Ritchie JL. Am J Cardiol 58:152-156, 1986. Used by permission of the American Journal Cardiology.)

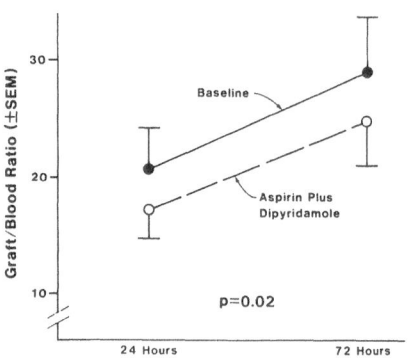

ASPIRIN PLUS DIPYRIDAMOLE
Tomographic Graft/Blood Ratio

Fig _9_

A combination of aspirin plus dipyridamole significantly reduced the tomographically determined graft/blood ratio on chronic grafts. (From Stratton JR, Ritchie JL. Circulation 73:325-330, 1986. Used by permission of the American Heart Association.)

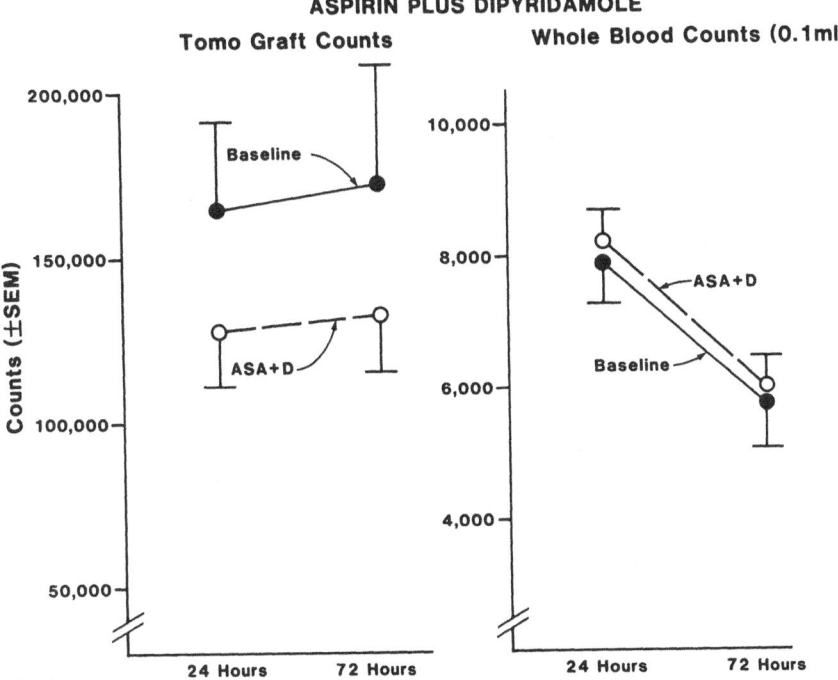

Fig <u>10</u>

The reduction in the graft/blood ratio induced by aspirin plus dipyridamole was due entirely to a decrease in the graft region counts as shown in the left panel. The whole blood counts were unchanged during the two phases of the study. ASA + D = aspirin plus dipyridamole.

deposition in the older grafts as well. The magnitude of the reduction in deposition was greater, however, among the patients with more recently implanted grafts. Surprisingly, there was some evidence to suggest that the prostacyclin effect persisted following discontinuation of the infusion.

In general, results of drug therapy in patients with chronically implanted grafts have been much less impressive than in patients with recently implanted prostheses.d We have assessed the effects of three additional agents in patients with chronically implanted grafts (>9 months old). In randomized placebo controlled cross-over studies, neither suloctidil (200 mg tid) (Figure 11) nor ticlopidine (250 mg bid) (Figure 12) caused a significant reduction in platelet uptake onto the surface of chronic grafts (8, 21). In another study, sulfinpyrazone (200 mg qid) also failed to reduce platelet uptake on chronically implanted grafts (22).

COMPARISONS OF VARIOUS GRAFT MATERIALS

There are limited data in humans comparing different types of graft materials. On one study, recently implanted Dacron popliteal grafts and PTFE femoro-popliteal grafts had significantly higher thrombogenicity indices than autologous vein grafts in patients who were receiving no antithrombotic medications (19). The mean deposition index in the Dacron group early after implantation was 0.25, in the PTFE group 0.16, and in the vein group 0.03. There were 7,6 and 10 patients respectively in each group. Thus, the thrombogenicity index in autologous vein grafts was much lower than in either type of prosthetic material.

We compared 10 studies in patients with DeBakey Dacron grafts, which are of a relatively smooth surface construction, with 10 studies in patients with Sauvage grafts, which are of a relatively irregular velour construction. There was no significant difference in the planar measured graft/blood ratio between the two graft types (7).

In a randomized trial, DeBakey Dacron grafts were compared to knitted Meadox Dacron grafts with a thrombogenicity index being determined at 2 weeks and again at 6-9 months following implantation (16). There were twelve patients in each group. There was no difference at either the early or late imaging times in the throbogenicity index between the two types of Dacron graft materials.

MISCELLANEOUS STUDIES

Platelet deposition at vascular access sites was assessed by Ritchie and colleagues (d23). Nineteen hemodialysis patients were imaged 2-48 hours following dialysis. Ten patients had bovine grafts, 4 had arterial venous fistula and 5 had PTFE grafts. Positive images were seen in 13 of 19 patients (3 of 4 patients with AV fistula,

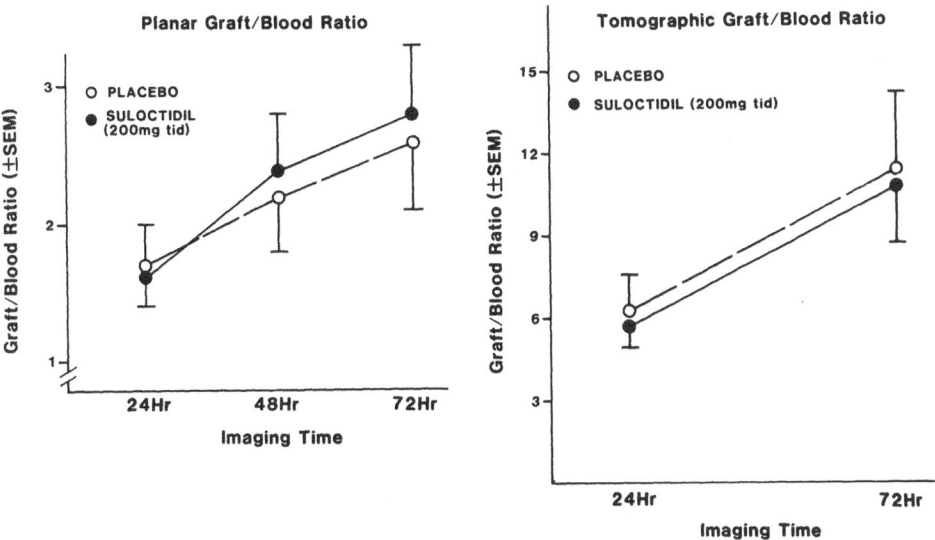

PLANAR AND TOMOGRAPHIC IMAGING RESULTS

Fig <u>11</u>

Suloctidil (200mg tid) failed to reduce either the planar or tomographically
determined graft/blood ratio in patients with chronically implanted Dacron
aortic grafts. (From Stratton JR, Ritchie JL. Am J Cardiol 58:152–156, 1986.
Used by permission of the American Journal of Cardiology.)

TICLOPIDINE EFFECTS ON PLATELET DEPOSITION
Individual Graft/Blood Ratios

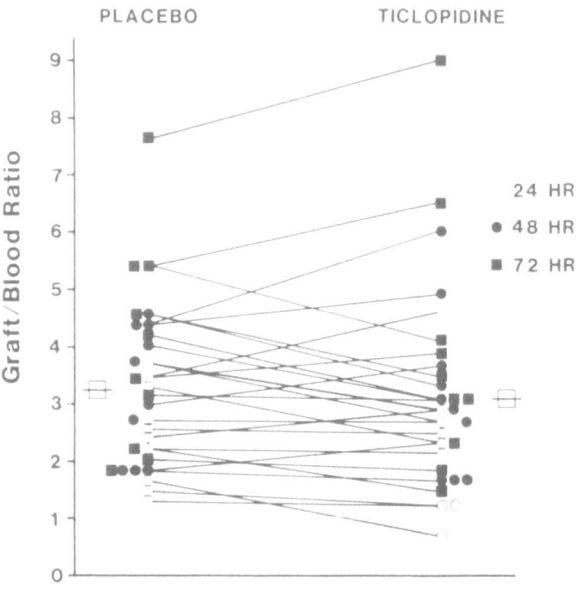

Fig 12

Ticlopidine (250mg bid) did not reduce the graft/blood ratio in patients with chronically implanted grafts. The individual values obtained at 24, 48 and 72 hour imaging times on placebo and on ticlopidine are displayed. The mean of all graft/blood ratios was 3.1 on placebo and 3.0 on ticlopidine.

7 of 10 with Bovine grafts and 3 of 5 with PTFE grafts).
Sulfinpyrazone (200 mg tid) in 6 patients led to a definite
decrease in deposition in three and a probable decrease in
two. There was no clear relationship in this study between
image positivity and a history of prior graft occlusion. One
study (24) has demonstrated platelet uptake onto vascular
catheters in humans. Another study has noted that no
definite platelet uptake was detectable in patients with
mechanical heart valves (11), possibly due to the limited
resolution of the imaging technique. The kinetics of
labelled platelets during cardiopulmonary bypass have been
studied in four patients. During cardiopulmonary bypass,
Indium-III platelet activity in the blood decreased by 46%,
due mostly to hemodilution (25). Overall, 11% of the
labelled platelets were sequestered in the pump oxygenator.

SUMMARY AND CONCLUSIONS

Platelet deposition on prosthetic arterial grafts has
been present on all materials studied in humans. By semi-
quantitative techniques, deposition is greatest early
following graft implantation. Over the first few months
following implantation, deposition does decrease. However,
detectable deposition appears to remain present indefinitely
in most, if not all, patients.

Deposition has been decreased in both recently and
chronically implanted grafts by the combination of aspirin
plus dipyridamole. Prostacyclin has also reduced deposition
on both acutely and chronically implanted grafts, although
it must be given intravenously. On chronically implanted
grafts, sulfinpyrazone, ticlopidine, suloctidil and
sulfinpyrazone have failed to reduce deposition. Deposition
may be less on PTFE than on Dacron grafts, although this
observation needs to be verified. Deposition is less on
autologous vein grafts compared to either PTFE or dacron
grafts.

Indium-III platelet imaging, by its ability to semi-
quantitatively evaluate platelet uptake on vascular grafts,
is a useful new technique to evaluate strategies designed to
reduce thromboembolic complications of prosthetic materials.
This technique has shown considerable promise in evaluating
materials and drugs in animal models, and there is a growing
body of information in humans. Improved methods of
quantitation need to be developed, and some standardization
of quantitative techniques would be desirable.

Platelet imaging will continue to have a very important
research role in the evaluation of new materials and drugs
in man. Whether platelet imaging findings in an individual
patient will be useful in making clinical decisions
regarding initiation of alteration of antithrombotic drug
therapy remains to be determined.

REFERENCES

1. Stratton J.R.(d1985) Platelet kinetics and imaging of prothetic materials In Heyns A. Dup., Badenhorst P.N., Lotter M/.G. (eds.) : Platelet Kinetics and Imaging. Boca Raton, Fla. CRC Press, vol. 2, pp 21-44.

2. Goldman M., Norcott H.C., Hawker R.J., Hail C., Drolc Z., McCollum C.N. (1982) Femoropopliteal bypass grafts - an isotope technique allowing in vivo comparison of thrombogenicity. Br. J. Surg. 69: 380-382.

3. Pumphrey C.W., Chesebro J.H., Dewanjee M.K., Wahner H.W., Hollier L.H., Pairolero P.C., Fuster V. (1983) In vivo quantitation of platelet deposition on human peripheral arterial bypass grafts using Indium-III-labelled platelets: Effect of dipyridamole and aspirin. Am. J. Cardiol. 51: 796-801.

SCINTIGRAPHY OF PLATELET ADHERENCE IN PROCESSED DERMAL SHEEP COLLAGEN (PDSC) GRAFTS

J. Bannenberg, K.Breuker, M.R. Hardeman, J.Feijen, P.J. Klopper

SUMMARY

We designed a method to test the thrombogenicity of coatings on vascular prosthetic material. The platelet adherence in small diameter (3mm) vascular grafts made of Processed Dermal Sheep Collagen (PDSC) was monitored during the fist two hours after restoring the blood flow following implantation.

Platelets and red blood cells were distinctly labelled, with Indium-111 and technetium-99 respectively and monitored with a gamma-camera which then distinguished the labelled platelet adherence to the graft surface from non-specific background radiation. As a result from this preliminary series we noted that a plateau-phase in platelet adherence is reached after twenty minutes. Moreover, upon inspection after two hours the platelet deposition did not show a consistent pattern.

INTRODUCTION

The search for good prosthetic material for small diameter vascular grafts is still on. Up till now the autologous vein gives by far the best results, namely when implanted in the femoropopliteal position, a patency rate of 70% in a 5 year follow-up is seen. This is in contrast to the 20% patency rate of prosthetic grafts in the same study (4). Currently, many new materials are investigated which could serve as a potential better alternative.

In our department a new biomaterial was developed. Processed Dermal Sheep Collagen (PDSC). In a 3.5 years follow-up an accumulated patency rate of 100% is reached for PDSC grafts implanted in aorta of mongrel dogs. The accumulated patency rate of small diameter PDSC grafts is 20% in a 3 months follow-up. However, when systemic antiplatelet therapy is used, the accumulated patency rate is 60% for a 3 months follow-up and can even become 80% when systemic antiplatelet therapy is combined with endothelial cell seeding (2)

The aim of our study is to improve the patency rate of the PDSC small diameter grafts. To achieve this goal we tried to make the grafts less trombogenic by coating the PDSC with various anticoagulant substances. In order to assess the efficiency of these coatings the adherence of platelets to the coated PDSC grafts has been calculated by

Ch. Kessler et al. (eds.), Clinical Application of Radiolabelled Platelets, 235–241.
© 1990 *Kluwer Academic Publishers.*

labelling the platelets with Indium-111 and labelling the red blood cells with Technetium-99. Previous studies indicated that labelling with just Indium-111 gave unreliable results. In this paper we will report only the preliminary results of the model for testing the efficiency of the material under consideration and not on the material itself. Further we followed the kinetics of platelets in the first minutes to hours after the first contact of blood with the material was established because these first interactions are of great importance for the long-term patency of the graft.

MATERIALS AND METHODS

PDSC is a biomaterial which consists of the split-skin of the sheep treated with pretanning procedures as used in the production of shammy leather followed by tanning in a glutaraldehyde (0.625%) solution.

The sterilised collagen fiber matrix thus obtained has great tensile strength comparable to industrially processed chamois leather. Previous research has shown the following features: induction of fibroblast invasion, biodegradability and bio-inertion (7).

PLATELET LABELLING

Platelet isolation and labelling was performed according to the technique described by Thakur (10) and modified by Hardeman (8). Whole blood (50ml) was taken and added to 10ml acid citrate dextrose (ACD). This was mixed and centrifuged for 20 min at 130 g. The supernatant platelet-rich plasma (PRP) was removed and pH of the PRP was adjusted to 6.5 using ACD. Next, this was centrifuged for 10 min at 500 g. Following, the solution was allowed to rest for 30-45 min. The supernatant was removed and the platelets were resuspended in 2 ml phosphate-buffered saline. 150 μCu 111 Indium Tropolonate was added and allowed to label for 15 min. Labelling efficiency was measured and when more than 90% the labelled solution was used.

ERTHROCYTE LABELLING

Erythrocyte labelling was performed according to the technique described by Vyth (11). First the dogs were injected intravenously with 2 ml of a stannous chloride solution (1mg/ml). After 10 min 4 ml blood was withdrawn and mixed with a ml citrate. This was centrifuged for 5 min at 500 g. Next, the plasma and white blood cells were removed. 1 mCi technetium-99m was added and allowed to label for 10 min. When the efficiency was more than 90% the labelled erthrocytes were used.

EXPERIMENTAL MODEL

Four mongrel dogs (A.B,C and D) weighing 20-25 kg were anaesthetized with 0.5-1.0 gram thiopentotal intravenously as an introduction, and administered Halothane (r) after intubation. Normal saline was administered for fluid replacement. No antiplatelet therapy or systemic heparin was given. Before operation whole blood was withdrawn for platelet and erythrocyte labelling (50 ml and 4 ml) respectively. In two dogs (A and B) a coated PDSC graft was implanted in the left carotid artery while in the right carotid artery an uncoated PDSC graft was implanted. A third dog (C) received in both carotid arteries uncoated PDSC graft. In the fourth dog (D) an uncoated PDSC graft was implanted while on the contralateral side 3 cm of carotid artery was taken out and reimplanted immediately. All PDSC grafts were 3 cm long with a 3mm internal diameter.

10 min before restoring the blood flow through the grafts Indium-111 labelled platelets and Technetium-99m labelled erythrocytes were returned to the dog.

SCINTIGRAPHY AND SUBTRACTION

Radiation activity was followed by a gamma-camera for 2-hours starting 1 minute after clamp release of all grafts were stored in a computer. If thrombus formation at the distal part of the graft growing down-stream occurred the thrombus was considered as originating from the graft area itself.

Subtraction techniques were used according to the following formula. The ratio of the activity of the labelled platelets and the labelled erythrocytes is determined in a bloodpool (In_{bp}/Tc_{bp}). The excessive Indium-111 radiation (In-ex) was quantified by subtraction of the adjusted Technetium-99m radiation (Tc-roi) from the Indium-111 radiation in the region of interest (In-roi)

$$In_{ex} = \frac{In_{roi} - In_{bp} \times Tc_{roi}}{Tc_{bp}}$$

Inex = Indium-111 in excess
Inroi= Indium-111 in region of interest
Inbp = Indium-111 in bloodpool
Tcbp = Technetium-99 in bloodpool
Tcroi= Technetium-99 in region of interest

RESULTS

Figures 1,2 and 3 show two grafts in the carotid

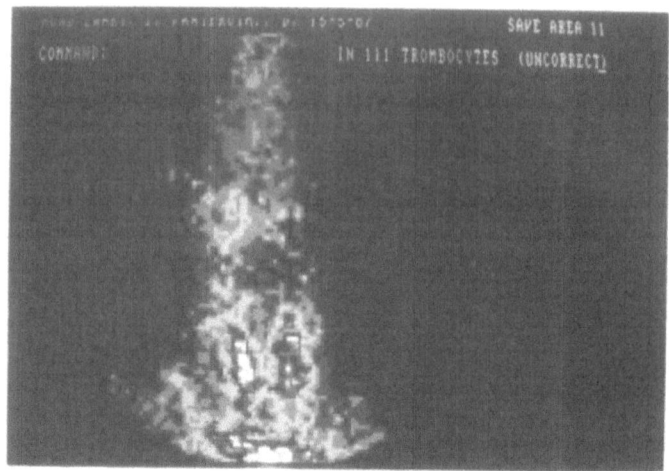

Fig 1. Carotid arteries in neck of dog A.
Indium-111 radiation not corrected.

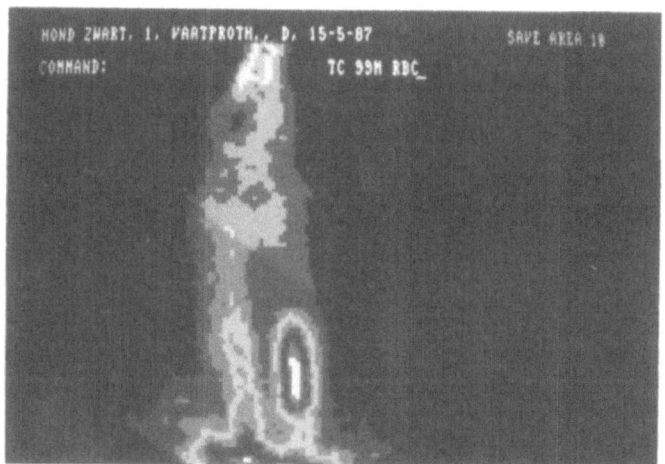

Fig 2. Carotid arteries in neck of dog A.
Technetium-99 radiation only.

position in dog A as seen on a gamma camera. Figure 1 shows what is seen when only the Indium-111 radiation is counted. When the exact place of the grafts are located and the total counts are calculated it is clear, as shown in Figure 1, that the experimental graft, which is implanted in the left carotid artery, is only slightly better than the control one. Figure 2 shows the labelled erythrocytes only, indicating a pool of blood around the coated graft in the left carotid artery. Figure 3 shows the excessive Indium-111 radiation only. It is evident that the experimental graft is less thrombogenic than the control one. The same results could be subtracted from dog B.

Both uncoated grafts in dog C had nearly equal radiation. The results from dog D showed that the operation itself has only little effect on the adherence of platelets.

Evaluation of the platelet adherence to the graft versus time showed that after approximately 20-minutes a plateau phase was reached (Fig.4). During that phase the number of adherent platelets was constant for the time of the measurement. In some experiments a tendency for a diminished radiation was seen at the end of the monitoring time.

Preliminary results of the PDSC grafts, taken out after the 2 hours blood flow, showed that there was no consistent pattern of labelled platelets on the grafts surface.

DISCUSSION

Scintigraphy of the adherence of labelled platelets in the first minutes after clamp release can only be done by labelling the blood pool too, because of the effect of blood loss which occurs after clamp release. This model can be used successfully to test different coatings of PDSC grafts.

Adherence of labelled platelets to a PDSC graft reaches a plateau-phase in 20 minutes and after approximately two hours a diminishing trend in radiation can be seen. This could suggest two different processes: a static or a dynamic turnover of adherent platelets. Several other investigators showed similar characteristics of platelet kinetics (5,9). Because of these results it is likely that the future predictions can be made on the ability of new materials to function as a vascular graft by studying the kinetics of platelet adherence in the first few hours after blood-restoring.

Platelet deposition was not as we expected. Other investigators (1,3,6) mentioned a uniform deposition high deposition on the proximal side, less in the midsection of the graft and the highest deposition on the distal side. The factors responsible for these differences are still unknown and further studies on these factors has to be done.

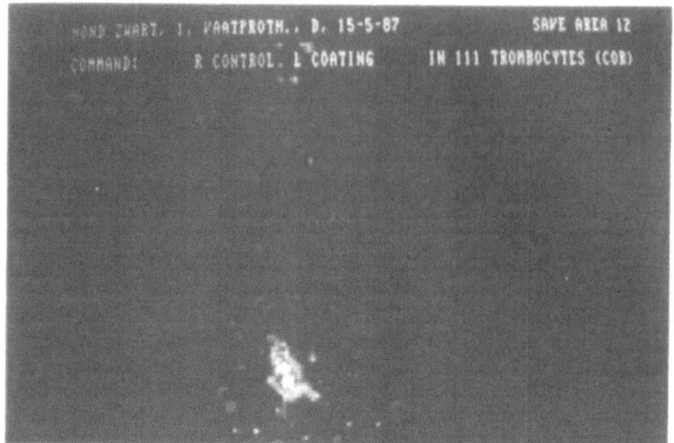

Fig 3.   Carotid arteries in neck of dog A.
         Indium-111 radiation after subtraction.

Platelet kinetics in PDSC grafts

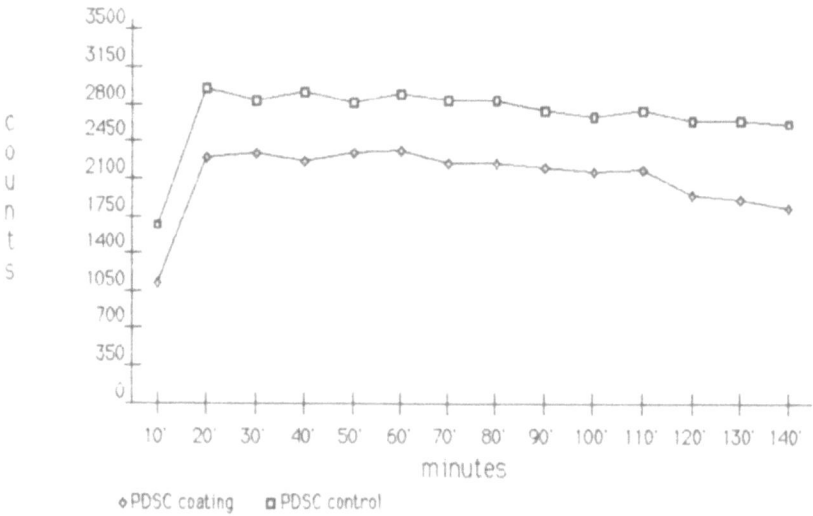

Fig 4.   As seen in dog A.

REFERENCES

1. Allen BT, Mathias CJ, Sicard GA, Welch MJ,Clark RE. Platelet deposition on vascular grafts. Ann Surg 302: 318-328

2. Bannenberg JJG, Breuker K, Wal A v/d, Feijen J, Klopper PJ. Processed dermal sheep collagen (PDSC) as a small diameter vascular graft. Eur Surg Res 1987, 19 (S1) 69

3. Christenson JT, Arvidsson D, Qvarfordt P,Dashti HM, Strand SE, Sjoberg T. The early platelet uptake and distribution of platelets in small diameter polytetrafluoroethylene (PTFE) vascular grafts in vivo. Eur J Nucl Med 1985. 10:160-164

4. Darling RC, Linton R. Durability of femoropopliteal reconstructions. Am.J.Surg.1972, 123: 472-479

5. Dewanjee MK. Cardiac and vascular imaging with labelled platelets and leukocytes. Sem.Nucl Med 1984,14: 154-187

6. Fuster V, Dewanjee MK, Kaye MP, Non-invasive radio-isotope technique for detection of platelet deposition in coronary artery by-pass grafts in dogs and it reduction with platelet inhibitors. Circulation 1979,60: 1508-1512

7. Gulik TM van. Processed Sheep Dermal Collagen as a biomaterial, a functional study. Thesis Amsterdam 1981

8. Hardeman MR, Eitjes van Overbeek EGJ, Velzen AJM, Rovekamp MH. Labelling techniques of granulocytes and platelets with 111 In-oxinate In: Blood cells in nuclear medicine, part 1. Hardeman MR and Najen Y (eds.) Martinus Nijhoff Publishers, The Hague.

9. Lipton MJ, Doherty PW, Goodwin DA, Bushberg GT, Prager R, Meares CF. Evaluation of catheter thrombogenicity in vivo with Indium labelled platelets. Radiology 1980, 135: 191-194

10 Thakur ML, Welch MJ, Joist JM, Coleman RE. Indium-111 labelled platelets: studies on preparation and evaluation of in vitro and in vivo functions. Thromb Res 1978,9: 345-353.

11 Vyth A, Raam CFM, Schoot JB v/d. Semi in vitro labelling of red blood cells with 99m-Tc: a comparison with the in vivo labelling. Pharmaceutisch Weekblad Scientific Edition 1981, 3: 1302-1304.

RADIOLABELLED PLATELET DEPOSITION PREDICTS PSEUDOINTIMAL HYPERPLASIA IN ARTERIAL PROSTHESES

A.C. Meek. D.A.J. Galvin, R.A. Harper, C.N. McCollum

INTRODUCTION

The lack of a secretory endothelium in vascular prostheses results in the adherence of thrombus onto the luminal surface of the graft. The progressive deposition of platelets, red blood cells and fibrin produces a pseudo intima which can lead to stenosis and thrombotic occlusion (4). Until recently there has been no accurate method by which in vivo thrombus formation could be measured. However, the use of 111-Indium, a high energy gamma emitter for radiolabelling of blood cells, has lead to external detection of platelet thrombus being possible by probe counting and gamma camera imaging (5). We studied 111-Indium platelet uptake on prosthetic grafts in a canine model and investigated the relationship between platelet accumulation and the subsequent development of pseudointimal growth.

MATERIALS AND METHODS

In thirty female greyhounds a 6 cm length of superficial femoral artery was excised and replaced with 6mm thin-walled polytetrafluoroethylene (Goretex), using a continuous 6.0 prolene (Ethicon) suture for both anastomoses/ A sham operation only mobilising the artery was performed on the contralateral side. On the 5th postoperative day autologous platelets from 17mls blood were labelled with 200 Ci111-Indium oxine with the method described by Wilkinson et al (6). Radioactivity was measured daily for 7 days over the graft using a highly collimated sodium iodide crystal and rate meter and compared to the contralateral femoral artery. The daily increase in the rate of activity of the graft over reference artery was calculated by linear regression and termed the Thrombogenicity Index (2).

Assessment of graft patency was performed daily by palpation and confirmed by ultrasound when necessary. At 60 days the grafts were excised and sectioned at the midpoint and 5 mm from each anastomosis. Under light microscopy using a micron grid. the degree of intra luminal pseudo-intimal hyperplasia was expressed as a percentage of the overall cross sectional area (Fig.1). This was then compared to the previous thrombogenicity measurements in the

Ch. Kessler et al. (eds.), Clinical Application of Radiolabelled Platelets, 242–247.

first week.

Measurement of Luminal Thrombus

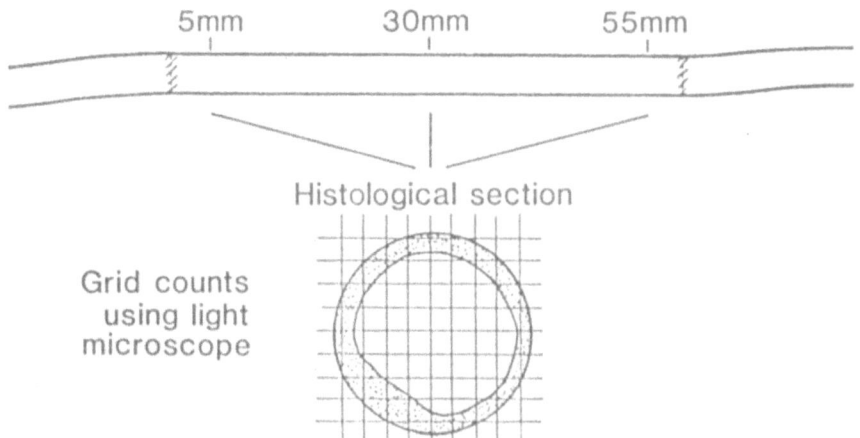

Fig 1   Measurement of graft stenosis by grid microscopy

RESULTS

All dogs tolerated surgery but in 3 animals the grafts became infected before measurements of thrombogenicity was complete and these have been excluded from the analysis. Mean (+/- sem) postoperative Thrombogenicity Index (TI) was 0.08 +/- 0.02. At two months after implantation, 7 grafts had developed pseudointimal narrowing in excess of 50% with 4 of these totally occluded. Mean TI in the 7 narrowed grafts of 0.22 +/- 0.03 was significantly higher than 0.03 +/- 0.02 in the 20 which maintained wide patency (p<0.02) (Fig.2). TI was highest in the 4 grafts which occluded at 0.31 +/- 0.09 compared to 0.04 +/- 0.02 in the 23 that remained patent (p<0.01) (Fig.3). There was a highly significant linear correlation (r=0.69) between the rate of platelet deposition against time in the early post-operative period measured as TI and the later development of pseudo-intimal hyperplasia (p<0.0001) (Fig.4).

DISCUSSION

In vivo animal models can accurately assess the incorporation of radiolabelled platelets into developing pseudo intimal hyperplasia in vascular grafts. This study has identified early postoperative platelet deposition as

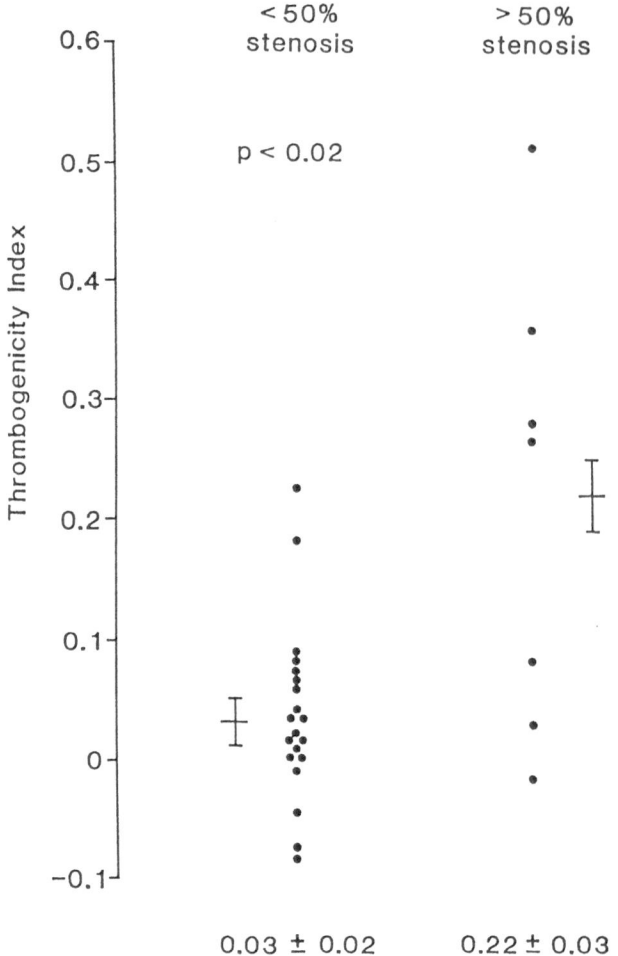

Fig 2   Comparison of thrombogenicity in grafts with less
         than and greater than 50 percent stenosis

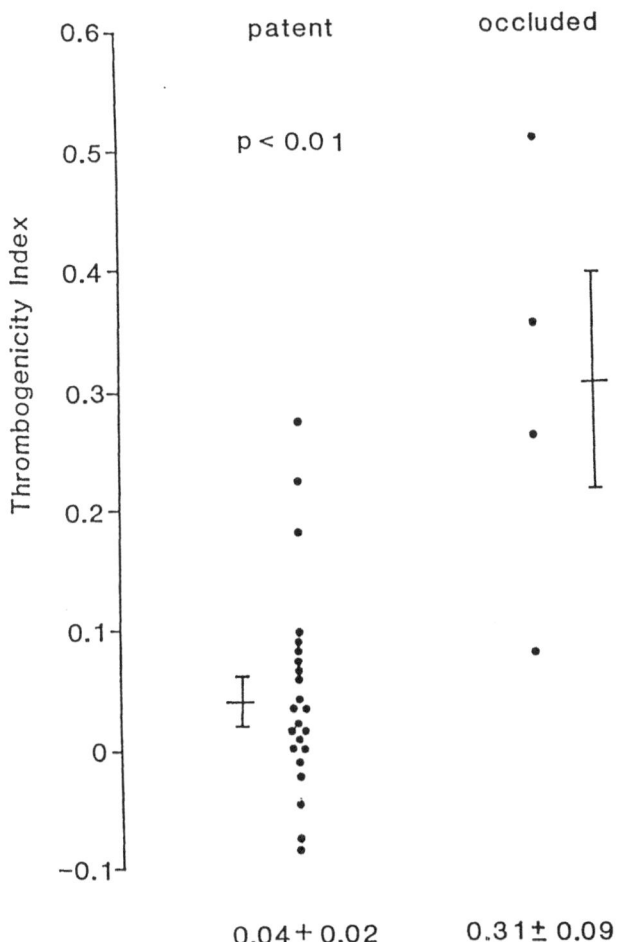

Fig 3   Comparison of thrombogenicity in occluded grafts
               and those remaining patent at 60 days

246

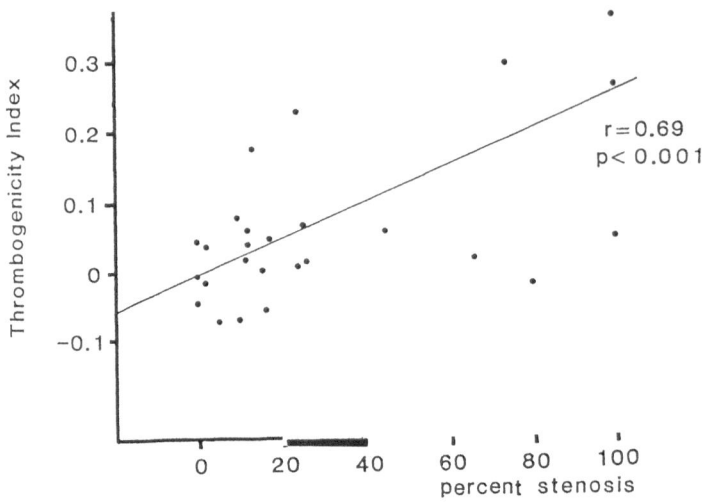

Fig 4   Linear correlation between Thrombogenicity Index
             and luminal stenosis

being at least a contributory factor to the progressive
thrombotic narrowing which leads to the occlusion of these
grafts.   This allows the intensity and duration of platelet
deposition on these artificial surfaces to be assessed and a
rational approach   to   platelet inhibitory therapy is
possible.   Unlike autogenous tissue such as saphenous vein
which recovers a secretory endothelium following arterial
bypass, a pseudo-intima forms on the luminal surface of
prosthetic materials.   The fibrin, platelets and red cells
which make up this layer continue to interact with
circulating blood and without the inhibitory effects of
endothelial prostacyclin will become progressively thicker
and result in graft occlusion.   Although studies of late
platelet uptake have yet to be reported in small calibre
grafts, there is evidence to suggest that mature Dacron
grafts in the aorto-bifemoral position in patients continue
to   show   appreciable   platelet   uptake   10-years   after
implantation (3).   If this is the case, platelet inhibitory
therapy is indicated in all patients with vascular
prostheses and is especially appropriate in small calibre
grafts in the femoro-popliteal position (1).
     This study suggests that the degree of platelet
deposition measured in the early postoperative period may
indicate the likelihood of graft stenosis and thrombosis.   A
reduction in platelet accumulation by inhibitory therapy may
result in improved long-term patency.

REFERENCES

1. Goldman M, McCollum CN: A prospective randomised study of aspirin plus dipyridamole on the patency of femoro-popliteal grafts. Vasc Surg. 1982; 18: 217-221

2. Goldman M, Norcott HC, Hawker RJ, Hail C, Drolc Z, McCollum CN: Femoro-popliteal Bypass Grafts - an isotope technique allowing in vivo Comparison of Thrombogenicity. Br.J.Surg. 1982; 69: 380-382

3. Goldman M, Norcott HC, Hawker RJ, Drolc Z, McCollum CN: Platelet accumulation on mature Dacron grafts in man. Br.J.Surg. 1982; 69 (Suppl): 538-540

4. Imparato AM, Bracco A, Kim GE, Zeff R: Intimal and neointimal fibrous proliferation causing failure of arterial reconstruction. Surgery 1972; 72: 1007-1017

5. Thakur ML, Welch MJ, Joist JH, Coleman RE: Indium-111 labelled platelets: studies on preparation and evaluation of in vitro and in vivo functions.Thromb Res 1976: 9; 345-357

6. Wilkinson AR, Hawker RJ, Hawker LM: 111-Indium labelled canine platelets. Thromb Res 1978; 13: 175-182

111-INDIUM LABELED PLATELETS IN THROMBOCYTOPENIC PURPURA. SURVIVAL AND BIODISTRIBUTION STUDIED WITH SCINTILLATION CAMERA. A REVIEW OF 485 PATIENTS.

MOISAN A, LE PRISE PY, LE CLOIREC J, LEGALL E, GHANDOUR C, LE BLAY R, HERRY JY
Service de Médicine Nucléaire, Centre Eugène Marquis-RENNES CHR RENNES

Since 1980, we have been studying the kinetics of 111-In-oxine labeled platelets in a reduced plasma medium. The advantages of 111-In over 51Cr are well known (4, 6, 8,). The method can be used in auto transfusion, regardless of the severity of the thrombocytopenia (5.10^9 pl/1), and the sites of platelet destruction visualised with a scintillation camera peaked for 173 and 245 kev with a 20 % window. The aim of our study is to evaluate the contribution of this method to the diagnosis of thrombocytopenic mechanism in diverse disorders and to assess its value in selecting patients clinically suitable for splenectomy.

Normal autologus 111-In labeled platelet distribution was tested in 6 volunteer controls. Fifteen patients underwent a double exploration. One with autologus 111-In labeled platelets and the other with donor 51Cr labeled platelets. Between 1980 and 1986, 485 platelet kinetics were investigated in 190 cases of ITP (Idiopathic Thrombocytopenic Purpura) and 295 thrombocytopenic purpuras secondary to haematologic disorders (3) such as lupus erythematosus. Waldenström's disease, acute or chronic leukemia.

METHOD

Fifty milliliters of blood were collected and acidified with an acid citrate dextrose solution (ACD A) at 20%. Platelet rich plasma (PRP) was obtained from this blood by slow centrifugation (150 G, 20°) and transferred to a conical plastic tube for centrifugation at 900 G and 20° C. The platelet poor plasma (PPP) was removed. 3 to 5 MBq of 111-Indium oxine was added dropwise to the platelet pellet in the reduced plasma volume (1 ml). After incubation at room temperature for 5 to 10 min, the platelet solution was washed with 10 ml of PPP (acidified at pH 6,5 with ACD A) and then resuspended in 5 ml of PPP for reinjection (9). Survival time was determined in 5 to 10 blood samples from 30 min after injection until activity in the blood had completely disappeared. In the first 30 min after injection,

248

Ch. Kessler et al. (eds.), Clinical Application of Radiolabelled Platelets, 248–257.
© 1990 Kluwer Academic Publishers.

the amount of 111-In radioactivity in the liver, spleen and heart was measured from the posterior view, with a large field of view gamma camera, peaked for 173 and 245 kev, and interfaced with a data processing system. At the 30th min post injection and daily thereafter the organs of interest were imaged and the count rates obtained using the data processor. The splenic platelet pool (SPP) was measured by the ratio of splenic activity at the 30th min to the total activity injected. The depth of the spleen was calculated from a lateral view.

The following ratios S and L were used to evaluate late sequestration:

-S   represents late splenic sequestration which was equal to the ratio of radioactivity of the spleen on the last day over the radioactivity of the spleen at the 30th minute.

- L   represents late liver sequestration which was equal to the ratio of radioactivity of the liver on the last day over the radioactivity of the spleen at the 30th minute. Late sequestration was considered normal when S and L = 1 ± 0.2. Late sequestration was called "pure spleen" when S > 1.2, "pure liver" when L > 1.2, and "mixed" when S and L > 1.2 (10).

RESULTS

No significant differences (5% threshold) were seen between In-111 and Cr-51 survival times in 10 of 15 patients investigated with both methods (table 1). In one case of isoimmunisation (case n 11), lifespan measured with In-111 autologus platelets was 5 days vs 1 day with the Cr-51 method using homologous platelets. In 4 cases of familial thrombocytopenia, survival of the homologous platelets labeled with Cr-51 was 6 to 7 days vs 2 to 5 days for autologous platelets labeled with In-111.

We obtained a high labeling efficiency in plasma medium which allowed autologus investigation of platelet kinetics however severe the degree of thrombocytopenia. The recovery of circulating platelets, obtained from count rate of the 30-minute blood samples averaged 71 % (1 SD:10%) in the healthy volunteers. 32 ± 5% in the hypersplenic patients, 55 ± 14% in the ITP patients (who showed a wide range of variability depending on the degree of thrombocytopenia) and 54 ± 11% in the patients with marrow hypoplasia. Platelet survival was calculated according to ICSH recommendations (23). Mean platelet lifespan for the healthy controls was 8.7 ± 0.8 d, vs 8.2 ± 1.4 for bone marrow failure patients, 6.1 ± 1.1 d for the hypersplenic patients, and only 2.5 ± 1.2 for the ITP (table 2).

Scintigraphic imaging techniques give a precise description of the early kinetics of hepato-splenic pooling (Fig 1).

TABLE 1 : SURVIVAL TIMES AND SEQUESTRATION SITES ASSESSED BY DONOR
51 CR LABELLED AND AUTOLOGOUS 111-IN LABELLED PLATELETS

PATIENTS	LIFESPAN (DAYS)		SEQUESTRATION*	
	IN-111	CR-51	IN-111	CR-51
1 ITP	1.7	1.5	S+	S+
2 ITP	1.2	1	S+	S+
3 ITP	1.2	1	S+	S+
4 ITP	1.2	1.3	S+H+	S+H+
5 ITP	2.3	2.5	S+	S+
6 ITP	2.3	2	S+H+	S+H+
7 ITP	1.4	1	S+H+	S+H+
8 ITP	1.7	1.3	S+	S+
9 ITP	2.3	2	S-	S-
10 hypersplenism	7	7	S-	S-
11 marrow hypoplasia	5	1	S+	S-
12 familial	2	7	S+	S-
13 familial	3	6	S+	S-
14 familial	6	8	S+	S-
15 familial	6	8	S+	S-

*S : splenic sequestration   H : hepatic sequestration

Table 2.

111IN-LABELLED PLATELET SURVIVAL AND EARLY DISTRIBUTION

PATIENTS	LABELLING EFFICIENCY %	% RECOVERY AT 30 MIN	LIFESPAN (days)	SPLEEN INDEX %
CONTROLS (6)	80 ± 10*	71 ± 10	8,7 ± 0,8	23 ± 2
primary and secondary ITP (246)	68 ± 18	55 ± 14	2,5 ± 1,2	25 ± 4
marrow hypoplasia (105)	56 ± 15	54 ± 11	8,2 ± 1,4	25 ± 4
hypersplenism (134)	52 ± 18	32 ± 5	6,1 ± 1,1	45 ± 6

* mean ± 1SD

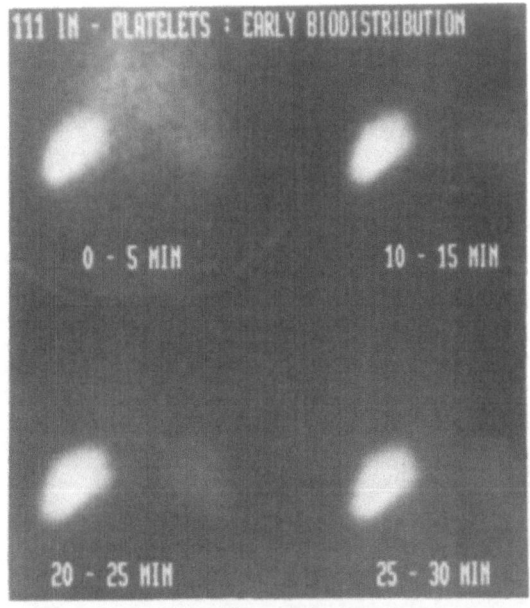

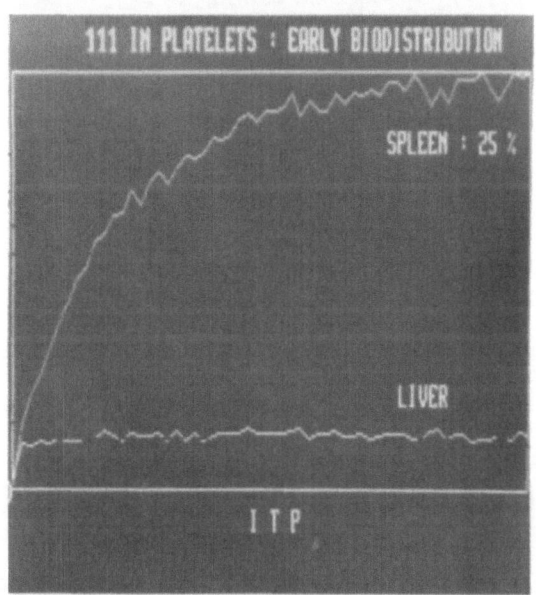

Fig 1. Example of early distribution in a case of ITP. This is useful when making a differential diagnosis between thrombocytopenic purpura and hypersplenism. They also enable the relative importance of the destruction sites to be assessed: in this study purely splenic uptake is observed in 90 % of primary ITP cases (Fig 2) and 79 % in secondary ITP (table 3)

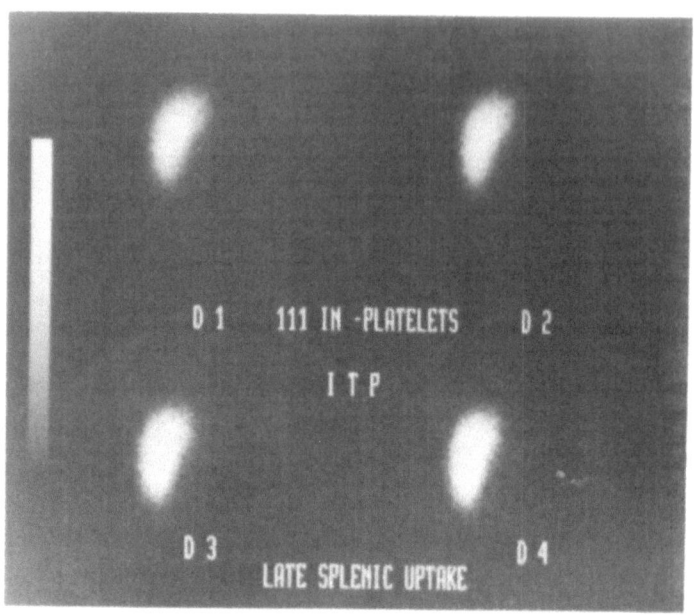

Fig 2. Pure splenic uptake in a case of ITP.

Eighty of the patients included in this study underwent splenectomy. Remission was achieved in most of the other patients either by a course of corticosteroid therapy or by one of Vincristine. The follow-up period is at least 6 months. Splenectomy was successful in 55 cases of auto-immune TP with purely splenic sequestration (table 4). It failed in one case: an accessory spleen was visualised one month after surgery. It failed also in 6 of 8 cases of hepatic or hepatosplenic uptake. In 16 cases of secondary thrombocytopenic purpura, splenetomy was effective in 11 of 14 cases of pure spleen uptake, was a partial failure in 2 cases of pure splenic uptake and failed in 2 cases of mixed sequestration (11, 12).

Table 3 :

111IN-LABELLED PLATELET : LATER SEQUESTRATION IN ITP		
SEQUESTRATION	primary ITP n = 190	secondary ITP n = 56
SPLEEN	171 (90 %)	44 (79 %)
LIVER and SPLEEN	16 (8 %)	7 (12 %)
LIVER	3 (2 %)	5 (9 %)

Table 4 :

RESULTS OF SPLENECTOMY IN 80 THROMBOCYTOPENIC PATIENTS INVESTIGATED WITH 111IN AUTOLOGOUS PLATELETS				
	N=64 PRIMARY ITP		N=16 SECONDARY ITP	
UPTAKE	SUCCESS	FAILURE	SUCCESS	FAILURE
SPLEEN	55	1*	11	(2) + 1
SPLEEN + LIVER	2	3	0	2
LIVER	0	3	0	0
1* accessory spleen				

DISCUSSION

Most authors (13) agree that thrombocytopenia with 8.10^{10} platelets/1. constitutes the threshold below which the results of 51-Cr autologus platelet kinetics can no longer be analyzed. Donor platelets are then usually required to continue investigation. In our study, donor platelets would have been necessary in two-thirds of cases. Thakur's work prompted us to develop a 111-In-oxine labelling method (22) which could be used whatever the degree of thrombocytopenia. We opted for incubation in a plasma medium so that the platelets were preserved in the best conditions possible. For platelet concentrations in the region of 10^9 /1., we obtained a labelling efficiency of between 20 and 50 %. Even when platelet concentrations were 10^{10} /1., labelling efficiency was high (70 % - 90 %). When labelling is carried out in a plasma medium, a greater quantity of blood must be drawn in severe cases of thrombocytopenia.

The results for the controls compared well with the 51-Cr method (2, 20). The normal 111-In life span we obtained was comparable to the one calculated for 51-Cr-labeled platelets (15). For the 10 patients (out of 15) who were investigated with both methods, the results concorded (Table 1) (19). Five discrepancies were observed in these results and were easily explained. The first concerned a case of isoimmunisation (case 11) and illustrates that whatever the degree of thrombocytopenia, an autotransfusion test is useful. 4 others involved cases of corpuscle disorders due to congenital thrombocytopenia (cases 12 to 15). The use of both 111-In and 51-Cr means a double labelling test can be performed which may be invaluable in understanding thrombocytopenic mechanisms. (7).

The use of a gamma-camera linked to a data processor in the study of platelet sequestration in preference to scintigraphic probes eliminates problems of localization: with scintigraphic imaging of liver and spleen, areas of interest may be easily selected. An injection of 2 MBq is sufficient for satisfactory statistical analysis of the counts.

Precise information concerning platelet distribution during the first 30 minutes post injection can be obtained once the computer has provided the first curves. Like Heyns (5), we would suggest that the splenic index be established at 30 minutes to assess the splenic pool. With this parameter, we are able, in our study, to distinguish hypersplenic forms of thrombocytopenia from other forms. The size of the spleen can also be measured with scintigraphic imaging.

The importance of the destruction sites of Cr-51-labeled platelets in ITP has been discussed by several authors (1, 5, 16, 17, 18). We are of the same opinion as Najean (14) : pure splenic uptake is a predictive factor for successful splenectomy. Our results show a success rate of

100 % in cases of pure splenic sequestration and of only 20 % in hepato-splenic or pure liver sequestration. Radionuclide investigation with 111-In labeled platelets is, in our opinion, an important contribution to the discussion as to whether splenectomy should be performed, especially in cases of primary ITP.

CONCLUSION

In conclusion, indium platelet kinetics seem useful in studying thrombocytopenic mechanisms when they are not clearly established by clinical investigation. The 111-Indium sequestration site appears a predictive factor of successful splenectomy in patients with peripheral thrombocytopenic purpura.

REFERENCES

1. Aster RH, Keene WR : Sites of platelet destruction in iopathic thrombocytopenic purpura. Brit J Haemat,1969, 16,61.
2. Bautista AP, Buckler PW, Towler HMA, Dawson AA, Bennett B: Measurement of platelet life-span in normal subjects and patients with myeloproliferative disease with indium oxine labeled platelets. British Journal of Haematology, 1984, 58:679-687.
3. Efira A, Cauchie P, Rauis M, de Martelaere E: Platelet survival in myelodysplatic syndromes. Acata haemat 1986, 76:124-126.
4. Heyns A DuP., Lotter MG, Badenhorst PN, van Rheenen OR, Pieters H, Minnaar C, Retief FP: Kinetics, distribution and sites of destruction of 111-indium-labeled human platelets. British journal of haematology 1980, 44, 269-280.
5. Heyns A DuP, Lotter MG, Badenhorst PN, de Kick F, Pieters H, Herbst C, van Reenen OR, Kotze H, Minnaar PC: Kinetics and sites of destruction of 111-indium oxine labeled platelets in idiopathic thrombocytopenic purpura: a quantitative study. American journal of hematology 1982, 12:167-177.
6. Heyns A DuP, Badenhorst PN, Wessels P, Pieters H, Kotze HF, Lotter MG : Indium-111 labeled human platelets : a method for use in severe thrombocytopenia. Thromb haemostas 1984, (stuttgart)52(3), 226-229.
7. Heyns A DuP, Badenhorst PN, Lotter MG, Pieters H, Wessels P, Kotze H : Platelet turnover and kinetics in immune thrombocytopenic purpura : results with autologous 111 in-labeled platelets and homologous 51cr-labeled platelets differ. blood 1986, 67, 1, 86-92.
8. Klonizakis I, Peters AM, Fitzpatrick ML, Kensett MJ, Lewis SM, Lavender JP : Radionuclide distribution following injection of 111 indium labeled platelets.

British journal of haematology 1980, 46, 595-602.

9.   Moisan A, Le Cloirec J, Herry JY: Marquage des plaquettes et des granulocytes par l'oxine-indium 111. J biophys et med nucl 1983, 7, 3, 113-115.

10. Moisan A, Herry JY, Le Cloirec J, Le Prise PY : 111-Indium labeled platelets in thrombopenic purpura : Survival and in-vivo distribution scintillation camera. European journal of nuclear medicine 7, a496, 1984 (abstract of the european nuclear medicine congress, Helsinki, August 1984, oral communication).

11. Moisan A, Herry JY, Le Prise PY: Platelet destruction sites in itp (176 cases) studied by 111-in labeled platelets, follow-up of 61 splenectomised patients. the British journal of radiology 1985, 58, 925 (proceedings of the british institute of radiology).

12. Moisan A, Ghandour C, Le Gall E, Daurac C, Grosbois B, Herry JY, Le Prise PY : Correlation between the results of splenectomy and the type of sequestration of autologous indium-111 oxine-labeled platelets in thrombocytopenic purpura. International congress world federation of nuclear medicine and biology. buenos aires. 1986. abstracts of scientific communications p 64.

13. Najean Y, Ardaillou N, Caen J, Larrieu MJ, Bernard J : Survival of radiochromium-labeled platelets in thrombocytopenias. blood, 1963, 22, 718.

14. Najean Y, Ardaillou N :The sequestration site of platelets in idiopathic thrombocytopenic purpura. its correlation with the results of splenectomy. British journal of haematology, 1971, 21, 153-164.

15. Peters AM, Lavender JP : Platelet kinetics with indium-111 platelets: comparison with chromium-51 platelets. Seminars in thrombosis and hemostasis, 1983, 9, 2, 100-114.

16. Peters AM, Saverymuttu SH, Wonke B, Lewis SM, Lavender: The interpretation of platelet kinetic studies for the identification of sites of abnormal platelet destruction. British journal of haematology 1984, 57, 637-649.

17. Peters AM, Saverymuttu SH, Bell RN, Lavender JP : The kinetics of short-lived indium-111 radiolabeled platelets. Scand J haematol 1985, 34:137-145.

18. Richards JDM, Thompson DS : Assessment of thrombocytopenic patients for splenectomy. Journal of clinical pathology, 1979, 32, 1248-1252.

19. Schmidt KG, Rasmussen JW: Kinetics and distribution in vivo of 111-in-labeled autologus platelets in idiopathic thrombocytopenic purpura. Scand j haematol, 1985, 34, 47-56.

20. Schmidt KG, Rasmussen JW, Rasmussen AD : Kinetics of 111-in-labeled platelets in healthy subjects. Scand j haematol 1985, 34, 370-277.

21. Stoll D, Cines DB, Aster RH, Murphy S ; Platelet kinetics in patients with idiopathic thrombocytopenic

purpura and moderate thrombocytopenia. blood 1985, 65, 3, 584-588.

22. Thakur ML, Walsh L, Malech HL, Gottschalk A : Indium-111-labeled human platelets : improved method, efficacy, and evaluation. J nucl med 1981, 22:381-385.

23. Recommended methods for radioisotope platelet survival studies. by the panel on diagnostic application of radioisotopes in hematology, international committee for standardization in hematology. Blood 1977, 50, 6.

USE OF 111-IN-FRAGMENTED PLATELETS IN THE DETECTION OF
OCCULT SEPSIS

Ruth A. Harper BSc
W.Th Goedemans PhD
Alan C Meek FRCS
Charles N. McCollum MD. FRCS

Department of Surgery,
Charing Cross & Westminster Medical School,
at Charing Cross Hospital,
London U.K.

and

Mallinckrodt Diagnostica BV,
Patten,
The Netherlands.

INTRODUCTION

   Delay in reaching the diagnosis of localising pus is
the major cause of morbidity and mortality in abdominal
sepsis (1).
   Following abdominal surgery, septic foci are often
missed by both ultrasound and computerised tomography
especially among the loops of bowel which normally contain
fluid and gas which may be confused with that of abscess
(2). III-Indium labelling of leukocytes was first described
in 1976 and their clinical value reported three years later
(3,4). However, the cell labelling process is time
consuming and requires both specialist facilities and
technical expertise. As a result, this accurate and
valuable technique is confined to a few hospitals with the
necessary facilities. A simpler, less time consuming
labelling technique which effectively localises in abscesses
would be of more widespread use.
   III-In-fragmented platelets were evaluated as a result
of an accident. A patient following renal and pancreatic
transportation was included in a study evaluating the use of
radiolabelled platelets to diagnose transportation
rejection. The III-In-platelets were accidentally injected
outside the vein, yet marked accumulation in the necessary
pancreas was seen. We can only assume that the platelets
were being taken up by phagocytic cells and therefore
accumulating in the developing abscess. Radiolabelled
fragmented platelets were compared to the usual III-In-
Oxine labelled mixed leukocytes, used as a "standard" for
comparison. The purpose being to test the possibility that a
labelled material could be prepared which could be used "off

258

Ch. Kessler et al. (eds.), Clinical Application of Radiolabelled Platelets, 258–263.
© 1990 *Kluwer Academic Publishers.*

the shelf" for detecting occult sepsis in patients.

METHOD

Animals

A reproducible chronic abscess model was developed in rats based on the method described by Goldman et al (5). Forty 200g Wistar rats underwent laparotomy during which a 800mm^3 polyester sponge placed intraperitoneally in the region of the right iliac fossa and inoculated with 0.1ml of a bacterial cocktail prior to closure. This bacterial inoculum contained E.Coli 3 x 10^9 Klebsiella sp 10^6 viable organisms/ml grown as pure cultures from rat faeces. Following recovery from anaesthesia the animals were maintained for 14 days and in every case a chronic abscess developed.

LABELLING PROCEDURES

III-In-mixed leucocyte: For each group of 12 rats, 10-15mls of blood was taken into 2mls heparinised saline from a syngeneic donor. An equal volume of Haemaccel was added prior to sedimentation for 60 minutes at room temperature. The supernatant leucocyte rich plasma was removed and centrifuged at 160g for 10 minutes. The platelet rich plasma was then discarded and the leucocyte pellet resuspended in 10mls Haemaccel containing 10 units of Heparin and re-centrifuged at 160g for 10 minutes. The resulting washed pellet was resuspended in 3mls heparinised Haemaccel and incubated with 200μCi of 111-In-oxine for 2 minutes at room temperature. Following further centrifugation at 160g, the labelled mixed leucocytes were resuspended in 6mls heparinised Haemaccel and 0.5mls was administered to each rat via the tail vein.

111-In-fragmented platelet: For each group of 12 rats 10-15mls of blood were taken into 2mls of acid citrate from a syngeneic donor. The labelling procedure is based on that described by Robert Hawker (6). The citrated blood is spun slowly (160g) to produce a platelet rich plasma fraction. This fraction is then spun rapidly (580g) to concentrate a platelet pellet. The washed and resuspended pellet is then incubated with 200μCi of 111-In-oxine for 2 minutes at room temperature. Following further centrifugation toe resuspended radiolabelled platelets are fragmented by alternate submersion in liquid nitrogen and warm water, this is performed a total of 3-times and the resuspended platelets are then ready for re-injection.

ABSCESS AND CRITICAL ORGAN RADIOACTIVITY MEASUREMENTS

Two weeks following the induction of the chronic abscess, 40 rats were randomised in batches to either 111-in-mixed leucocytes or 111-In-fragmented platelets. At 48 hours following the injection of radiolabelled cells the abscess, liver and spleen were excised and counted in a well-crystal. This activity was expressed as a percentage of the total body count measured by counting the homogenised carcass in the same crystal. Gamma camera studies were performed to confirm that abscess imaging was adequate for visualisation.

DATA ANALYSIS

Abscess, hepatic and splenic radioactivity calculated as percent injected activity per gram of tissue was compared between the mixed leucocyte label and the fragmented platelet technique using the Student' unpaired t-tests. All results are expressed as mean ±.

RESULTS

The 40 animals were randomised into two equal groups. In the 20 animals labelled with the "standardised" mixed leucocytes the mean percentage activity found per gram of abscess was 0.41±0.033 which was significantly lower than the 0.58±0.040 found in the 20 animals labelled with 111-In-fragmented platelets (p<0.01) (Figure 1a)

On gamma imaging, uptake was visualised around the region of the abscess in both cases, an example of which is shown in Figure 2.

Clinical evaluation of these techniques depend both on the abscess uptake and the dose that can be administered which is limited by the dose to the critical organs. The critical organ for 111-In-mixed leucocytes was the spleen and in this rate model, 11.81±4.472 percent of the injected activity accumulated per gram of spleen. In the fragmented platelet group the accumulation was surprisingly low with a mean value of 5.27±0.0.450 percent/gram, (p<0.02) (Figure 1b) On studying other possible sites of fragmented platelet uptake it was found that there was increased accumulation in the liver with mean values of 2.10±0.065 compared to 1.26±0.108 percent/gram in the mixed leucocyte rats (p<0.001) (Figure 1c).

DISCUSSION

In this study, invivo leucocyte labelling by using fragmented platelets labelled with 111-In-oxine surprisingly achieved significantly higher abscess accumulation than leucocytes labelled with the same isotope. Direct intravenous administration of 111-Indium oxine or 111-In-chloride may produce low levels of abscess uptake but renal excretion is high and tends to obscure the images (7).

The sensitivity of these techniques depend in part on the dose of isotope that can be administered which is limited for radiolabelled leucocytes by splenic radiation (8). Fragmented platelets reduced splenic uptake by 2 fold, but at the cost of an increased hepatic accumulation

Fig 1

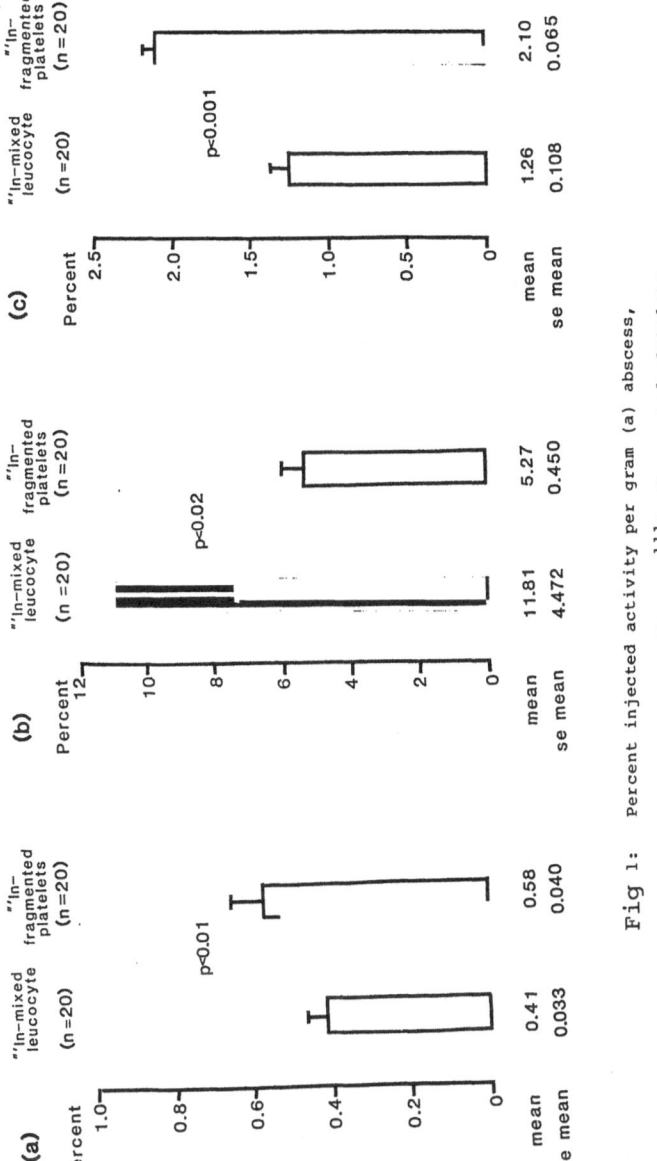

Fig 1: Percent injected activity per gram (a) abscess,
(b) spleen, (c) liver. 111In-fragmented platelets
are compared to the mixed leucocyte label using a
student unpaired t-test.

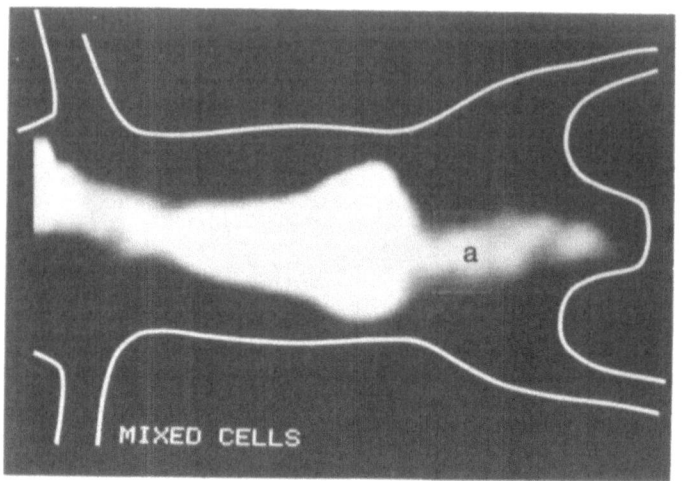

Fig 2:   Gamma image showing uptake of radioactivity in the
          abscess (a) 48 hours following administration of
          ^{111}In-mixed leucocytes.

presumably due to metabolisation of radiolabelled proteins from the fragmented cells. However, though the increase is significant in absolute terms it is small in terms of radiation dosimetry. Technical expertise and sterile facilities are still required but this labelling technique is simpler, reduces the time required for labelling from 3 hours to 1 hour, and reduced the volume of blood used from 60 to 20ml. Although this may be considered sufficient reason for some centres to take up this method perhaps the real promise lies in the possibility that a radiolabelled protein may be identified which could be manufactured and administered directly "off the shelf" to diagnose abscess in any hospital equipped with a gamma camera.

REFERENCES

1. Dry DE, Garrison RN, Heitsch RC, Calhoun K, Polk HC. Determinants of death in patients with intraabdominal abscess. Surgery 1980. 88: 517-523
2. Doust BD, Quiroz F, Stewart JM. Ultrasonic distinction of abscess from other intraabdominal fluid collections. Ultrasound 1977. 125: 213-217
3. Thakur ML, Coleman RE, Mayhall CG, Welsh MJ. Preparation and evaluation of 111-In-labelled leukocytes as an abscess imaging agent in dogs. Radiology 1976. 119: 731-732
4. Ascher NL, Ahrenholz DH, Simmons RL et al. Indium 111 autologous tagged leukocytes in the diagnosis of intraperitoneal sepsis. Arch Surg 1979. 114: 386-392
5   Goldman M, Gunson B, Ambrose NS, McCollum CN. A low mortality rat model for studying pyogenic abdominal abscess. Surg.Res.Comm. 1987. 1: 13-15
6   Hawker RJ, Hawker LM, Wilkinson AR. Indium 111-In labelled human platelets. Optimal method. Clin.Sci.1980. 58: 243-248
7   Goedemans WTh, Hardeman MR, Belfer AJ. Comparison of Indium-111 oxinate labelled autologous granulocytes with Indium-111 oxinate and Indium-111 chloride as abscess scanning agents. An experimental study in an animal model. Eur.J.Nucl.Med.1980. 5: 63-68.
8   Busemann Sokole E, Hengst D, Rovekamp MH. Radiation dosimetry of 111-In-oxinate labelled leucocytes. Nucl.Med.Bull. 1982. 4: 14-16

THE CLINICAL UTILITY OF INDIUM-111 LABELED PLATELET
SCINTIGRAPHY IN THE DIAGNOSES OF RENAL TRANSPLANT REJECTION

Gary V. Desir MD*, Margaret Bia MD, Robert C Lange Phd,
Eileen O Smith BS, Wayne Flye MD, Phd, Michael Kashgarian
MD, Martin Schiff MD and Michael D. Ezekowitz MD, PhD*,
Departments of Medicine, Radiology, Surgery and Pathology,
Yale University School of Medicine.

Indium-111 labeled platelet scintigraphy, kidney transplant
rejection.

Acknowledgements:
Grant Support
*National Institute of Health PPG No. 2 PO1 HL 17812-07
*Veteran Administration Merit Review Grant
*Robert Wood Johnson Foundation

INTRODUCTION

Acute rejection, which often threatens graft survival
in kidney transplant recipients, should be diagnosed and
treated urgently. There is indirect evidence that the
earlier treatment is initiated, the better are the chances
of preserving graft function (1). At present, allograft
rejection is best diagnosed histologically (2). Since kidney
biopsy is an invasive procedure which carries a small but
significant risk of major complications (3) it is usually
obtained only when acute rejection is strongly suspected on
clinical grounds, that is after renal damage has already
occurred. In the first month following transplantation, when
the incidence of acute rejection is very high, clinical
parameters, namely graft pain, tenderness and enlargement
and fever, are often not helpful since acute rejection can
occur in their absence, especially in patients maintained on
cyclosporine (4). Moreover, rejection is notoriously
difficult to diagnose clinically in the setting of post
operative acute tubular necrosis since urine output is
decreased and since serum creatinine, the single most
diagnostic biochemical parameter, is already markedly
elevated. For these reasons, a non invasive test that
detects rejection before it is clinically apparent is very
much needed.
Several non invasive methods have been tested as
diagnostic tools for renal allograft rejection. Immunologic
methods using monoclonal antibodies to T cell subsets,
endothelial cells and more recently to adenosine deaminase
binding protein (ABP) have been evaluated (5-9). Many of

Ch. Kessler et al. (eds.), Clinical Application of Radiolabelled Platelets, 264–277.

these tests though accurate require complicated and time consuming immunologic assays that do not readily lend themselves to widespread clinical use (10). Various radiologic techniques have also been used to detect acute rejection. Technetium-99m-DTPA scintigraphy lacks in both sensitivity and specificity (11,12). Iodine-131-hippurate scanning is accurate but of limited usefulness since it only detects well established rejection (13). Pulsed doppler duplex scanning, a technique in which real time ultrasonographic imaging is combined with blood flow characterization by pulsed doppler, has a low sensitivity, detecting only vascular rejection (14).

Platelets and fibrin deposition in rejection renal transplants has been documented (15-17). Platelet accumulation is expected to occur in both cellular and vascular rejection since platelet activating factor, a potent platelet aggregating factor, is released by both lymphoid and endothelial cells during inflammatory processes (18). Several tests that detect or reflect platelet and fibrin deposition in renal allografts have been evaluated. Urinary thromboxane B2 (a stable metabolite of thromboxane A2), released from platelets, lymphocytes and granulocytes is increased in graft rejection (19). The assay is non specific and cannot differentiate thromboses in the kidney and elsewhere from graft rejection. In addition, the test cannot be used in anuric patients. I-125 labelled fibrinogen can accurately detect kidney allograft rejection (20). It is limited by being a count based, non imaging method. Thus, extra renal activity, particularly isotope excreted in the urine, can complicate the interpretation of the test. 123-I, an excellent imaging agent, may potentially be used to label fibrinogen. This poses logistic difficulties since the isotope has a short half life, requires cyclotron production and is not readily available (21).

Indium-111 labeled platelet scintigraphy does not carry the same drawbacks. The isotope is short lived (2.8 days) and possesses physical characteristics suitable for imaging. In addition, labeling platelets with indium-111 does not significantly alter their function (22). Imaging with a gamma camera is possible for up seven days following a single injection of labeled platelets. Quantitative, in vivo, measurements of sites of platelet accumulation can be achieved by computer assisted image processing. Thus, indium-111 labeled platelet scintigraphy has been used successfully to detect deep venous thrombosis and intracardiac thrombi (23-28).

In earlier reports, autologous platelets labeled with indium-111 oxine were shown to accumulate in acutely rejecting renal transplants (29-32). The present study demonstrates that indium-111 labeled platelet scintigraphy is a highly accurate test for detecting acute untreated renal allograft rejection. More importantly, it shows that changes in platelet uptake can precede signs and symptoms of rejection by at least 48 hours.

MATERIAL AND METHODS

PLATELET LABELING

Platelets are labeled according to the method of Thakur et al (22) as modified by Heaton et al (33) and Ezekowitz et al (34). Forty three ml of autologus whole blood is drawn in 7 ml of Squibb Modified Acid Citrate Dextrose (ACD), through a 19 gauge needle. Platelets are harvested by gentle centrifugation, washed in ACD saline and incubated at room temperature for 20 minutes in ACD saline with indium-111 oxine (Amersham). Platelets are then washed with plasma to remove free and loosely bound indium-111. Contamination by erythrocytes and leukocytes was minimal.

Labeling efficiency, calculated as the ratio of radioactivity in the platelet pellet over the activity in the original incubation media was $88 \pm 3\%$ (mean $\pm$ SEM). Prior to reinjection, platelets are suspended in citrated plasma. In this study 200 ± 5 μCi of indium-111 labeled platelets was injected. This amount is within the guidelines established by the Federal drug administration. The labeling procedure is usually complete within one hour.

SCINTIGRAPHY

Fifteen minute images are obtained in the supine position on a wide field of view scintillation camera fitted with medium energy collimator. Imaging is performed by centering on the gamma ray of peaks of 173 and 247 keV, with 20% symmetrical windows. The first image was obtained 16 ± 2 hours following platelet injection and then once a day thereafter for a maximum of seven days. The platelet uptake index (PUI) is calculated as the ratio of counts over the transplant to that of a contralateral area of similar size (Fig 1). For each patient, the areas of interest were manually defined on the first scan and were then used for the remainder of the study. The platelet uptake index was determined on line using Gamma-11 (Digital Equipment Corp.) dedicated computer.

PATHOLOGY

All renal biopsies were read by pathologist (M.K.) without knowledge of the results obtained by indium-111 labeled platelet scintigraphy. Tissue was prepared for light, electron and immunofluorescence microscopy. Each rejection episode was classified as cellular, vascular or mixed. Cellular rejection was characterized by the presence of interstitial edema and infiltration with lymphocytes, plasma cells, macrophages and granulocytes. Vascular

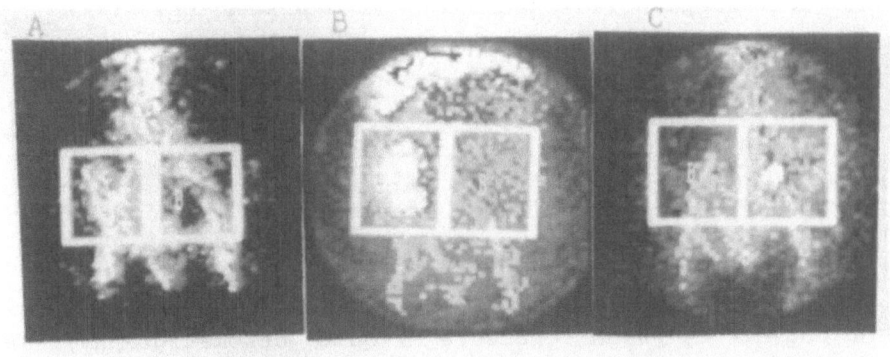

Fig 1:
     Platelet   scan of a patient with normal transplant
function. The platelet uptake index (PUI=1.16) is calculated
as the ratio of counts over the transplant (Left panel)
against a contralateral area of similar size (Right panel).
1B: Platelet scan of a patient with acute untreated
rejection. Platelet uptake in the transplanted kidney (Left
panel) is homogeneous and the PUI is 1.55. 1C: Platelet scan
of a patient with no clinical or biochemical evidence of
rejection. Platelet deposition in the graft (Right panel) is
nonhomogeneous. The PUI is 1.52. This probably represents a
perirenal hematoma.

rejection was diagnosed in the presence of vasculitis, vascular necrosis, intravascular thrombosis or severe glomerulo-endothelial swelling. Mixed rejection had features of both cellular and vascular rejection. Acute tubular necrosis was diagnosed in the presence of interstitial edema and tubular epithelial necrosis and regeneration.

IMMUNOSUPPRESSIVE PROTOCOL

Until November of 1983, maintenance immunosuppressive therapy was identical in both living and cadaveric renal transplant recipients and consisted of azathioprine, 2mg/kg/day, plus prednisone, starting at a dose of 2-4 mg/kg/day and tapered to 0.4 mg/kg/day by the first month post transplant. Since November 1983, cadaveric renal transplant recipients have been treated with cyclosporine (at a dose designed to maintain serum trough levels at 50-150 ng/ml by high pressure liquid chromatography) and prednisone, starting dose of 4 mg/kg/day then tapered to 0.25 mg/kg/day by the first month post transplant. Acute rejection episodes unresponsive to intravenous solumedrol (7 mg/kg/day for 3 days) were treated with intravenous anti thymocyte globulin (Upjohn) at 15 mg/kg/day for 2 weeks.

PATIENT POPULATION

All adult patients undergoing renal transplantation at Yale New Haven Hospital were eligible to participate in the study. Written consent was obtained prior to participation and the protocol was approved by the Yale Human Investigation Committee. Preliminary studies revealed that patients injected with indium-111 labeled platelets 2 days post transplant surgery had elevated platelet uptake index (1.8 ± 1) which steadily decreased with time until day 7 (1.38 ± 07). This was probably due to platelet deposition in the transplant bed and in perfusion damaged capillaries. Therefore, all patients reported in this study were injected at least one week after transplant surgery. Of the sixty four patients studied 13 were excluded from the analysis for the following reasons: In 7 patients the concomitant administration of 131 I-hippurate precluded accurate analysis of the indium-111 images; 3 patients had 2 transplanted kidneys and a contralateral area was not available for computing the platelet uptake index. One had markedly decreased blood flow through the iliac artery on the contralateral side which provided a low background and could not be used to calculate the platelet uptake index. The last 2 patients excluded had marked localized platelet uptake in the hilum of the graft. These most likely represented perirenal thrombi complicating surgery. The remaining 51 patients were analyzed as described. Diagnostic and therapeutic decisions were not made on the basis of indium-111 labeled platelet scintigraphy results.

CONTROL PATIENTS

The mean and the upper limit of normal of the platelet uptake index were established. Intra patient variability of the platelet uptake index over 7 days was also examined. Fifty seven scans were performed in 14 patients (5 females and 9 males). They all had stable renal function, serum creatinine of 2 3mg/dl, and no evidence of rejection (kidney biopsy in 3). They had undergone renal transplantation 1 to 110 weeks prior to study. Immunosuppressive therapy consisted of prednisone plus azathioprine in 6 and prednisone plus cyclosporine in 8.

PATIENTS WITH RENAL DYSFUNCTION

Thirty seven patients with graft dysfunction were studied. The platelet uptake index values reported were obtained during the first day of imaging or within 24 hours of a kidney biopsy.

Nineteen patients (11 females and 8 males) had acute untreated rejection. They had been transplanted 1-20 weeks prior to study. The serum creatinine concentration was 5 ± 1 mg/dl and maintenance immunosuppressive therapy consisted of prednisone plus azathioprine in 12 and cyclosporine in 7. Rejection was diagnosed on the basis of clinical parameters namely graft pain, tenderness and enlargement, fever and deterioration of graft function as indicated by changes in the serum creatinine and in urinary output. The diagnoses was confirmed histologically in 18 of the 19 patients (insufficient renal tissue in 1). The patient however, had an excellent clinical response to anti-rejection treatment (serum creatinine concentration falling from 6.2 to 2.1mg/dl in one week).

Studies were also performed in 8 patients (1 female and 7 males) who were already under treatment (7 ± 1 days) for biopsy proven rejection at the time the first scan was obtained. They had been transplanted 4-10 weeks prior to study. The serum creatinine concentration was 5 ± 1.5 mg/dl. Rejection therapy was as described above.

Seven male patients had primary graft nonfunction. They had been transplanted 1-2 weeks prior to study. Immunosuppressive therapy consisted of prednisone in all plus azathioprine in 3 and cyclosporine in 4. The diagnosis of acute tubular necrosis was established by biopsy in 3 patients and by restoration of normal renal function without specific treatment in the remaining 4.

Finally, 3 female patients with acute cyclosporine nephrotoxicity were evaluated. They had been transplanted 1-12 weeks prior to study and all had an acute decline in renal function (serum creatinine concentration of 2.6 ± 1

mg/dl). Serum cyclosporine levels as determined by high pressure liquid chromatography was 350 ± 12 ng/ml (normal 50-150 ng/ml). Renal function improved in all over 3 ± 0.5 days following a reduction of the cyclosporine dose and a decrease in serum cyclosporine level to 86 ± 10 ng/ml.

PROSPECTIVE EVALUATION

To determine if changes in platelet uptake index preceded signs and symptoms of acute rejection, a subset (n=18) of the 51 patients described above were analyzed. In all 18 patients, indium-111 labeled platelet scintigraphy was begun 1 week post transplantation surgery, before there was clinical or biochemical evidence of rejection. Imaging was continued for 7 days. Immunosuppressive therapy of prednisone in all with either azathioprine in 8 or cyclosporine in 10. The diagnoses of stable renal function, acute tubular necrosis or acute rejection were made on the basis of their clinical course and histologic findings (biopsy in 6). These diagnoses were then compared to the results obtained by indium-111 labeled platelet scintigraphy. Diagnostic and therapeutic decisions were not made on the basis of indium-111 labeled platelet scintigraphy results.

Table 1. Daily Platelet Uptake Index (PUI) in 14 Control Patients

Day*	Scans**	PUI (mean±SEM)***
	14	1.23±0.02
	11	1.25±0.03
	11	1.30±0.02
	8	1.29±0.02
	5	1.28±0.04
	4	1.20±0.05
	4	1.12±0.04

* Represents time following injection of labeled platelets that images were acquired.

** Total number of scans performed on the designated day.

*** No significant difference in PUI from day 1 to 7

one way ANOVA).

RESULTS

Control patients

In the control group, there was no significant difference in the platelet uptake index values from day 1 to 7 of scanning, (Table 1) and the interday variation in the values was minimal. The mean platelet uptake index for the first day of scanning was 1.23 0.02 and no patient had a platelet uptake index greater than 1.38. Furthermore, there was no significant difference in platelet uptake index in patients on prednisone and cyclosporine (1.23 ± 0.03) versus those on prednisone plus azathioprine (1.23 ± 0.03). For diagnostic purposes, a platelet uptake index > 1.4 was considered the upper limit of normal.

PATIENTS WITH RENAL DYSFUNCTION

In patients with acute untreated rejection (n=19) platelet uptake index was significantly greater than in controls:1.66 ± 0.12 vs 1.23 ± 0.02 ($p< 0.05$, Dunnett's test), (Figure 2). In all but 3, platelet uptake index was equal to or greater than 1.4. Both patients with cellular (n=10,PUI=1.42 ± 0.04) and with acute vascular or mixed rejection (n=8 PUI=1.95 ± 0.25) had significantly higher platelet uptake index than controls (PUI=1.23 ± 0.02),$p< 0.005$ and 0.0001 respectively. Patients with vascular or mixed rejection (n=8) had significantly higher platelet uptake index than those with only cellular rejection (n=10), 1.95 ± 0.25 versus 1.42 ± 0.04 respectively ($p< 0.025$, simple t-test). Indium-111 labeled platelet scintigraphy correctly identified all patients with vascular rejection and 70% of those with cellular rejection.

In contrast, patients (n=8) who had begun treatment for rejection before the first scan had platelet uptake index in the normal range: 1.21 ± 0.04 (range 1.1-1.3). The lower platelet uptake index did not correlate with favorable clinical outcome or with improving renal function at the time of study since 4 of these patients sustained permanent graft dysfunction.

In patients with acute tubular necrosis and cyclosporine nephrotoxicity, platelet uptake index was 1.21 ± 0.03 (range 1.15-1.32) and 1.14 ± 0.04 (range 1.07-1.22) respectively. Thus, none of the patients with acute tubular necrosis or cyclosporine nephrotoxicity had a platelet uptake index above 1.32 (Figure 1). Using a platelet uptake index of 1.4 above as abnormal, and using the biopsy and the clinical outcome as the reference standard, indium-111 labeled platelet scintigraphy detects untreated renal allograft rejection with a sensitivity of 84% (16/19) and specificity of 100% (24/24).

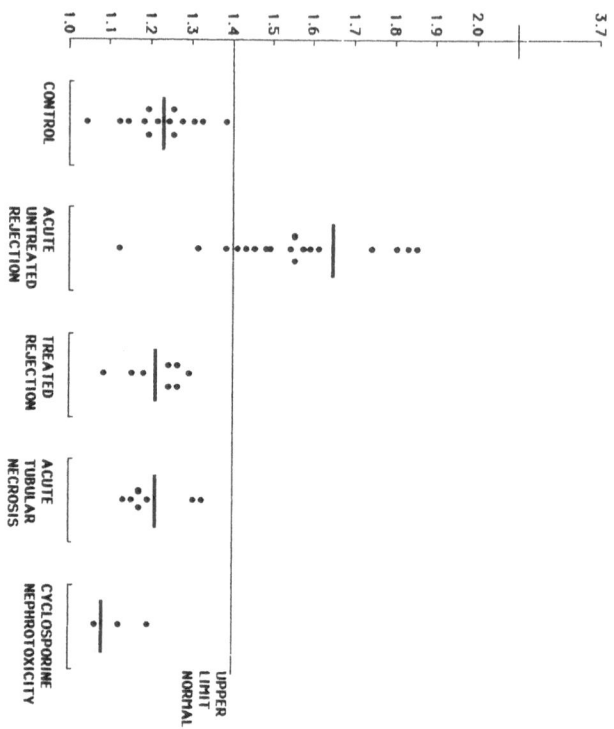

Figure 2:
    Comparing acute untreated rejection, treated rejection
acute tubular necrosis and cyclosporine nephrotoxicity
against control. PUI in acute untreated rejection is
significantly higher than in control, treated rejection, and
acute tubular necrosis, (p<0.005 one way ANOVA and p<0.05,
Dunnett's test). Using a PUI> 1.4 as the upper limit of
normal indium-111 labeled scintigraphy detects acute
rejection with a sensitivity of 84% and a specificity of
100%.

PROSPECTIVE EVALUATION

Of the subset of patients evaluated prospectively, n=18, 8 had normal transplant function and all had platelet uptake index in the normal range:1.24 ± 0.02 (range 1.21-1.38). Four had uncomplicated acute tubular necrosis and the platelet uptake index was 1.03 ± 0.03.

Six developed biopsy proven acute rejection during the study period (5 in the setting of post operative acute tubular necrosis). All 6 patients with acute rejection had platelet uptake indices above the normal range, 1.78 ± 0.2 (range of 1.56-2.06), 2-5 days before the diagnoses was clinically suspected. In the 5 patients with acute rejection and acute tubular necrosis, indium-111 labeled platelet scintigraphy identified rejection (platelet uptake index >1.4), 3.5 ± 1 days before it was clinically suspected. Therapeutic decisions were not made on the basis of indium-111 labeled platelet scintigraphy results and none of those patients were treated before rejection was suspected clinically and confirmed by biopsy. Four of these 6 patients had permanent graft dysfunction due to rejection and 3 underwent transplant nephrectomy.

DISCUSSION

Indium-111 labeled autologus platelets accumulate in the transplanted kidney. From day 2 to 7 following transplantation, significant platelet accumulation can occur in the absence of rejection. If rejection does not develop, platelet deposition decreases progressively, reaching a steady state approximately 1 week post transplantation. And in patients without rejection, who undergo platelet scintigraphy at least 1 week after surgery, the upper limit of normal for the platelet uptake index was 1.4 (Figure 2).

Sixteen of 19 patients with acute untreated rejection had platelet uptake index above the normal range. False negative results (n=3) occurred only in patients with mild to moderate cellular rejection probably because platelet accumulation is not the predominant histologic finding in cellular rejection. Platelet accumulation can still be detected in 70% of patients with cellular rejection. All patients with acute tubular necrosis or cyclosporine toxicity had platelet uptake indices in the normal range. Because of the small sample size, the data related to cyclosporine nephrotoxicity must be interpreted with]caution.

Indium-111 labeled platelet scintigraphy can diagnose acute rejection with a sensitivity of 84% (16/19) and a specificity of 100% (24/24). More importantly, indium-111 labeled platelet scintigraphy can detect rejection 2-5 days before the diagnoses is clinically suspected. This is particularly true of patients with post operative acute tubular necrosis in whom the clinical diagnosis of acute rejection is often delayed and therapy instituted only after extensive renal damage has already occurred.

Although indium-111 labeled platelet scintigraphy accurately detects untreated rejection, it cannot assess the efficacy of treatment. Indeed, in the present study, the platelet uptake index was in the normal range in all treated patients even though 50% of them did not respond to therapy and sustained permanent graft dysfunction. Changes in platelet count could not explain this finding and we conclude that a decrease in platelet uptake index after rejection therapy has begun does not necessarily predict a favorable clinical outcome.

Our results lend support to the concept that significant platelet deposition occur in renal allografts in acute rejection. In vascular rejection, which is often characterized by intravascular thromboses there is greater platelet deposition than in cellular rejection. In this Study, the mean platelet uptake index was significantly higher in patients with vascular as compared to those with cellular rejection (1.95 ± 02 vs 1.42 ± 0.04, p<0.025).

In summary, platelets can be readily labeled with indium-111. A single injection of labeled platelets (200 Ci) allows daily monitoring of the graft for approximately 7 days. If clinically indicated, additional platelet injections can be given. The transplanted kidney can be imaged with a gamma camera and potential false positive results such as localized thrombosis or perirenal hematoma can be excluded. The major limitations of this technique are that it cannot be used in the first week following transplantation because of nonspecific platelet uptake in the transplant area and that is not accurate in confirming rejection once therapy has begun. In addition, factors involving the contralateral reference area, such as second transplants or reduced vascular activity, interfere with the calculation of the platelet uptake index. The major advantages are that it is accurate in untreated patients detecting both cellular and vascular rejection and may allow institution of therapy earlier than was previously possible.

Acknowledgments

We thank Dr Paul Hoffer for supplying imaging facilities and the transplant team members for their cooperation.

REFERENCES

1. Strom T, Garavoy M: Clinical and experimental aspects of renal allograft rejection. American J Kidney Disease 1981;1:5-14.
2. Finkelstein FO, Siegel NJ, Bastl CR, Forrest JN, Kashgarian M: Kidney transplant biopsies in the diagnosis and management of acute rejection reactions.

Kidney Inter.1976;10:171-73

3. Ginsgurg JC, Fransman SL, Slinger MA et al: Use of computerized tomography to evaluate bleeding after renal biopsy. Nephron 1980; 26:240-43.

4. Cohen D, Loertscher R, Rubin MF, Tilney NL, Carpenter CB, Strom TB: Cyclosporine a new immunosuppressive agent for organ transplantation. Ann. Inter. Med. 1984: 101 667-76

5. Paul LC, van Es LA, van Rood JJ, van Leeuwen A, Brutel de la riviere G, de Graeff J: Antibodies directed against antigens on the endothelium of peritubular capillaries in patients with renal allograft rejection. Transplantation 1979:27:175-79.

6. Gailiunas P, Suthanthiran M, Person A et al: Post transplant immunologic monitoring of the renal allograft recipient. Transplant \proc 1978;10:609-11.

7. Vessella RL, Pierce GE, Barth RF et al: Correlation of spontaneous leukocyte blastogenesis with human allograft rejection. Transplantation 1977;23:227-31.

8. Cosimi AB, Colvin RB, Button RC, Rubin RH, Goldstein G, Kung PC, Hansen WP, Delmonico FL, Russell PS: Use of monoclonal antibodies to T cell subsets for immunologic monitoring and treatment in recipients of renal allografts. N Engl J Med. 1981;305:308-14.

9. Tolkoff-Rubin NE, Cosimi AB Delmonico FL, Russell PS, Thompson RE, Piper DJ, Hansen WP, Bander NH, Finstad CL, Cordon-Cardo C, Klotz LH, Old LJ and Rubin RH: Diagnosis of tubular injury by a urinary assay for a proximal tubular antigen, the adenosine-deaminase-binding protein. Transplantation 1986; 41:593-97.

10. Kahan BD: Immunologic monitoring. Utility and limitations. Transplantations Proc. 1985;17:1537-45

11. Kim YC, Massari PU, Brown ML: Clinical significance of 99m Technetium sulfur colloid accumulation in renal transplant recipients. Radiology 1977;124:745-48.

12. Leonard JC, Baumann WE, Pederson JA et al :99m Technetium sulfur colloid scanning in diagnosis of renal transplant rejection. J Urology 1980;123:815-18

13. Diethelm AG, Dubowsky EW, Whelchel JD et al : Diagnosis of impaired renal function after kidney transplantation using renal scintigraphy, renal plasma flow and urinary excretion of hippurate. Am Surg. 1980;604-16.

14. Rigsby CM, Tailor KJW, Weltin G, Burns PN, Bia M, Pricenthal RA, Kasgarian M, Flye MW: Renal allograft in acute rejection. Evaluation using duplex sonnography. Radiology 1986;158:375-78.

15. Williams GM, Hume DM, Hudson RP, Morris RJ, Kano K, Milgrom F: Hyperacute renal homograft rejection in man. N Engl J Med.1968; 279:611-18.

16. Busch GJ, Reynolds ES, Galvanek E, Braun WE, Dammin GJ: Human renal allografts. The role of vascular injury in early graft failure. Medicine 1971; 50:79.

17. Kincaid-Smith P: Histological diagnosis of rejection of renal homografts in man. Lancet 1967; 11:849-52.

18. Rosam Ac, Wallace JL, Whittle BJR: Potent ulcerogenic actions of platelet activating factor on the stomach. Nature 1986;319:54-56.
19. Foegh ML, Zmudka M, Colley C, Winchester JF, Helfrich GB, Ramwell PW: Urine i-TXB in renal allograft rejection. Lancet 1981; 2:431-34.
20. Salaman JR: Use of radioactive fibrinogen for detecting rejection of human renal transplants Br Med J 1970;2:517-   21.
21. Yeboah ED, Shackman R, Chisholm GD: The use of radioactive fibrinogen for detecting of human renal transplants. Br J Surg. 1972; 59:311-15.
22. Thakur ML, Welch MJ, Joist JH, Coleman RE: Indium-111 labeled platelets. Studies on preparation and valuation of in vitro and in vivo function. Thromb Res. 1976; 9:345-57.
23. Moser KM, Spragg RG, Bender F, Konopka R, Hartman MT, Fedullo P: Study of factors that may condition scintigraphic detection of venous thrombi and pulmonary emboli with Indium-111 labeled platelets. J Nucl Med. 1980; 21:1051-58.
24. Davis HH, Siegel BA, Sherman LA, Heaton WA, Welch MJ: Scintigraphy with 111-In-labeled autologus platelets in venous thromboembolism. Radiology 1980; 136:203-07.
25. Fenech a, Hussey JK, Smith FW, Dendy PP, Bennett B, Douglas AS: Diagnoses of deep vein thrombosis using autologous indium-111-labeled platelets. Br Med J. 1981;282:1020-21.
26. Ezekowitz MD, Pope CF, Sostman DH et al : Indium-111 platelet scintigraphy for the diagnoses of acute venous thrombosis. Circulation 1986; 73:668-74.
27. Stratton JR, Ritchie JL, Hamilton GW, Hammermeister KE, Harker LA: Left ventricular thrombi: in vivo detection by indium-111-platelet imaging and two dimensional echocardiography. Am J Cardiol. 1981; 47:874-81.
28. Ezekowitz MD, Wilson DA, Smith EO, Burow RD, Harrison LH, Parker DE, Elkins RC, Peyton M, Taylor FB: Comparison of Indium-111 platelet scintigraphy and two-dimensional echocardiography in the diagnosis of left ventricular thrombi. N Engl J Med. 1982; 306:1509-13.
29. Smith N, Chandler S, Hawker RJ, Hawker LM, Barnes AD: Indium labeled autologous platelets as diagnostic aid after renal transplantation. Lancet 1979; 2:1241-42.
30. Fenech A, Nicholls A and Smith FW: Indium (111-In)- labeled platelets in the diagnosis of renal transplant rejection: preliminary findings. Br J Radiology 1981; 54:325-27.
31. Jurewicz WA, Dykes JGA, Gunson ST, Chandler RJ, Hawker RJ, Barnes AD: Indium-111 labeled platelets as a diagnostic aid in post transplant monitoring of renal allograft in human Transplantation Proc. 1984; 16:1481-83.
32. Grino JM, Alsina J, Martin M, Roca M, Castelao A, Romero R and Caralps A: Indium-111 labeled autologous

platelets as a diagnostic method in kidney allograft rejection. Transplantation Proc. 1982; 16:198-200.

33. Heaton WA, Davis HH, Welch MJ, Mathias CJ, Joist JH, Sherman A, Siegel BA: Indium-111, a new radionuclide for studying human platelet kinetics. Br J Haematol. 1979; 42:613-22.

34. Ezekowitz MD, Leonard JC, Smith EO, Allen EW, Taylor FB: The identification of left ventricular thrombi in man using Indium-111 labeled autologus platelets: a preliminary report. Circulation 1981; 63:803-10.

PLATELET LABELLING WITH 111 IN - MERC-USEFULNESS IN RENAL TRANSPLANTATION.

C. Piera; M.Roca; J.Martin-Comin*; F.Lomena; J.Mora*; L.Sanchez; M.Ramos* and J. Setoain
* Radiochemical Centre, Amersham

INTRODUCTION

In 111-oxine labelled platelets are routinely used in our department to monitor kidney grafted patients (1-3). The labelling is performed in non-plasma media which are believed not to affect cell function. However, there is a general agreement that L=ct labelling in plasma may better preserve platelet functionability. Recently Thakur et al have published their experience with a new labelling agent (4); the sodium salt of 2-Mercaptopyridine-N-oxide (Merc) which permits 111-In cell labelling in a plasma medium.

The purpose of this study is to present our experience in the platelet labelling with this new agent and its clinical application in human transplantation.

MATERIAL AND METHODS

In each case (patient or donor) 49 ml of venous blood was obtained. Thirty-four ml over 6 ml of anticoagulant A (25.0 mg of dihydrated trisodium citrate and 14.9 mg of monohydrated citric acid per ml of solution) and 15 ml over 1.5 ml of anticoagulant B (3.8 % Na-citrate). Cell separation was carried out as described by Thakur et al (5). Thereafter the basic labelling procedure was (Fig.1):

The platelet bottom was resuspended in 0.5 ml of platelet poor plasmas (PPP-A) and 2.5 μg of Merc in 10 μl of an aqueous solution was added. The tube was incubated for 10 min. at room temperature.

Subsequently 200-400 μCi of 111-In* μl of 111-InCl3 dissolved in 0.04 N HCl and 25 μl of citrate buffer IM pH 6.5) was added to the cell suspension and the mixture was incubated for 20- mins at 37° C.

The tube was centrifuged 10 min at 1000 g to eliminate with unbound indium activity and the platelet bottom was washed with PPP-A and subsequently resuspended in 4 ml of PPP-B.

- A sample was withdrawn for aggregation studies.
- The cell suspension was reinjected to the patient when indicated.

The labelling efficiency was calculated as usual.

278

Ch. Kessler et al. (eds.), Clinical Application of Radiolabelled Platelets, 278–292.
© 1990 Kluwer Academic Publishers.

LABELING PROCEDURE

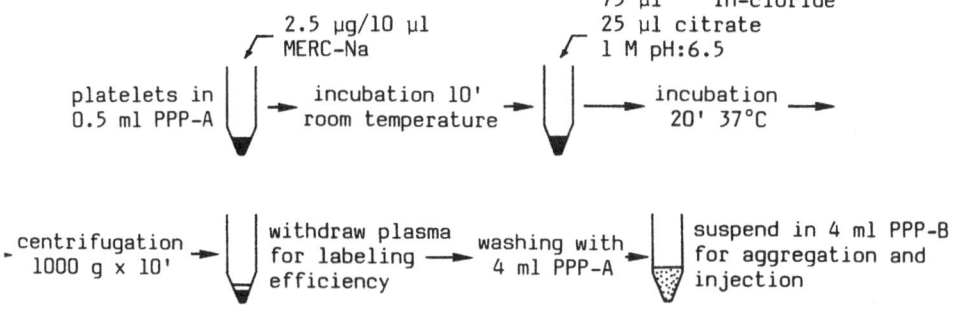

Fig.1. Platelet labelling with Merc-Na

The influence of several parameters on the labelling efficiency was tested in a variety of experimental sets.

1. Influence of Merc concentration from 2.5 to 40 μg.
2. Influence of 111-In incubation time from 5 to 30 min.
3. Influence of 111-In incubation temperature at 25°C and 37°C
4. The stability of the Merc solution stored in darkness in vacuum glass tubes was tested weekly up to 3-weeks. The number of labelled platelets ranged from 1.0 to 3.1 x 10^9.

Aggregation Studies

The platelet aggregation capacity was measured before and after labelling using the turbidimetric method of Born (6). In 15 cases it was measured with 4 μM ADP or collagen 5 μg/ml and in 10 cases with 10 μM epinephrine.
In 15 normal volunteers 61 ml of venous blood was obtained. 34 ml over 6 ml of anticoagulated A and 27 ml over 3 ml of anticoagulant B. Cell separation was performed as described above. The platelet rich plasma (PRP) was separated into 2 equal alliquotes and centrifuged at 1000 g for 10-min. The first platelet pellet was labelled with In-111-oxine in Modified Tyrode Solution (MTS) as described by Thakur et al (5) and the second one was labelled with Merc as described before. The In-111 activity used in both cases was 90-110 μCi.
The number of platelets labelled with each method was 1.1 +/- 0.4 x 10^9.
The labelling efficiency was calculated as unusual in both procedures. The platelet aggregability was also measured in both platelet pellets using the turbidimetric method of Born (6). The stimulating agents used were : ADP 5 μM; epinephrine 12.5 μM; collagen 20 μg/ml, sodium arachidonate 1.5 mM and ristocetine 1.5 ng/ml.

Patient Studies

In 31 kidney graft recipients labelled platelets were reinjected and the patient was scanned daily for a maximum of one week. Details of patient management and activity index calculations are described elsewhere (1-3). The results were compared with those previously reported with In-111-oxine labelled platelets (1-3).

RESULTS

Labelling efficiency decreased dramatically from 70% to less than 40% when Merc concentration was increased from 2.5 to 5 μg. The use of increasing Merc amounts reduced the labelling yield even more (Fig.2).
The labelling efficiency increased with an incubation time from 5 up to 20 min. Incubation times longer than 20

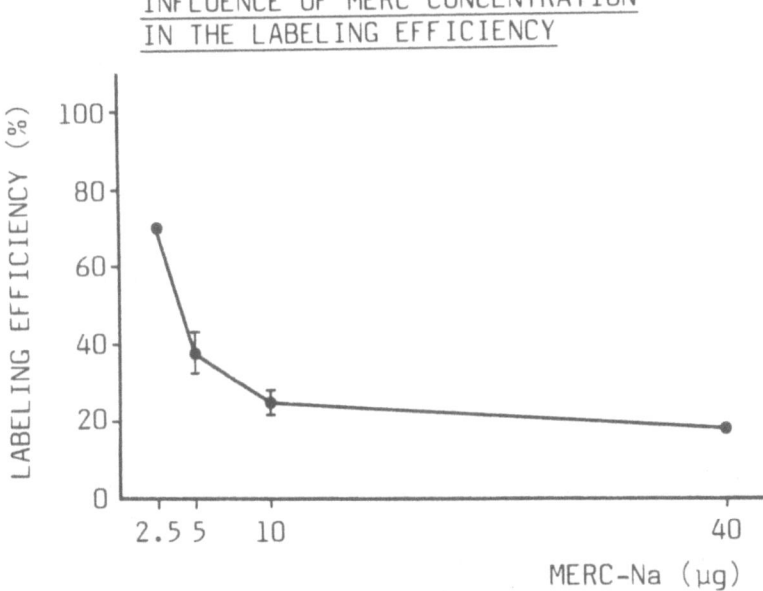

Fig.2.   Influence of Merc concentration on
           labelling efficiency

min. did not modify it significantly (Fig.3).

The influence of incubation temperature was, however, small. A slight increase of labelling efficiency was observed when labelling was performed at 37°C (Fig.4).

Merc stability showed a slight decrease from the first to the 5th week but at that time it was still within an acceptable range (Fig.5).

Using the basic labelling method described, mean labelling efficiency calculated in 50 cases was 65.5 +/- 7.0%.

In the 15 volunteers the labelling efficiency was 83.5 +/-9.2 in the case of oxine and 58.7 +/- oxine and 58.8+/- 7.7 when Merc was used.

Aggregation Studies

Platelet aggregability measured before and after labelling is shown in Table 1.

In the 15 normal volunteers studies, mean platelet aggregability was significantly lower with Oxine than with Merc with all the stimulant agents used but one (ristocetine) (Fig.6). When the aggregation velocity was measured the difference only was significant in the case of ADP and epinephrine (Fig.7).

Patient Studies

In 29 scans performed in 9 non-rejecting patients mean activity index value was 1.2 +/- 0.2 (in only one case out of the 29 the activity index was over 1.50. Mean index value was similar in 14 scans performed in 5 patients in which renal biopsy was consistent with nephrotoxicity (1.1 +/- 0.1). Activity index was significantly higher in the 37 scans performed in 11 patients showing acute rejection 2.9 +/- 1.8. (renal biopsy showed acute rejection signs in all cases/ In all but 3 scans the activity index was over 1.5 and in 19 out of the 37 scans performed the activity index was over 2 (Fig.8).

Four patients suffered from a cytomegalovirus infection as shown by clinical signs and serum titer, mean index value in them was 1,2 +/- 0.1 (0.9-1,5). Two patients were excluded because a final diagnosis was not obtained.

Considering 1.5 as the upper normal level sensitivity was 97% specificity was 90% and accuracy was 94%. When compared with Oxine results, no significant differences were observed between non-rejecting or nephrotoxic patients. However, in acutely rejecting patients the difference was statistically significant (p<o.001) as shown in Fig.9). The distribution range in the case of Merc was wider than in the case of Oxine. Activity index values with Merc and Oxine are shown in Table 2.

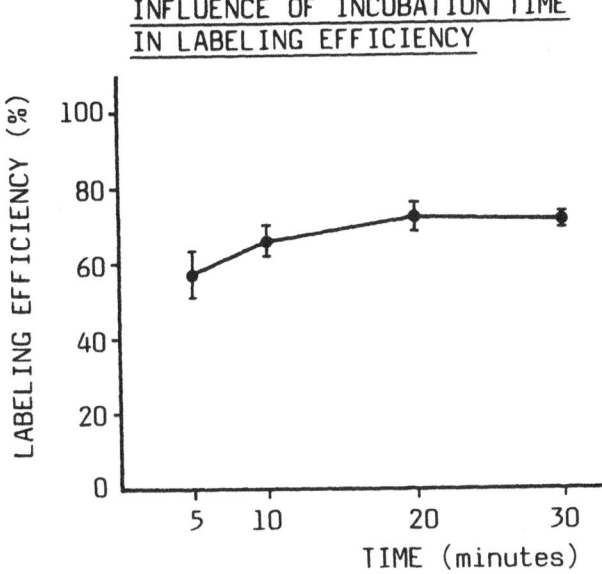

INFLUENCE OF INCUBATION TIME
IN LABELING EFFICIENCY

Fig.3   Influence of 111-In incubation time on labelling
          efficiency

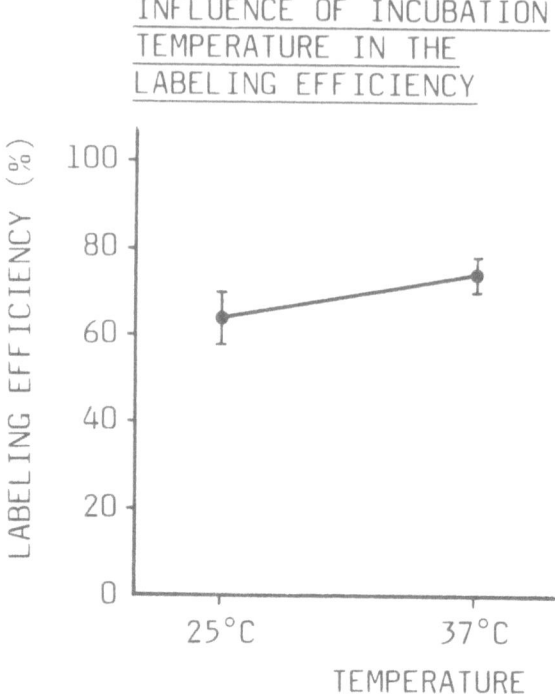

Fig.4   Influence of incubation temperature on labelling
         efficiency

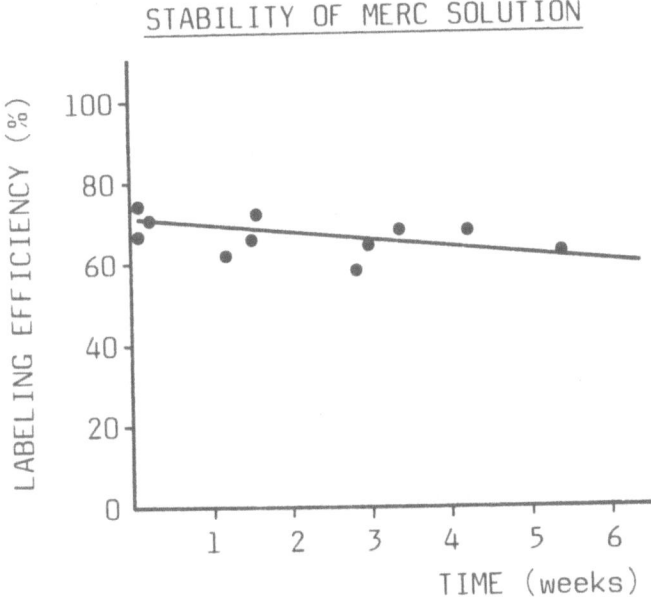

Fig.5   Merc-Na aqueous solution (2.5 $\mu g/\mu l$) storage
          stability

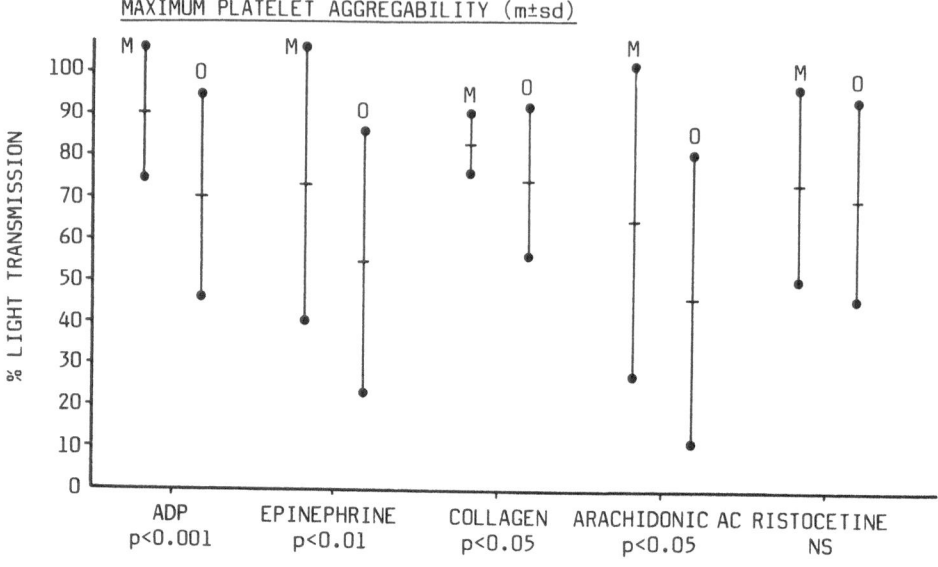

Fig.6   Maximum platelet aggregability with Merc and Oxine

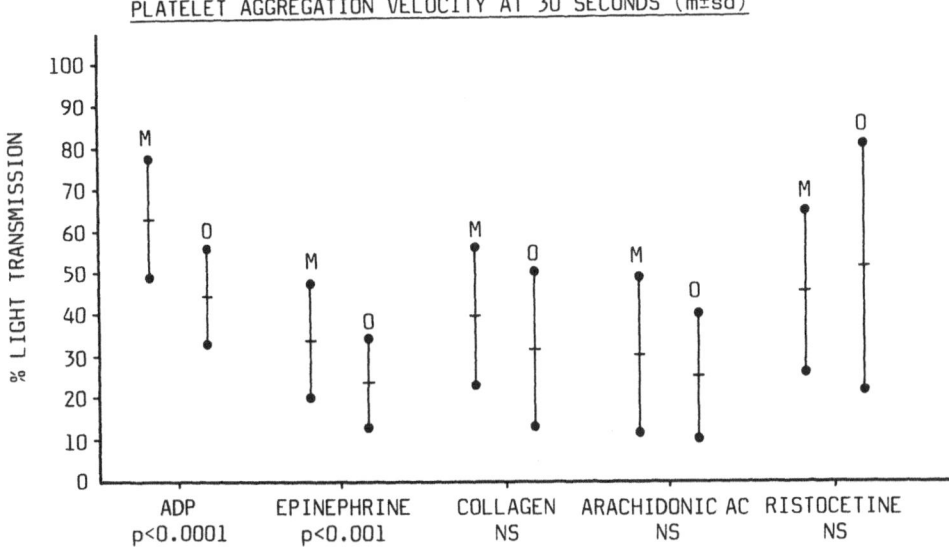

Fig.7   Platelet aggregation velocity at 30 seconds with Merc and oxine

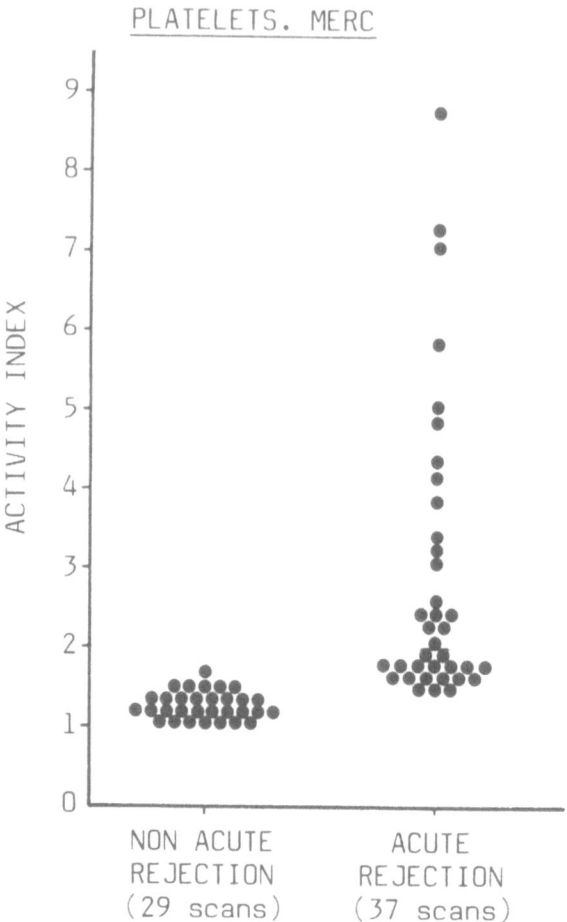

Fig.8   Platelet activity index distribution with Merc in
             kidney graft recipients

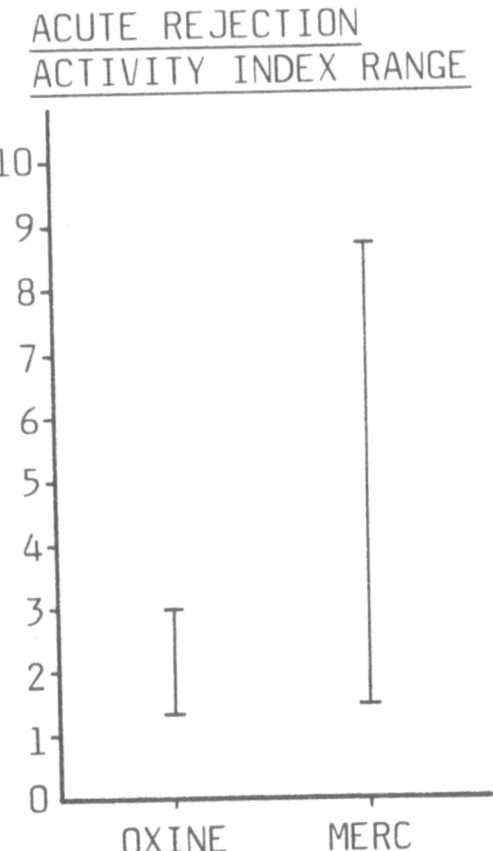

Fig. 9   Platelet activity index distribution range with
            Merc and Oxine in acute rejection

TABLE 1

Platelet aggregability before and after labelling with 200-400 μCi of 111-Merc.

AGENT	N	BEFORE LABELLING $\overline{X} \pm$ s.d.	AFTER LABELLING $\overline{X} \pm$ s.d.
ADP 4 μM	15	79.3 ± 17.2	67.1 ± 20.2
Collagen 5 μg/ml	15	82.3 ± 14.3	74.7 ± 19.5
Epinephrine 10 μM	10	75.9 ± 17.4	69.1 ± 15.6

==
N: number of platelet labelling procedures

TABLE 2

Activity index values with Merc and Oxine

	MERC N	MERC $\overline{X} \pm$ s.d	OXINE N	OXINE $\overline{X} \pm$ s.d
No rejection	29	1.2 ± 0.2	151	1.1 ± 0.1 n.s.
Nephrotoxicity	14	1.1 ± 0.1	22	1.0 ± 0.1 n.s.
Acute rejection	37	2.9 ± 1.8	41	1.8 ± 0.3 p<0.001

==
N: number of scans

DISCUSSION

According to our results Merc is a suitable agent for labelling platelets with 111-In in plasma. When prepared and stored as described it keeps its activity at least for 5 weeks.

Similar to the results reported by Thakur et al (4) we found the maximal labelling efficiency using 2,5 μg of Merc. This small quantity is less toxic to platelets than the concentration usually employed of other chelates (Oxine, Tropolone). However using 5 μg these authors observed only a slight decrease in the labelling efficiency while we found a sharp decrease. The difference may be due to the higher number of platelets (9×10^9) used by this team.

Incubation time should be between 15-20 min. longer times are not necessary as they do not increase labelling efficiency. A satisfactory labelling yield is obtained by incubating at room temperature (25°C), however, we prefer to do it at 37°C which slightly increases the labelling efficiency, it is a more physiological temperature for platelets.

Aggregation capacity is an expression of platelet functionability (7). It was significantly better maintained when platelets were labelled with Merc in plasma than when they were labelled in MTS with Oxine. That is in agreement with the clinical results obtained. The activity index in non-rejecting or nephrotoxic patients was similar with both agents (Merc and Oxine). Nevertheless, in acutely rejecting patients, when platelets are actually acting in the kidney, the index was significantly higher when the labelling agent was Merc. This may be due to the better preservation of platelet function with this agent. Moreover, there was agreement between observers that liver activity with Merc was lower than with Oxine though unfortunately it has not been quantified in this study.

In summary, the method is suitable for labelling platelets, preserves cell function better than Oxine does and may, in our experience, be used for Kidney graft monitoring.

REFERENCES

1. J.Martin-Comin et al 111-In-oxine labelled platelets in renal transplantation. Value in cyclosporine therapy. Contributions to Nephrology. In press.
2. J.Setoain et al. Platelet labelling in renal transplantation. Proc.111 World Congress Nucl.Med.and Biology Paris 1982.pp 1583-1585.Pergamon Press,Paris 1982.
3. J.Martin-Comin. Kidney graft rejection studies with

labelled platelets and lymphocytes.Nucl.Med.and Biology.13:173-181, 1986.

4. M.L.Thakur et al. Simplified and efficient labelling of human platelets in plasma using 111-In-2-mercaptopyrridine-N-oxide: preparation and evaluation. J.Nucl.Med. 26:510-517, 1985.

5. M.L.Thakur et al. 111-In labelled human platelets: Improved method, efficacy and evaluation. J.Nucl.Med. 22: 381-385, 1981.

6. G.V. Born. Aggregation of blood platelets by adenosine diphosphate and its reversal. Nature 192: 927-9229, 1962.

7. H.J. Day et al. Evaluation of platelet function. Sem.in Hematology. 23:89-101, 1986.

INDEX

Developments in Nuclear Medicine

1. P.H. Cox (ed.): *Cholescintigraphy.* 1981   ISBN 90-247-2524-0
2. P.H. Cox (ed.): *Progress in Radiopharmacology.* Selected Topics. Proceedings of the 3rd European Symposium (Noordwijkerhout, The Netherlands, April 1982). 1982
    ISBN 90-247-2768-5
3. M.H. Jonckheer and F. Deconinck (eds.): *X-Ray Fluorescent Scanning of the Thyroid.* 1983   ISBN 0-89838-561-X
4. K. Kristensen and E. Nørbygaard (eds.): *Safety and Efficacy of Radiopharmaceuticals.* 1984   ISBN 0-89838-609-8
5. A. Bossuyt and F. Deconinck: *Amplitude/Phase Patterns in Dynamic Scintigraphic Imaging.* With a Foreword by A. Bertrand Brill. 1984   ISBN 0-89838-641-1
6. M.R. Hardeman and Y. Najean (eds.): *Blood Cells in Nuclear Medicine, Part I.* Cell Kinetics and Bio-distribution. 1984   ISBN 0-89838-653-5
7. G.F. Fueger (ed.): *Blood Cells in Nuclear Medicine, Part II.* Migratory Blood Cells. 1984   ISBN 0-89838-654-3
8. H.J. Biersack and P.H. Cox (eds.): *Radioisotope Studies in Cardiology.* 1985
    ISBN 0-89838-733-7
9. P.H. Cox, G. Limouris and M.G. Woldring (eds.): *Progress in Radiopharmacology 1985.* 1985   ISBN 0-89838-745-0
10. P.H. Cox, S.J. Mather, C.B. Sampson and C.R. Lazarus (eds.): *Progress in Radiopharmacy.* 1986   ISBN 0-89838-823-6
11. H. Deckart and P.H. Cox (eds.): *Principles of Radiopharmacology.* 1987
    ISBN 0-89838-774-4
12. W.-D. Heiss, G. Pawlik, K. Herholz and K. Wienhard (eds.): *Clinical Efficacy of Positron Emission Tomography.* 1987   ISBN 0-89838-898-8
13. G.B. Gerber, H. Métivier and H. Smith (eds.): *Age-related Factors in Radionuclide Metabolism and Dosimetry.* 1987   ISBN 0-89838-953-4
14. K. Kristensen and E. Nørbygaard (eds.): *Safety and Efficacy of Radiopharmaceuticals 1987.* 1987   ISBN 0-89838-986-0
15. C. Beckers, A. Goffinet and A. Bol (eds.): *Positron Emission Tomography in Clinical Research and Clinical Diagnosis.* Tracer Modelling and Radioreceptors. 1989
    ISBN 0-7923-0254-0
16. M. De Schrijver: *Scintigraphy of Inflammation with Nanometer-sized Colloidal Tracers.* 1989   ISBN 0-7923-0272-9
17. Ch. Kessler, M.R. Hardeman, H. Henningsen and J.-N. Petrovici (eds.): *Clinical Application of Radiolabelled Platelets.* 1990   ISBN 0-7923-0729-1

Kluwer Academic Publishers - Dordrecht / Boston / London